AF849081

PULMONARY AND RESPIRATORY DISEASES AND DISORDERS

RESPIRATORY VENTILATORY STRATEGIES IN ACUTE AND CHRONIC RESPIRATORY FAILURE IN IDIOPATHIC PULMONARY DISEASES

A PRACTICAL APPROACH

PULMONARY AND RESPIRATORY DISEASES AND DISORDERS

Additional books and e-books in this series can be found
on Nova's website under the Series tab.

PULMONARY AND RESPIRATORY DISEASES AND DISORDERS

RESPIRATORY VENTILATORY STRATEGIES IN ACUTE AND CHRONIC RESPIRATORY FAILURE IN IDIOPATHIC PULMONARY DISEASES

A PRACTICAL APPROACH

ANTONIO M. ESQUINAS, MD, PHD
EDITOR

nova
Medicine & Health
New York

Copyright © 2020 by Nova Science Publishers, Inc.

All rights reserved. No part of this book may be reproduced, stored in a retrieval system or transmitted in any form or by any means: electronic, electrostatic, magnetic, tape, mechanical photocopying, recording or otherwise without the written permission of the Publisher.

We have partnered with Copyright Clearance Center to make it easy for you to obtain permissions to reuse content from this publication. Simply navigate to this publication's page on Nova's website and locate the "Get Permission" button below the title description. This button is linked directly to the title's permission page on copyright.com. Alternatively, you can visit copyright.com and search by title, ISBN, or ISSN.

For further questions about using the service on copyright.com, please contact:
Copyright Clearance Center
Phone: +1-(978) 750-8400 Fax: +1-(978) 750-4470 E-mail: info@copyright.com.

NOTICE TO THE READER

The Publisher has taken reasonable care in the preparation of this book, but makes no expressed or implied warranty of any kind and assumes no responsibility for any errors or omissions. No liability is assumed for incidental or consequential damages in connection with or arising out of information contained in this book. The Publisher shall not be liable for any special, consequential, or exemplary damages resulting, in whole or in part, from the readers' use of, or reliance upon, this material. Any parts of this book based on government reports are so indicated and copyright is claimed for those parts to the extent applicable to compilations of such works.

Independent verification should be sought for any data, advice or recommendations contained in this book. In addition, no responsibility is assumed by the Publisher for any injury and/or damage to persons or property arising from any methods, products, instructions, ideas or otherwise contained in this publication.

This publication is designed to provide accurate and authoritative information with regard to the subject matter covered herein. It is sold with the clear understanding that the Publisher is not engaged in rendering legal or any other professional services. If legal or any other expert assistance is required, the services of a competent person should be sought. FROM A DECLARATION OF PARTICIPANTS JOINTLY ADOPTED BY A COMMITTEE OF THE AMERICAN BAR ASSOCIATION AND A COMMITTEE OF PUBLISHERS.

Additional color graphics may be available in the e-book version of this book.

Library of Congress Cataloging-in-Publication Data

Names: Esquinas, Antonio M., editor.
Title: Respiratory ventilatory strategies in acute and chronic respiratory failure in idiopathic pulmonary diseases: a practical approach / Antonio M. Esquinas, editor.
Description: New York: Nova Science Publishers, [2020] | Series: Pulmonary and respiratory diseases and disorders | Includes bibliographical references and index. | Summary: "Idiopatic pulmonary fibrosis (IPF) represents one of the most important devastating diseases that affects the lungs. Traditionally, the development of acute or chronic respiratory failure in disio represents an important dilemma for pulmonologists, intensivists, internists and anesthesiologists, due to the limited respiratory and functional reserve of these patients. In the last decade, we have witnessed a novel development of non-invasive mechanical ventilation and high flow oxygenation systems, representing an attractive option for patients compared to those patients with well-known poor results of invasive mechanical ventilation. In this book, we analyze all the options of non-invasive mechanical ventilation, indications, ventilatory modes, protocols, technology, equipment and applications in acute and chronic phase of patients with IPF, in addition to an exhaustive approach of all complementary techniques that optimize the application of these procedures. There are no previous descriptions or updates that incorporate this comprehensive analysis. This book, thus, serves as an updated scientific and practical reference for the knowledge of all spectrum respiratory failure presentations in idiopathic pulmonary fibrosis"-- Provided by publisher.
Identifiers: LCCN 2020016168 (print) | LCCN 2020016169 (ebook) | ISBN 9781536178470 (hardcover) | ISBN 9781536178487 (adobe pdf) Subjects: LCSH: Pulmonary fibrosis--Patients--Rehabilitation. | Pulmonary fibrosis--Complications. | Respiratory insufficiency--Treatment. | Respiratory therapy.
Classification: LCC RC776.F5 R47 2020 (print) | LCC RC776.F5 (ebook) | DDC 616.2/4--dc23
LC record available at https://lccn.loc.gov/2020016168
LC ebook record available at https://lccn.loc.gov/2020016169

Published by Nova Science Publishers, Inc. † New York

CONTENTS

PREFACE

Idiopatic pulmonary fibrosis (IPF) represents one of the most important devastating diseases that affects the lungs. Traditionally, the development of acute or chronic respiratory failure in disiorepresents an important dilemma for pulmonologists, intensivists, internists and anesthesiologists, due to the limited respiratory and functional reserve of these patients.

In the last decade, we have witnessed a novel development of non-invasive mechanical ventilation and high flow oxygenation systems, representing an attractive option for patients compared to those patients with well-known poor results of invasive mechanical ventilation.

In this book, the authors analyze all the options of non-invasive mechanical ventilation, indications, ventilatory modes, protocols, technology, equipment and applications in acute and chronic phase of patients with IPF, in addition to an exhaustive approach of all complementary techniques that optimize the application of these procedures. There are no previous descriptions or updates that incorporate this comprehensive analysis. This book, thus, serves as an updated scientific and practical reference for the knowledge of all spectrum respiratory failure presentations in idiopatic pulmonary fibrosis.

Chapter 1 - Interstitial lung diseases (ILD) are a heterogeneous group of pathologies that have in common the involvement of the pulmonary interstitium. Although they share similar clinical, radiological, physiological or pathological characteristics, its prognosis or response to specific drugs is completely different, so a correct classification will be very important to assess the better management. Mainly ILD are classified in two groups, those where the ILD was developed by a known cause (organic, inorganic agents, drugs, connective tissue diseases…) or by unknown origin. Among the latter there is a group of them with a poorly defined processes like sarcoidosis, langerhans cells hystiocitosis, lymphangioleiomyomatosis or pulmonary eosinophilias, and another group of idiopathic interstícial pneumonias that used to be subclassified among those that develop lung fibrosis, those associated with smoking or those with an acute/subacute evolution.

Chapter 2 - Idiopathic Pulmonary Fibrosis (IPF) is a rare disease with limited literature regarding epidemiology, because of the relatively few number of cases, along with varying definitions that have evolved over time. Geographically, IPF is more prevalent in industrialized nations, specifically in Europe and the United States; data from Asia is relatively limited at this time, but new information is emerging. Men, older patients, and Caucasians have been noted to have a great predisposition towards IPF. Additionally, several environmental exposures have been implicated in the pathogenesis of IPF. The most common risk factors for IPF include smoking and gastroesophageal reflux disease (GERD). Additional high-risk exposures include but are not limited to wood dust, metal dust, and agriculture. In rare case, familial genetic alterations have also been identified. The mortality in IPF is high, rivaling that in aggressive neoplasms in some cases. IPF exacerbations are associated with high utilization of healthcare resources, in association with high morbidity. In the future, more research is needed to elucidate epidemiology and risk factors, in order to develop more effective treatments, and to implement more preventative measures.

Chapter 3 - In Idiopathic Pulmonary Fibrosis there is typically recognizable restrictive ventilatory pattern: in this pattern the static expiratory pressure – volume (P-V) curve of the lung is moved down and to the right compared with normal subjects. Lung recoil is increased over the entire range of the reduced inspiratory capacity and both vital capacity (VC) and total lung capacity (TLC) are reduced. The causes of decreased lung compliance in ILD are multifactorial and involve leak of lung volume, decreased alveolar distensibility, alterations in the elastic properties and raised alveolar surface tension. Lung diffusing capacity is nearly always reduced in subjects with IPF. DLCO decrease come out from parenchymal and vascular damages. Pulmonary hypertension (PH) is usually associated with higher mortality in subjects with IPF. The causes of pulmonary hypertension in IPF are still not known. Latest data offer a multifactorial etiology (e.g., primary lesions of vessels and vasoconstriction).

Chapter 4 - The role of the immune system in idiopathic pulmonary fibrosis (IPF) pathogenesis has been debated, with seemingly contradictory results between promising experimental data and disappointing clinical trials. As the understanding of the paramount role of the epithelium in the disease arose, the concept that immunity and inflammation influence rather than drive fibrosis developed. Immune cells involved in both innate and adaptive immunity have been implicated in experimental fibrosis development and display alterations in idiopathic pulmonary fibrosis, shaping a pro-fibrotic environment. Accordingly, the levels of several cytokines with a pro-fibrotic potential, such as IL-4, IL-13, IL-1β, TNF-α and IL-17A are elevated in IPF patients. Additionally, the interplay with cellular stress components such as danger associated molecular patterns and infectious alarm signals under the form of pathogen associated molecular patterns is an area of ongoing investigation. Finally, recent advances in sequencing techniques have unraveled a potential role for viruses and bacteria.

Chapter 5 - Idiopathic pulmonary fibrosis is a noninfectious chronic disease of unknown cause of progressive and often fatal character, which has as its most striking feature the reduction in the ability to perform gas exchange. Although this disease is known to be limited to the respiratory system, patients with IPF are often affected by various alterations in other systems, such as the nervous system, cardiovascular system and skeletal muscular system, which may be determinant in the prognosis of these patients.

Chapter 6 - Lung fibrosis is characterized by the progressive replacement of lung alveoli by a fibrotic scar tissue. The disease is considered as epithelial-derived: repeated lung injury or sustained inflammation leads to the destruction of alveolar epithelial cells, which reside at the forefront of the interface between lung and environment. This epithelial injury is followed by type 2 alveolar cell hyperplasia and dysfunction, along with the recapitulation of developmental pathways. Impaired cell differentiation is also a key characteristic of lung fibrosis, and the way the balance between epithelial repair and fibrosis is regulated still remains partially unexplained. Interestingly, epithelial remodeling and cell turnover provide opportunities for biomarkers. Finally, currently available drugs, as well as novel treatments, exert, at least partially, their function through epithelial cell regulation.

Chapter 7 - Pulmonary hypertension (PH) is commonly present in patients with idiopathic pulmonary fibrosis (IPF) and classified as group III PH due to chronic lung diseases and hypoxemia. PH should be suspected in patients with rapid clinical worsening, progressive exercise limitation and/or gas exchange abnormalities which are not deemed attributable to ventilatory impairment. Echocardiography and enlarged main pulmonary artery ratio are non-invasive modalities for screening PH. Right heart catheterization (RHC) is the gold standard test for the measurement of pulmonary artery pressure. It should be performed in patients in whom severe PH is suspected and the patient's management will likely be influenced by RHC results. Currently there is no specific therapy for IPF associated PH. Supplemental oxygen is prescribed for hypoxemic patients. PH targeted therapy is not typically indicated in IPF patients. It may be considered in patients with severe PH which cannot be explained with the underlying lung disease. These patients should be referred to specialized centers experienced in the management of PH for possible enrollment in clinical trials.

Chapter 8 - Idiopathic pulmonary fibrosis (IPF) is a chronic, progressive and a form of interstitial pneumonia leading to fibrosis and loss of function of the lung. It is usually diagnosed in elderly population after excluding the known causes of interstitial lung diseases, the presence of the radiological findings and histopathology patterns of usual interstitial pneumonia (UIP). The fact that etiology is unknown makes it difficult to understand the complexity of the pathogenesis behind the disease, develop new treatment options, foresee the clinical outcome of different patients and the way they will respond to the available therapies. Taking in consideration the complexity of the disease the identification of biomarkers would help not only in determining the predisposition of patients for the disease, but also classify them according to the prognosis, choose the right treatment for specific groups and help in their follow-up. Many studies in the last 2 decades have been focused in identification of the ideal biomarker for IPF, but as a result of what these studies have shown it is yet unclear if any of the numerous potential biomarkers can be used in clinics.

Chapter 9 - Gastroesophageal Reflux Disease (GERD) is an important consideration as the direct cause or a contributing factor in patients presenting with pulmonary symptoms. This chapter aims to look at several different pulmonary diseases affected by GERD ranging from upper airway including chronic cough, vocal cord dysfunction, lower airway diseases including COPD, asthma, and bronchiolitis obliterans syndrome, down to parenchymal diseases such as interstitial lung diseases. The chapter will also discuss the potential mechanisms leading to pulmonary disease associated with GERD, the diagnostic approach and different treatment options.

Chapter 10 - Idiopathic pulmonary fibrosis (IPF) is usually characterized by a progressive disease course, during which multiple complications may arise that cause significant morbidity and mortality. The most severe complication is idiopathic acute exacerbation of IPF (AEx) which accounts for nearly 40% of mortality in IPF. AEx is characterized by acute worsening of dyspnea with associated radiographic findings and lacks effective treatment. Patients with IPF are also at significantly increased risk of lung cancer, likely due to multiple shared pathogenetic pathways between fibrosis and tumor formation and proliferation. Additional common complications include pneumothorax, pneumomediastinum, bacterial and viral respiratory infections, and thromboembolic disease such as acute coronary syndrome and deep vein thrombosis. In IPF patients presenting with a decline in respiratory status, it is important to consider these entities as they carry important implications for both medical management and clinical outcomes.

Chapter 11 - Lung function tests in patients with Idiopathic Pulmonary Fibrosis (IPF) show a characteristic restrictive pattern with a decrease of Diffusing Capacity for Carbon Monoxide (DLCO) and moderate hypoxemia and hypocapnia at rest, which, in the more advanced stages, develops into persistent respiratory failure. International recommendations on IPF remark the importance of lung function testing in the control of this disease. Clinical trials testing new drugs for the treatment of IPF have adopted Forced Vital Capacity (FVC) and DLCO as primary variables for confirming clinical efficacy. FVC was a standard spirometric measure of pulmonary function in IPF for many decades. Change over time in serial measures of FVC is a widely accepted reflection of disease progression and several studies have identified change in predicted FVC as an independent predictor of mortality in patients with IPF. A reduction in static (Total Lung Capacity) and dynamic lung volumes is typical in patients with IPF as in other Interstitial Lung Diseases. In patients with IPF, the DLCO and the value of gas exchange per unit of lung volume (KCO) are both reduced, because of the coexisting alterations on alveolar membrane and on capillary vessels. In addition, the 6-minute walking test and the distance assessed during exercise represent mortality predictors.

Chapter 12 - Interstitial lung diseases are a heterogeneous group of chronic lung diseases. Several hundred disorders are known to cause interstitial lung disease. Overall approximately one third of ILDs have known etiologies but the majority are idiopathic. Epidemiologic data, derived primarily from patient registries, suggest that the prevalence of ILD in the U.S.s ranges from 67 per 100,000 in women to 81 per 100,000 in men. However, there are significant variations in prevalence among different geographic populations, likely reflecting a combination of genetic and environmental differences. Certain risk factors, including exposure to cigarette smoke or environmental toxicants (asbestos, silica, coal dust, and air pollution), genetic mutations, and single nucleotide polymorphisms, have all been associated with developing interstitial lung disease. While the cause of the interstitial lung disease may vary, common characteristics include impaired alveolar gas exchange and symptoms of breathlessness and a non-productive cough. Patients with ILD are prone to the development of acute respiratory failure, which is an acute exacerbation of the underlying lung disease. The combination of pre-existing lung impairment combined with a superimposed acute injury can often be fatal. In this chapter, the authors review the definition of an acute exacerbation, discuss the underlying pathophysiology, and highlight salient features related to the diagnosis and treatment of acute interstitial lung disease exacerbations.

Chapter 13 - Idiopathic pulmonary fibrosis (IPF) is a form of interstitial lung disease that may be worsened by chronic respiratory failure (CRF) as the disease progresses into advanced stages. Many pathophysiological mechanisms underlying CRF occur with IPF over time, including reduced lung compliance and volume from airway obstruction and capillary surface destruction, resulting in impaired diffusion capacity and ventilation-perfusion mismatch. These complex physiological changes affect all lung functions and compartments and worsen the underlying disease. Consequently, in the majority of these cases, CRF develops as a secondary cause of IPF progression.

Chapter 14 - Idiopathic Pulmonary Fibrosis (IPF) is an incurable condition in which progressive pulmonary fibrosis causes progressive respiratory failure, resulting ultimately in death. Despite the introduction of the first drugs to treat this condition, no agent has been proven yet to reduce mortality. IPF patients commonly have sleep complaints, and obstructive sleep apnea (OSA) has been found to be prevalent among IPF patients. OSA is a condition that results in significant morbidity, and, with certain patients, increased mortality. OSA was first described in the 1960s using nocturnal polysomnography. It is estimated to occur in anywhere from 4% to 20% of adults, depending on the population, and is most common in age 60 to 69. Unlike IPF, OSA is treatable, resulting in reduced morbidity and mortality in OSA patients. OSA appears to play an important role in quality of life and potentially, mortality in IPF patients. Treatment of OSA in patients with IPF appears to provide patients with better lung function, fewer symptoms, and possibly, improved survival. This raises the possibility of OSA being an important modifiable factor in IPF patients. In this chapter, the authors discuss physiologic interactions between OSA and IPF as well as the clinical presentation, diagnosis, and treatment of OSA in IPF patients.

Chapter 15 - When evaluating respiratory failure severity in Idiopathic Pulmonary Fibrosis (IPF), there are two forms that should be distinguished and analyzed separately. In this chapter the authors will focus on both acute and chronic respiratory failure.

Chronic respiratory failure and hypoxemia in IPF may be a combination of many mechanisms – mainly ventilation/perfusion mismatch, shunt, and diffusion limitation. Several tests and exams support this assessment, namely pulmonary function tests, 6-minute walk test, cardiopulmonary exercise test and high-resolution chest CT scan. Acute respiratory failure is linked to acute exacerbations of the disease, often requiring hospital admission. In this chapter the authors will characterize risk factors for exacerbation, and the authors will describe a staging system that allows identification of prognostic groups. The authors will also briefly describe the treatment options in IPF patients with respiratory failure.

Chapter 16 - *Purpose of review*: Idiopathic pulmonary fibrosis (IPF) is a relentless progressive parenchymal lung disease [1]. Among the idiopathic interstitial pneumonias (IIPs), IPF is the most common disease and most difficult to manage. Therefore, the purpose of this chapter is to show practical diagnostic approaches for IPF such as serum biomarker, chest radiogragh, chest high resolution computed tomography (HRCT) and broncho-alveolar lavage (BAL).

Chapter 17 - Idiopathic pulmonary fibrosis (IPF) is a progressive form of interstitial lung disease of unknown cause. Comprehensive history, physical examination and noninvasive diagnostic testing are required to exclude other causes of interstitial lung diseases. Diagnosis of IPF may be established based on usual interstitial pneumonia (UIP) characteristic findings on high-resolution CT scan and compatible clinical history. Lung biopsy is required to establish a diagnosis when HRCT pattern is suggestive of probable UIP, indeterminate for UIP or an alternative diagnosis. The potential values of establishing the diagnosis of IPF include discontinuation of harmful medications such as systemic steroid, starting recently Food and Drug Administration (FDA) approved medications and timely referral to lung transplant centers. It also has prognostic value given the average life expectancy is similar to many advanced cancers. Bronchoscopic transbronchial lung biopsy using forceps and / or cryoprobe and surgical lung biopsy are the main modalities for obtaining lung tissues for the diagnosis of IPF.

Chapter 18 - Patients with Fibrotic Interstitial Lung Disease have a poor prognosis and have symptoms that destroy quality of life. Patients usually develop hypoxemia due to multiplied physiologic derangements, including diffusion limitation, ventilation-perfusion mismatching, and abnormalities of the pulmonary vasculature. Many patients will require supplemental oxygen at some point in the course of their disease, and although it can increase blood oxygen and symptoms, it also creates physical and emotional challenges for patients and their cherished ones. Oxygen supplementation is typically use in patients with advanced lung disease with resting hypoxemia; however, there is a paucity of evidence guiding the use of supplemental oxygen in ILD, and significant heterogeneity in clinical practice. It rests unclear whether supplemental oxygen improves clinically significant outcomes, and the role of ambulatory oxygen supplementation in isolated exertional hypoxemia is not yet explicit today.

Chapter 19 - Interstitial lung diseases (ILD) comprise a group of pulmonary diseases characterized by inflammation and fibrosis of the lung parenchyma. Associated with respiratory failure and dyspnoea, these are chronically evolving entities marked by acute exacerbations (AE-ILD) with further decreases in pulmonary function, hypoxemia and ultimately, higher mortality. The mainstay of treatment for AE-ILD consist of oxygen therapy, which mainly included invasive mechanical ventilation, non-invasive ventilation and conventional oxygen therapy. The first two options have not shown clinical benefit, being the latter the recommended initial approach. In the last few years, another focus has been placed on the high-flow nasal cannula oxygen therapy (HFNC), a non-invasive method that provides heated and humidified air-oxygen mixture with flow rates up to 70 L/min. HFNC enables the correction of more severe degrees of hypoxemia, better mucociliary clearance, washout of anatomic dead space gasses, creating a PEEP effect, but most importantly, leading to improving patient comfort and tolerance to treatment. When compared to previous methods, HFNC also reduced mortality risk and need for intubation in cases of acute respiratory failure. Consequently, HFNC can be regarded as an excellent option for AE-ILD refractory to low-flow conventional oxygen therapy.

Chapter 20 - Background and objectives: Acute respiratory failure (ARF) in patients (pts) with idiopathic pulmonary fibrosis (IPF) is associated with poor prognosis, therefore a non-invasive approach, such as noninvasive ventilation (NIV) may represent a good option to turn to. NIV modes: continuous positive airway pressure (CPAP) in spontaneous breathing (SB) (range 8-10 cmH_2O level) is applied in the absence of respiratory acidosis in order to treat hypoxemia with tachypnea. Inspired oxygen fraction (FiO_2) is set at the lowest value to keep PaO_2 at more than 60mmHg. Hypercapnia, hypoventilation and respiratory fatigue are treated in assisted/controlled ventilation by face-mask (FM) in pressure support ventilation (PSV). Pressure support (PS) and positive end-expiratory pressure (PEEP) level are set respectively at 12-18 and 4-9 cmH_2O, titrated to provide a moderate tidal volume (TV) (6-8 ml/Kg of predicted body weight). When NIV-Helmet is applied, PS and PEEP baseline levels are respectively set at 10 and 5 cmH_2O, both raising in increments of 2–3 cmH_2O. FM advantages: higher efficacy in improving CO_2 elimination and reducing work of breathing while applying PSV in pts with high respiratory muscle load. Disadvantages: not tolerated in pts with prolonged MV necessity. Helmet advantages over FM: improved tolerability and lesser air leaks as with a new helmet that can be performed for prolonged periods of time. Disadvantages: because of its larger inner volume, standard helmet is characterized by less efficient rates of pressurization and triggering function, worsening patient–ventilator synchrony. In pts with high respiratory drive and intense inspiratory effort, the risk of patient self-inflicted lung injury (P-SILI) is highly considerable. Conclusions: NIV with helmet in CPAP mode and face-mask in PSV provides relief from dyspnoea and avoids endo-tracheal intubation (ETI).

Chapter 21 - Idiopathic pulmonary fibrosis (IPF) is a progressive interstitial lung disease. Patients may present with acute respiratory failure, named as acute exacerbation during follow-up, and they often require intensive care and mechanical ventilation support. While mechanical ventilation has been considered as futile treatment due to high mortality rates, recent studies have shown that prognosis is better in patients. However, there are no IPF-specific treatment strategies in mechanical ventilation. Because of the pathophysiological and clinical similarities with acute respiratory distress syndrome, it is considered that lung protective ventilation strategies with low-tidal volume can be applied in IPF. However, high positive end expiratory pressure is not recommended because of the low probability of recrutability due to lung damage.

Chapter 22 - Non-invasive ventilation may represent a valuable option in certain patients with idiopathic pulmonary fibrosis and respiratory worsening. Despite technical improvements, subject-ventilator asynchrony may occur, which is shown to be a major factor promoting failure of non-invasive ventilation and is associated with decreased survival. This chapter summarizes different asynchrony entities and their treatment during non-invasive ventilation in patients with idiopathic pulmonary fibrosis.

Chapter 23 - Indications for putting patient on NIV are well-defined but there are no established guidelines for weaning patients from NIV though it is very important to reduce the complications related to prolonged ventilation and hospital stay. There are several weaning criteria that need to be considered while withdrawing NIV. Current data on weaning strategies from NIV is limited. NIV withdrawal strategies include progressive weaning or immediate withdrawal. In progressive weaning strategies step wise reduction of NIV duration or ventilator pressure support is attempted while in immediate withdrawal strategy, NIV is discontinued abruptly as soon as patient meets weaning criteria. Stepwise reduction of NIV use seems reasonable and may be adopted in day to day practice. Well-designed randomized studies with adequate sample size are needed to find the best strategy for weaning from NIV that would shorten the length of hospital/ICU stay and improve outcome parameters.

Chapter 24 - Pulmonary hypertension (PH) is defined as an increase in mean pulmonary arterial pressure to values $\geq$ 25 mmHg at rest as assessed by right heart catheterization. Right ventricle (RV) failure is the most frequent cause of death in PH patients. Cardiovascular performance can be independently influenced by positive intrathoracic pressure due to a decrease in RV preload. Also both lung hyperinflation and lung volumes under functional residual capacity lead to increased pulmonary vascular resistance. PH is associated with an increased afterload on the RV, conditioning mechanical ventilation strategy and its weaning. Special attention is required to avoid hypoxia, hypercapnia and high PEEP (levels should be (<10 cmH_2O). Low tidal volume ventilation strategies are a good option, however $PaCO_2$ levels should be closely monitored. PH also hinders weaning from mechanical ventilation, since it worsens some of the weaning potential negative effects on cardiovascular function.

Chapter 25 - Preoperative evaluation is the indispensable component for caring for a surgical patient planned to undergo surgery. Although the practice is nearly universal now, a robust pathway is still lacking. The objective of preoperative evaluation is to assess the patient's disease and comorbid conditions, their impact on the different vital organ systems and functional reserve of the patient. The evaluation also aims to find out the different risk factors that can have an impact on the perioperative morbidity and mortality of the patients. The respiratory system is very critical for perioperative physicians, intensivists, and health care providers caring for surgical patients. Idiopathic pulmonary fibrosis is a progressive lung disease with hampered oxygen transport. As it can affect the morbidity and mortality of the patient during the perioperative period, it is essential to assess the patient, risk-stratify accurately, and optimize the patient before proceeding for elective surgery. This chapter briefly describes the preoperative evaluation and management approach to a patient with idiopathic pulmonary fibrosis planned for both thoracic and non-cardiac surgeries. A flow algorithm is also proposed to help the perioperative health care provider.

Chapter 26 - Idiopathic pulmonary fibrosis (IPF) constitutes progressive inflammation resulting in fibrotic areas in the lung parenchyma and causing chronic respiratory distress. These fibrotic areas disrupt the gas exchange and cause a decrease in compliance of the lungs and lung volumes. It is an invasive disease and progresses with acute worsening periods. The criteria and results of non-invasive or invasive mechanical ventilation for these patients have not been established yet. However, it is important not to delay mechanical ventilation. Patients with IPF should have high-resolution computed tomography examinations preoperatively. Early postoperative noninvasive mechanical ventilation may be required in patients with IPF after extubation. High oxygen concentration used in mechanical ventilation during general anesthesia (any oxygen concentration above 21% counts as high oxygen concentration), single lung ventilation, and ischemia-reperfusion injury may cause acute exacerbations and respiratory insufficiency in the postoperative period. Patients with IPF should be kept in negative fluid balance in the postoperative period to avoid disrupting gas exchange. Drugs such as "pirfenidone" and anticoagulants should be continued and lung protective measurements should be done in the perioperative period.

Chapter 27 - Acute respiratory failure is very common in interstitial lung diseases and optimal ventilatory management in this setting is still under investigation. The dismal prognosis of patients needing mechanical ventilation urged the search for alternative strategies, such as extracorporeal life support. Since its first use as a bridge to lung transplant, extracorporeal membrane oxygenation (ECMO) improved its technology and results. Despite available data on the topic mostly derive from small non-homogeneous case series or reports, usually with a single center setting and a retrospective design, the literature shows that the use of ECMO bridging transplants has risen. Clinical success is more related to appropriate candidacy and timely deployment rather than to device-specific complications. Anyway, further efforts need to be done to improve outcomes and to increase the bridge to transplant/bridge to no-where ratio.

Chapter 28 - Noninvasive ventilation is a treatment option in patients with acute respiratory failure who have declined tracheal intubation. Moreover, NIV may be considered questionable for patients with hypercapnic coma. NIV can relieve dyspnea, improve comfort, and serve as a rescue therapy that can facilitate hospital discharge for some patients who are terminally ill and want to go home. The impact of NIV on the clinical and health-related quality of life is not known. In the case of severe acute respiratory failure in patients with DNI orders, NIV may avoid the need for endotracheal mechanical ventilation.

Chapter 29 - Idiopathic pulmonary fibrosis (IPF) is the most prevalent of interstitial lung diseases (ILD). The disease consists in the replacement of lung alveoli by a fibrotic tissue. Median survival in the absence of treatment is 3 to 5 years. Pirfenidone and nintedanib, two recently approved antifibrotic drugs, are able to slow disease course and prevent IPF-related exacerbations. For all these reasons, proper diagnosis and management are mandatory. The American (ATS), European (ERS), Latin American (ALAT) and Japanese (JRS) respiratory societies published joined updated guidelines for IPF diagnosis end of 2018(1). Those guidelines clearly highlight the role of a multidisciplinary discussion (MDD)-based management. First step consists in ruling out concurrent diagnosis through an appropriate interpretation of clinical, biological and radiological features by the members of the MDD. Optimal and holistic IPF management includes pharmacological and non-pharmacological interventions.

Chapter 30 - Idiopathic pulmonary fibrosis (IPF) is an age-associated, progressive, and irreversible disease of unknown etiology. IPF is typically diagnosed in the sixth decade, and its incidence significantly increases with age. It is characterized by a progressive decline in lung function from an irreversible process of destruction of pulmonary architecture, and currently approved antifibrotic agents, nintendanib and pirfenidone, only slow the progressive decline in lung function without improving survival. Early recognition allows referral to a multidisciplinary approach with consideration to lung transplantation.

Chapter 31 - In 2011, clinical practice guidelines were established by a joint assembly of representatives from the American Thoracic Society (ATS), the European Respiratory Society (ERS), the Japanese Respiratory Society (JRS), and the Latin American Thoracic Association (LATA) to create recommendations for the treatment of Idiopathic Pulmonary Fibrosis (IPF). These guidelines were later updated in a 2015 statement published by the ATS. These official joint statements, along with numerous other studies, continue to build upon current best practices to attenuate the progression of IPF. As of 2019, only two anti-fibrotic drugs have demonstrated clinical efficacy by significantly reducing decline in forced vital capacity - pirfenidone and nintedanib. Current recommendations for the pharmacologic treatment of IPF are summarized within. Other approaches to management seek to optimize patient's other comorbidities while providing symptom relief, pulmonary rehabilitation, and palliative care. In this chapter, the authors will discuss the pharmacologic therapies recommended for use in IPF, as well as discuss potential new therapies currently being investigated.

Chapter 32 - Over the last decade advances in pulmonary radiology have led to an increased familiarity of interstitial lung disease (ILD). Among the ILDs, idiopathic pulmonary fibrosis (IPF) is the most studied *in terms of basic* pharmaceutical research. Following diagnosis, disease progression can be slowed and quality of life can be improved, however, despite the availability of promising new drugs, life expectancy is still 3 to 5 years after diagnosis. There is still no definitive evidence regarding the effect of long term oxygen therapy (LTOT) on prolonged survival of patients with IPF although patients mostly opt to use LTOT as it improves their level of comfort. Even acute state, high flow oxygen with a nasal cannula (HFO-NC) provides promising results with respect to patient's comfort and allowing them to feel better in their last days of life in hospital. Domiciliary continuous positive airway pressure (CPAP) and non-invasive mechanical ventilation (NIV) can provide respiratory support in the advanced stages of IPF. CPAP with LTOT shows a similar effect to that of HFO-NC. NIV can be helpful if in cases with hypercapnia. Regardless of this respiratory support, the involvement of lung parenchyma determines the outcome. In this review, the long term management of IPF with LTOT and CPAP/NIV are evaluated.

Chapter 33 - Several transformations are used to reduce more complex Ising models on two-dimensional lattices to known exact solutions. In this way one can greatly extend the variety of systems that could be analyzed without any approximation. The systems discussed are based on the standard square lattice, the more elaborate 4-6 lattice and the triangular lattice. Four examples of solvable models are studied that include pairwise interactions with nearest neighbours and also with some more distant spins, competing and frustrated interactions, higher spins and crossing bonds. One observes models with disordered ground states showing coexistence of order and disorder, a model with critical surface with singular critical point that affects the behaviour in the proximity of the neighbouring regular critical points in the parameters space. Re-entrance phenomenon is quite common and manifests itself in two different forms. Its appearance does not require minimal coordination number of four. One model mapped to the eight-vertex displays three transitions each of them having different sets of critical exponents. The same system has an ordered phase at higher temperatures while its ground state is disordered. Two ordered and two partially ordered phases are observed on a decorated triangular lattice.

Chapter 34 - Chronic respiratory diseases represent a burden for healthcare systems, demanding new solutions in monitoring and treating these patients. New technologies may have a role in this setting.The present chapter describes the main telemedicine platforms used in monitoring patients with respiratory diseases and the experience with idiophatic pulmonary fibrosis.

Chapter 35 - Idiopathic pulmonary fibrosis (IPF) is a well-known interstitial lung disease (ILD) and has the worst prognosis of all the ILDs. The median life expectancy is approximately 3-5 years after diagnosis. In the last decade new anti-fibrotic drugs have led to an improvement in the health-related quality of life (HRQoL) and a slowing of IPF disease progression. Despite advances in diagnostic technology and medical treatment there is still a high mortality rate, i.e., nearly 50%, in cases of acute exacerbation of IPF or infectious conditions due to immunosuppression therapy, which require intubation for mechanical ventilation in the intensive care unit. As IPF progresses, supplemental oxygen treatment is required (when pulse oxygen saturation is below 88% at rest and in room air) and these IPF patients' have a decreased life expectancy. IPF patients 60 years or older and with acute respiratory failure have a shorter survival and a higher mortality rate. IPF is a crucial health problem that requires further research and attention to prevent mortality.

Chapter 36 - Lung transplantation (LTX) is an established treatment for patients with end-stage lung disease. Since the first combined heart and lung transplants the authors assessed to an amelioration of survival rates in solid organ transplantation and for this reason an evaluation on long-term outcomes following transplant is needed. Pulmonary Rehabilitation (PR) is an exercise-based treatment that improves walking endurance, muscle strength, and functional recovery: it has been demonstrated that PR is beneficial for patients with Chronic Pulmonary Diseases. After lung transplant it has been observed that despite an improvement in lung function, exercise intolerance and reductions in quality of life could persist up to years after transplantation. Literature reported that Pulmonary Rehabilitation post-LTx increases physical exercise capacity and health-related quality of life (HRQL), but few studies are available and a clear consensus is needed.

Chapter 37 - Idiopathic pulmonary fibrosis (IPF) and other forms of fibrosing interstitial lung diseases (F-ILD) induce a very severe limitation to exercise, due to changes in mechanical lung properties, impaired gas exchange and vascular pulmonary disruption. Disease progression is associated with a progressive impairment of exercise capacity and mobility, as a consequence of dyspnoea and exercise-induced hypoxaemia. Deconditioning and muscle wasting contribute to the inactivity of these patients, worsening the age-related loss of muscle mass quality and strength Pulmonary rehabilitation is recognized as a core component in the management of individuals with chronic respiratory disease, able to alleviate respiratory and psychological symptoms in different fibrosing interstitial lung disease. Improvement in exercise tolerance, walking capacity and quality of life scores following rehabilitation have been described, as well as improvement in dyspnoea and anxiety. Clinically relevant improvements in exercise capacity, symptoms and quality of life have been observed in F-ILD of different aetiologies following pulmonary rehabilitation, as well as after lung transplantation. Given the positive impact on patient-centred outcomes, irrespective of disease severity, efforts should be made to increase the accessibility of symptomatic ILD patients to pulmonary rehabilitation.

Chapter 38 - Pulmonary rehabilitation (PR) is a common practice in many respiratory diseases but most of the available evidence is limited to studies in Chronic Obstructive Pulmonary Disease (COPD) patients. Thus, most centers have applied COPD programs to other respiratory diseases. Due to its different pathophysiology, as well as its rapid progression and poor prognosis, idiopathic pulmonary fibrosis (IPF) has a different evolution of COPD and certainly has different needs to a design of a PR program. Thus, the aim of this review was to gather some of the available evidence on the role of PR in IPF, its particularities and the impact of these studies on available guidelines.

Chapter 39 - Psychiatric and psychological disorders are very common in idiopathic pulmonary fibrosis. Although this topic is well-known among chronic lung diseases, specific reviews about patients suffering from idiopathic pulmonary fibrosis, are no very frequent. The present analyses were performed to review the main diagnostic and therapeutic approaches in the authors' patient population. The authors' final aim is to provide a better quality of life to their patients and it´s possible with current tools. However, further investigations are needed to in this area.

Chapter 40 - Idiopathic pulmonary fibrosis (IPF) is defined as a specific form of chronic, progressive fibrosing interstitial pneumonia of unknown cause. The first guideline on IPF management, published in 2000, is based on the consensus of an international group of experts in the field. The guideline, created by hard work by the American Thoracic Society (ATS), European Respiratory Society (ERS), Japanese Respiratory Society (JRS), and Latin American Thoracic Society (ALAT) in 2011, reviewed all available evidence, clarified the definition of IPF, provided precise diagnostic criteria, described the natural course of the disease, and provided evidence-based recommendations for treatment. In 2015, recommendations for the treatment of IPF were updated on the basis of new scientific evidence. No pharmacological intervention has received strong recommendations for treatment. Clinicians should make individualized decisions based on conditional recommendations in the treatment of patients with IPF.

In: Respiratory Ventilatory Strategies …
Editor: Antonio M. Esquinas
ISBN: 978-1-53617-847-0
© 2020 Nova Science Publishers, Inc.

Chapter 1

INTRODUCTION: CLASSIFICATION OF INTERSTITIAL LUNG DISEASES

Irene Nieto Codesido[1,*], MD and Pedro J Marcos[2,†], MD, PhD
Respiratory Section, Complejo Hospitalario Universitario de Ferrol (CHUF), Sergas, A Coruña, Spain
Respiratory Service, Instituto de Investigación Biomédica de A Coruña (INIBIC), Complejo Hospitalario Universitario de A Coruña (CHUAC), Sergas, Universidade da Coruña (UDC), A Coruña, Spain

ABSTRACT

Interstitial lung diseases (ILD) are a heterogeneous group of pathologies that have in common the involvement of the pulmonary interstitium. Although they share similar clinical, radiological, physiological or pathological characteristics, its prognosis or response to specific drugs is completely different, so a correct classification will be very important to assess the better management. Mainly ILD are classified in two groups, those where the ILD was developed by a known cause (organic, inorganic agents, drugs, connective tissue diseases…) or by unknown origin. Among the latter there is a group of them with a poorly defined processes like sarcoidosis, langerhans cells hystiocitosis, lymphangioleiomyomatosis or pulmonary eosinophilias, and another group of idiopathic intersticial pneumonias that used to be subclassified among those that develop lung fibrosis, those associated with smoking or those with an acute/subacute evolution.

* Corresponding Author's E-mail: irene.nieto.codesido@sergas.es.
† Corresponding Author's E-mail: pedro.jorge.marcos.rodriguez@sergas.es.

INTRODUCTION

Interstitial lung diseases (ILD) are a heterogeneous group of pathologies that have in common the involvement of the pulmonary interstitium, the anatomical space between the basal membranes of the alveolar epithelium and the capillary endothelium. Although the interstitium is mainly affected, these diseases can also affect the small airways and pulmonary vasculature. Interstitial lung diseases are a heterogeneus group of diseases, they share similar clinical, radiological, physiological or pathological characteristics. If the disease is not controlled, either by avoidance of the potential causative agent, or by targeted effective treatment, the trend is a progressive evolution to an irreversible fibrosis.

A complete physical history and examination will be essential for the diagnosis, paying special attention to the occupational, environmental and pharmacological history [1]. Since these diseases share symptoms with other diseases more prevalent in the general population, such as chronic obstructive pulmonary disease (COPD) or asthma, a delay in the diagnosis of ILD is frequently observed.

CLASSIFICATION

The reference point on the classification of the ILD was established by Liebow and Carrington when they published their histological classification of chronic interstitial pneumonia in 1969 [2]. This classification was subsequently modified in 1997, both by the Katzenstein [3] group and by the Müller and Colby [4] group. The most accepted and used classification worldwide is the one made by consensus between the American Thoracic Society (ATS) and the European Respiratory Society (ERS) in 2002 [5] and its subsequent update in 2013 [6]. In these guides, the "gold standard" historical histological diagnosis was replaced by a multidisciplinary approach, so that the final diagnosis must be established after a team consisting of a clinical pulmonologist, radiologist and an expert pathologist has analyzed the patient's clinical, radiological and pathological data.

The classification of ILD will be based on whether they are associated with a known cause. In the group of entities with no known cause, we distinguish the idiopathic interstitial pneumonia (IIP) section from other ILD associated with poorly defined processes [6] (Table 1).

Table 1. ILD classification

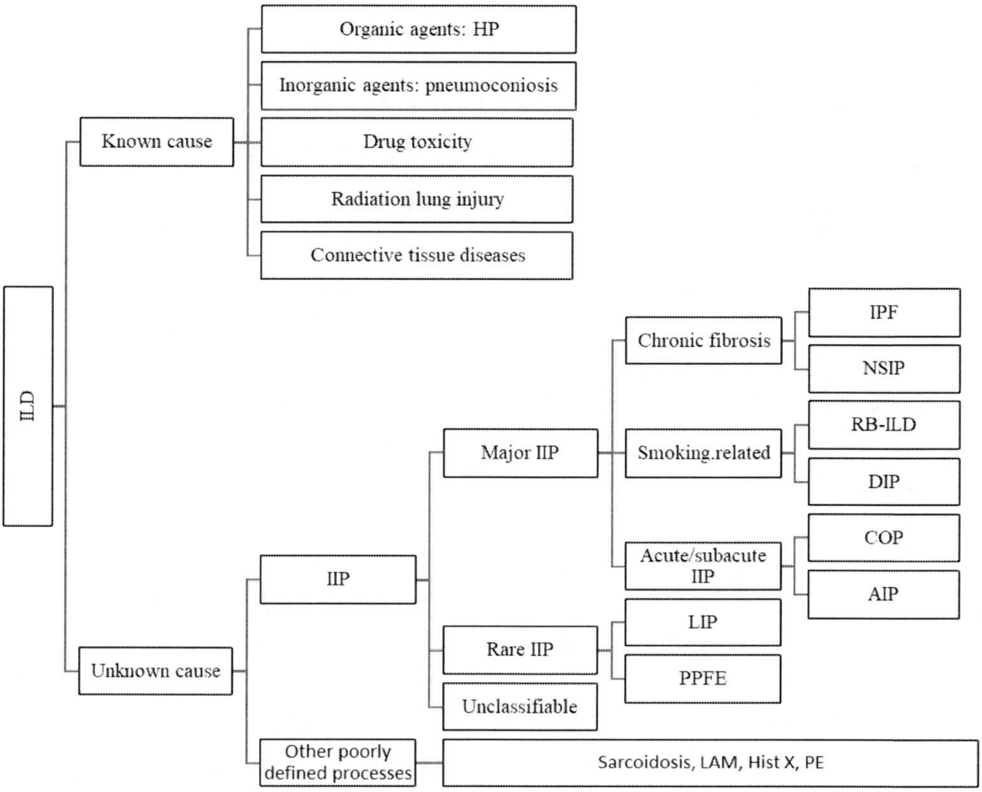

ILD: Interstitial lung diseases. HP: hypersensitivity pneumonitis. IIP: idiopathic interstitial pneumonia. IPF: idiopathic pulmonary fibrosis. NSIP: nonspecific idiophatic interstitial pneumonia. RB-ILD: respiratory bronchiolitis-interstitial lung disease. DIP: Desquamative interstitial pneumonia. COP: cryptogenic organizing pneumonia. AIP: acute interstitial pneumonia. LIP: lymphoid interstitial pneumonia. PPFE: pleuroparenchymal fibroelastosis. LAM: Lymphangioleiomyomatosis. Hist X: Hystiocitosis X. PE: Pulmonary eosinophilias.

Among the ILD of known cause, the most common are those secondary to exposure to occupational and environmental agents, mainly due to contact with inorganic (pneumoconiosis) or organic powders (hypersensitivity pneumonitis), and those due to drug-generated toxicity or radiation induced lung injury. There are also connective tissue diseases that can develop an ILD, such as polymyositis/dermatomyositis, rheumatoid arthritis, systemic lupus erythematosus, scleroderma or mixed connective tissue disease.

ILD with no known cause consists of a wide range from granulomatous diseases such as sarcoidosis to idiopathic interstitial pneumonia (IIP), within which there is another subclassification: major IIP, rare IIP and unclassifiable IIP.

Regarding the IIPs, on the one hand, we have the group of major IIP, which are grouped in chronic fibrosis (idiopathic pulmonary fibrosis and nonspecific idiophatic interstitial pneumonia), related to smoking (respiratory bronchiolitis-interstitial lung disease and interstitial pneumonia) and acute/subacute IIP (cryptogenic organizing pneumonia and acute interstitial pneumonia). On the other hand, it remains the idiopathic lymphoid interstitial pneumonia and idiopathic pleuroparenchymal fibroelastosis entities in the rare IIP section.

IIP with inadequate clinical, radiological or pathological data are included in the group of unclassifiable IIP, as well as cases of significant disagreement between clinical, radiological or pathological findings.

This includes the following situations [7]:

- Having received a previous treatment that modifies the radiological or histological findings, for example with steroids.
- The appearance of a new entity or an unusual variant of a recognized entity.
- Multiple high resolution CT and/or histological patterns that can be found in patients with IIP.

In the Consensus Classification of the IIP of the American Thoracic Society/European Respiratory Society [6] a classification according to disease behavior is also proposed. This is especially useful in those non-classifiable cases and those entities that can be associated with different behavior patterns. However, this classification still needs to be validated in clinical practice and is currently complementary to the classification of IIP, so in no case should it delay the performance of a surgical lung biopsy [7].

The five behavioral patterns of the disease described are the following [8]:

- Reversible and self-limited.
- Reversible disease with risk of progression.
- Stable with residual disease.
- Progressive, irreversible disease with potential for stabilization.
- Progressive, irreversible disease despite therapy.

REFERENCES

[1] Raghu G., Mageto Y. N., Lockhart D., Schmidt R. A., Wood D. E., Godwin J. D. The accuracy of the clinical diagnosis of new-onset idiopathic pulmonary fibrosis and other interstitial lung disease: a prospective study. *Chest* 1999; 116:1168-1174.

[2] Liebow A. A., Carrington C. B. The interstitial pneumonias. In: Simon M., Potchen E. J., LeMay M., editors. *Frontiers of Pulmonary Radiology,* 1st edition. New York: Grune & Stratton, 1969:102-141.

[3] Katzenstein A. L. A. *Katzenstein and Askin's surgical pathology of non-neoplasic lung disease.* Philadelphia: W. B. Saunders; 1997.

[4] Müller N. L., Colby T. V. Idiopathic interstitial pneumonias: high-resolution CT and histologic findings. *Radiographics* 1997; 17:1016-1022.

[5] American Thoracic Society, European Respiratory Society. American Thoracic Society/European Respiratory Society international multidisciplinary consensus classification of the idiopathic interstitial pneumonias. *Am J Respir Crit Care Med* 2002; 165:277-304.

[6] An official American Thoracic Society/European Respiratory Society statement: Update of the international multidisciplinary classification of the idiopathic interstitial pneumonias. *Am J Respir Crit Care Med.* 2013 Sep 15; 188(6):733-48.

[7] Ryerson C. J., Urbania T. H., Richeldi L., Mooney J. J., Lee J. S., Jones K. D., Elicker B. M., Koth L. L., King T. E. Jr., Wolters P. J., et al., Prevalence and prognosis of unclassificable interstitial lung diseases. *Eur Respir J* 2013; 42:750-757.

[8] Latsi P. I., du Bois R. M., Nicholson A. G., Colby T. V., Bisirtzoglou D., Nikolakopoulou A., Veeraraghavan S., Hansell D. M., Wells A. U. Fibrotic idiophatic interstitial pneumonia: the prognostic value of longitudinal functional trends. *Am J Respir Crit Care Med* 2003; 168:531-537.

In: Respiratory Ventilatory Strategies …
Editor: Antonio M. Esquinas
ISBN: 978-1-53617-847-0
© 2020 Nova Science Publishers, Inc.

Chapter 2

EPIDEMIOLOGY OF IDIOPATHIC PULMONARY FIBROSIS

Mohamed Y. Elnaggar*[1,2]*, MD
and Priyanka Heeru Teckchandani*[2]*, MD
[1]Department of Pulmonary, Critical Care, and Sleep Medicine,
University of California, Irvine, CA, US
[2]Department of Pulmonary, Critical Care, and Sleep Medicine,
Long Beach Veterans Affairs, Long Beach, CA, US

ABSTRACT

Idiopathic Pulmonary Fibrosis (IPF) is a rare disease with limited literature regarding epidemiology, because of the relatively few number of cases, along with varying definitions that have evolved over time. Geographically, IPF is more prevalent in industrialized nations, specifically in Europe and the United States; data from Asia is relatively limited at this time, but new information is emerging. Men, older patients, and Caucasians have been noted to have a great predisposition towards IPF. Additionally, several environmental exposures have been implicated in the pathogenesis of IPF. The most common risk factors for IPF include smoking and gastroesophageal reflux disease (GERD). Additional high-risk exposures include but are not limited to wood dust, metal dust, and agriculture. In rare case, familial genetic alterations have also been identified. The mortality in IPF is high, rivaling that in aggressive neoplasms in some cases. IPF exacerbations are associated with high utilization of healthcare resources, in association with high morbidity. In the future, more research is needed to elucidate epidemiology and risk factors, in order to develop more effective treatments, and to implement more preventative measures.

INTRODUCTION

Idiopathic Pulmonary Fibrosis (IPF), also known as Cryptogenic Fibrosing Alveolitis, is the most common type of Idiopathic Interstitial Pneumonia (IIP). IPF is defined as a spontaneously occurring specific form of chronic fibrosing interstitial pneumonia, typically associated with a pattern of Usual Interstitial Pneumonia (UIP) on High Resolution Computed Tomography (HRCT), or histologic appearance on surgical lung biopsy.

Although UIP is a distinct histologic lesion, this histologic pattern is not specific for IPF and can also be found in other diseases (ex: connective tissue diseases, asbestosis, and diseases related to diverse occupational, environmental, or drug exposures). A diagnosis of IPF can be established only when these and other alternative etiologies have been excluded.

In the United States (US), a rare disease is defined as a disease affecting fewer than 200,000 people. The epidemiology of IPF remains poorly described for many reasons, but complex diagnostic algorithms, and changes in definitions of IPF, have proven to be major challenges. IPF is rare, thus precise data regarding incidence and prevalence are lacking. There is global distribution of the progressive-fibrosing phenotype of all Interstitial Lung Diseases (ILDs), and yet there is significant paucity of data regarding prevalence and incidence of this type. Additionally, these studies in an already rare condition are limited by inclusion of those patients with access to healthcare in areas where research and epidemiologic studies are being conducted. Furthermore, the accuracy of the reported diagnoses of IPF is unknown, as most data has been retrospectively obtained from review of medical records, with variation in definitions, along with the evolution of coding practices over time. However, some of these limitations are overcome by using separate definitions, as described below. Numerous studies suggest that the prevalence of IPF is increasing, and that IPF is highly associated with advanced age, as well as complex interplay of environmental factors in the setting of genetic predisposition.

PREVALENCE AND INCIDENCE

Present literature suggests that IPF is the most common, or the second-most common type of ILD worldwide; variation has been noted by country. Most epidemiologic studies about IPF have been performed in the United States (US) and Europe (Italy, Greece, United Kingdom, Czech Republic, Norway, Finland, and Turkey), and very few studies performed in Asia thus far (Japan, Taiwan, China).

Europe

Overall in Europe, IPF prevalence ranged from 1.25 to 23.4 cases per 100,000, and the annual incidence ranged between 0.22 and 7.4 per 100,000.

A large study in Lombardy, Italy (population of approximately 10 million), by Harari et al. examined the epidemiology of IPF in detail, using "broad," "generic," and "narrow" definitions to define IPF. "Broad" categorization was defined as patients with at least one hospitalization or outpatient visit with IPF listed as a coded diagnosis. "Generic" diagnosis included the definition for "broad," in addition to having no outpatient or inpatient visit with "ILD" diagnosis on or after the date of IPF diagnosis. Finally, "narrow" was defined as including the requirements for "generic," plus either a surgical or transbronchial biopsy or a high-resolution computed tomography (HRCT) scan on or before the IPF diagnosis. IPF cases were identified based on inpatient and outpatient diagnosis codes from 2000-2010. Adjusting for age and sex, estimates were provided for prevalence and incidence from 2005-2010. The mean annual incidence was found to be 2.3 per 100,000 person-years using the narrow definition, and 5.3 per 100,000 person-years using the generic definition. Prevalence, on average, ranged from 12.6 and 35.5 per 100,000 depending on the definition used.

Annual incidence in Greece in the early 2000s was found to be approximately 0.9 per 100,000 person-years, and a prevalence of 3.4 per 100,000. In the United Kingdom, the IPF incidence in 2008 was 7.4 per 100,000 person-years. Prevalence in Norway was found to be 23.4 per 100,000, with an incidence of 4.3 per 100,000 person-years based on a study by von Plessen et al. from 1984-1998 in one hospital district. Similarly, Hodgson et al. studied hospital databases in Finland, and found prevalence to be approximately 16 to 18 per 100,000. Musselim et al. found a prevalence of 4.9 per 100,000 in Turkey from 2007 to 2009. Karakatsani et al. found a prevalence of 3.4 per 100,000 with an incidence of 0.9 per 100-000 person-years in Greece in 2004, significantly lower when compared to the US and the remainder of Europe.

United States

In the US, four large studies focusing on IPF have been performed. Raghu et al. have conducted multiple studies, including a landmark study in 2006. Additionally, Esposito et al. conducted a large study in 2015, wherein patient data was obtained from HealthCare Integrated Research Database, a nationwide private insurance claims database with linkage to medical records. Patients aged 50 years and older were evaluated from 2006 to 2012 using International Classification of Diseases (ICD)-9 codes to screen from more than 3.6 million individuals.

The study by Coultas et al. evaluated pathology reports, discharge diagnoses, autopsy reports, and death certificates from Bernalillo County, New Mexico, from 1988 to 1990. The definition used was for the former term of "idiopathic fibrosing alveolitis," estimating the prevalence of IPF in males to be 20.2 per 100,000 and in females to be 13.2 per 100,000. Raghu et al. examined IPF epidemiology by querying a database from a private health insurance claims database consisting of 20 patients from the year 2000. Prevalence in the US as studied by Raghu et al. was 14 and 42.7 per 100,000 using narrow and broad definitions respectively. Incidence was 6.8 and 16.3 per 100,000 person-years for the narrow and broad definitions respectively. Fernandez-Perez et al. evaluated patients in Olmsted County, Minnesota, from 1997-2005, using a country-wide medical record linkage system. Patients were screened initially based on diagnosis code, and then included based on revised IPF definitions. This study included 47 patients and estimated the prevalence of IPF in the US to be 27.9 and 63 per 100,000 using narrow and broad definitions respectively. Incidence was noted to be, on average, 17.4 per 100,000 person-years. Notably, this study only evaluated patients 55 years of age and older.

Asia

A study in Japan by Natsuizaka et al. found the prevalence in Japan to be much lower at 10 per 100,000, with incidence being 2.2 per 100,000 person-years. Ohno et al. evaluated medical benefit certificates for all idiopathic interstitial pneumonias (IIPs) in Japan in 2005, with data available for review in 35% of cases. The IIP incidence was 3.4 per 100,000 person-years, of which, 85.7% were categorized as IPF. A study by Lai et al. in Taiwan evaluated patients within the national health insurance system from 1997 to 2007, using similar definitions (for "narrow" and "broad") as denoted by Raghu et al. and Harari et al. as above. Prevalence was 0.7 to 6.4 per 100,000, and incidence was 0.6 to 1.4 per 100,000 person-years.

Trends

Raghu et al. reported that the prevalence of IPF in US patients ≥65 years of age in 2011 had more than doubled (494.5 cases per 100,000 people) from that found in 2001 (202.2 cases per 100,000 people), although the incidence had remained stable, suggesting that patients with IPF may be living longer. The study by Harari et al. also provided evidence that survival in IPF is increasing, based on the fact that the prevalence has been increasing while incidence has remained stable. Notably, incidence and prevalence of IPF in Europe and Japan are noted to be lower by comparison to the United States. However, some of these differences may relate to different definitions and varying criteria for subject selection, which could possibly account for some of the variation in observed rates of IPF.

VARIATION BY AGE

In the Harari et al. study, 63% of new incident cases occurred in patients between the ages of 65 years and 84 years. Incidence was 0.92 per 100,000 person-years in patients younger than 55 years of age, in contrast to 25.59 per 100,000 person-years in patients between the ages of 80 and 84 years. Prevalence (using the generic definition) in the Lombardi study was noted to rise with increasing age, increasing from 9.77 per 100,000 for patients under 55 years of age, to 143.71 per 100,000 for patients from 80-84 years of age. Notably, prevalence decreased to 99.20 per 100,000 for patients aged 85 and older. This trend in patients older than 84 years of age was similarly noted in a study in the United Kingdom by Gribbin et al. This trend has been attributed to clinical complexities and existence of various comorbidities in the elderly population.

VARIATION BY SEX

The consistent trend in epidemiologic studies evaluating prevalence of IPF notes a much higher rate of disease present in males, as compared to females. Some epidemiologic experts believe that the differences in rates of IPF among males and females may possibly correlate with the rates of smoking between the two groups. In the US, IPF is present with a male to female ratio that usually approaches 2:1. In the Harari et al. study, 60% of new incident cases were noted to occur in males; notably, this trend by sex was consistent regardless of the definition used. The prevalence of IPF in males by the narrow definition was 2.85 (confidence interval: 2.65-3.05), and in females was 1.84 (confidence interval: 1.65-2.00), and by the broad definition, was 4.63 (4.37-4.89) in males and 2.88 in females (2.69-3.08). Incidence in the Coultas et al. study for female was 7.4 per 100,000 person-years, and for males was 10.7 per 100,000 person-years.

Risk Factors

General Trends

Animal models have implicated repetitive alveolar epithelial stress due to a wide variety of possible inciting agents, contributing to the pathogenesis of IPF. Additionally, incidence and prevalence broadly appear to be higher in more industrialized countries; however, a large portion of the data available on IPF also stems from highly industrialized nations. Autopsies of patients with IPF in certain studies have shown an increased percentage of inorganic particles (such as silicon and aluminum) within the hilar lymph nodes of patients with IPF, as compared to the general population. Despite the associations described below, many patients with IPF do not appear to have any risk factors that have been linked to disease risk, and risk factors that have been identified require individuals to have genetic predisposition to develop pulmonary fibrosis in response to injury-inducing exposures.

Inhalants/Exposures

Smoking cigarettes has been identified repeatedly, consistently in multiple studies, to be a risk factor for IPF. A review of six case-control studies by Taskar and Coultar in 2006 evaluated patients from the US, UK, and Japan. This study found an association between IPF and agriculture/farming, hairdressing, bird exposure, animal/vegetable dust, livestock, wood dust, textile dust, mold, metal dust, stone, silica, sand, wood fires, and smoking. Notably, smoking was found to be associated with higher rates of IPF when adjusted for age and sex. As above, incidence in men is higher, which is possibly attributable to similarly higher smoking rates, including a higher risk for developing familial pulmonary fibrosis. Meta-analysis of two studies was suggestive of a dose-related response for exposure to metal dust and moderate smoking history. Notably, Gustafson et al. found no association between IPF and metal dust exposure or general wood dust exposure in Sweden. However, they did find an association specifically for men with hardwood dust exposure and birch exposure.

In Egypt, Awadalla et al. conducted a multicenter database analysis from 2010-2011, revealing associations with woodworking and petrochemicals among men, and birds and farming among women. A database search of the national death certificate registry from 1999-2003 was conducted by Pinheiro et al. using ICD-10 code J84.1 (other interstitial pulmonary diseases with fibrosis) with matched controls. They found a higher association between IPF and metal mining (2.34, 95% CI 1.3-4.0) and fabricated structural metal products (1.9, 95% CI 1.1-3.1).

GERD

A more recently implicated risk factor is the presence of pathologic gastroesophageal reflux disease (GERD), which may also play a role in acute exacerbation.

While a correlation between GERD and IPF has been identified, causality is yet to be proven. The pathogenesis of GERD in IPF has been proposed to involve microaspiration causing repetitive injury and inflammation, eventually inducing pulmonary fibrosis in predisposed patients. Notably, the prevalence of GERD in patients with IPF is about 67%-94%, and some retrospective studies associate GERD treatment with improved survival and reduced disease progression in IPF. Approximately half of IPF patients with GERD are found to be asymptomatic with regard to GERD symptoms, making this possibly preventable insult difficult to identify.

Genetics

Familial IPF has been defined as occurring in two or more members of the same biological family. Familial cases represent <5% of all IPF cases. Genes associated with familial IPF include telomerase-related genes (*TERT* and *TERC*), which account for approximately 18% of familial IPF. Additional genes include surfactant proteins C and A2 (*SPC* and *SPA2*), and *ELMOD2*. Interestingly, 25% of sporadic and 37% of familial cases without *TERT*/*TERC* mutations have short telomeres, possibly implicating shortening of telomeres in IPF pathogenesis. Finally, in families with the *TERT* mutation, development of IPF is age-related and associated with smoking. A common single nucleotide polymorphism in the promoter region of the mucin 5B gene (*MUC5B*) was discovered in 38% of sporadic IPF cases and 9% of controls. This association has been replicated in other cohorts.

HEALTHCARE RESOURCE UTILIZATION

Most of the healthcare utilization for IPF stems from acute hospitalizations. A large majority of hospitalizations related to IPF occur due to acute worsening of respiratory status in a period of less than 1 month, in the absence of other acute causes of respiratory failure, such as infection. Largely based on retrospective data, the annual rate of IPF exacerbations is estimated at around 5-20%, associated with a mortality rate ranging from 20-100%. Fernandéz-Peréz et al. showed that 79% of IPF patients required hospitalization with a rate of 0.13 hospitalizations per patient year. In the United Kingdom, Navaratnam et al. found a hospitalization rate of 14.5 per 100,000 person-years related to IPF, upon examining IPF-related hospitalization data from 1998-2010. The hospitalization rate was also found to increase by 5% per year. Men and older patients tended to have higher rates of admission; average length of stay decreased from 7.2 days to 5.1 days over the study period.

However, the associated healthcare cost increased from approximately £12 million to £16.2 million. Collard et al. performed a similar analysis in the US by performing a review of two insurance claims databases evaluating patients between 2001 and 2008. The inclusion criteria for their study included age >55 years and at least two claims of ICD-9 code 516.3 (idiopathic interstitial pneumonia) or one claim each with ICD-9 code 516.3 and 515 (post-inflammatory pulmonary fibrosis). Age- and sex-matched controls were used for comparison. The review found that all-cause hospitalization rate (0.5 per person-year), the days in hospital (3.1 days per person-year), and the outpatient visit rate (28 visits per person-year) were twice as high than in the control group, and similarly, inpatient mortality was more than three-fold higher in the IPF group. The average annual direct costs were approximately twice as high in IPF patients, which amounted to an annual cost of $12,124. Based on a prevalence of 89,000 patients with IPF in the United States, it was estimated that the aggregate incremental cost due to IPF was over $1 billion per year.

SURVIVAL RATES AND MORTALITY

Mortality within IPF is defined as death within the general population of patients in whom IPF considered to be the underlying cause, or an associated cause. Data is collected typically from national death certificate registries. These are often underreported due to either misclassification or under-recognition of IPF.

Despite attempts to attain accurate estimates of mortality and morbidity for patients with IPF, considerable variability in survival rates has been found. Studies also have found geographic variability, which suggests that ethnic background or environmental exposures may possibly account for these findings. One of the most remarkable findings is that IPF-related mortality is similar to that of many aggressive cancers.

Although IPF has been generally associated with a poor prognosis with a median survival that has been estimated at two to three years from the time of diagnosis, more recent studies suggest that median survival is three to five years following diagnosis. Raghu et al. reported a median survival of 3.8 years in US patients who were ≥65 years, with increased mortality risk for males and older age. Three studies evaluated mortality from IPF in the US, Canada, United Kingdom, Germany, Australia, and New Zealand from the 1970s to 1990s. Trends from those studies show that mortality rates are higher in men and in older patients. Similarly, Navaratnam et al. found higher rates of mortality in the United Kingdom in older patients and men, when they examined data from 1968 to 2008. Olson et al. conducted an investigation regarding mortality rates in IPF in the US from 1992 to 2003. The IPF mortality rate was found to be very similar to the contemporary incidence rate of IPF in this study, with a mortality of approximately 5.8 per 100,000 person-years, and a coinciding incidence rate of 6.8-8.8 per 100,000 person-years.

Mortality rates increased during the study period, most notably in women, presumably associated with the rise in smoking rates among women. Most patients were noted to die of IPF, rather than with IPF and from another cause such as ischemic disease.

Most deaths were noted in Caucasian patients. In another study, among all IPF-related deaths, 87.2% occurred in white patients, 5.1% in black patients, 5.4% in Hispanic patients, and 2.2% in other racial/ethnic groups. In the study by Navaratnam et al. in the UK, mortality was observed to increase from 0.92 per 100,000 person-years in 1968-1972 to 5.1 per 100,000 person-years in 2005-2008; additionally noted was an annual increase of 5% after controlling for age and sex.

Interestingly, Nathan et al. found that a substantial percentage (25% at 10 years following initial diagnosis) of patients with IPF have long-term survival without transplantation; these patients tend to have better preserved values for forced vital capacity (FVC) and diffusion capacity for carbon monoxide (DLCO) at the time of diagnosis.

CONCLUSION

Idiopathic pulmonary fibrosis is an uncommon disease, but its prevalence appears to be increasing, and may be higher than reported in the literature because of reporting and recognition bias.

The risk factors of developing IPF likely include both host and environmental factors. In general, IPF prevalence increases with age. There is a much greater prevalence of IPF in males than in females. There is yet a large deficit in knowledge regarding the epidemiology of the disease; at present, there are entire continents without any available data on the occurrence of IPF. Future research efforts to elucidate epidemiology of IPF further will need to focus on stricter definitions and further identification of predisposing risk factors.

References

Callahan, William P. "Acute Diffuse Interstitial Fibrosis of the Lungs." *Archives of Internal Medicine*, vol. 90, no. 4, 1952, p. 468, doi:10.1001/archinte.1952.00240100045005.

Coultas, D. B., et al. "The Epidemiology of Interstitial Lung Diseases." *American Journal of Respiratory and Critical Care Medicine*, vol. 150, no. 4, 1994, pp. 967-972, doi:10.1164/ajrccm.150.4.7921471.

Esposito, Daina B., et al. "Idiopathic Pulmonary Fibrosis in United States Automated Claims. Incidence, Prevalence, and Algorithm Validation." *American Journal of Respiratory and Critical Care Medicine*, vol. 192, no. 10, 2015, pp. 1200-1207, doi: 10.1164/rccm.201504-0818oc.

Harari, Sergio, et al. "Epidemiology of Idiopathic Pulmonary Fibrosis in Northern Italy." *PLoS One*, vol. 11, no. 2, 2016, doi:10.1371/journal.pone.0147072.

Ley, Brett, and Harold Collard. "Epidemiology of Idiopathic Pulmonary Fibrosis." *Clinical Epidemiology*, 2013, p. 483, doi:10.2147/clep.s54815.

Meyer, Keith C. "Pulmonary Fibrosis, Part I: Epidemiology, Pathogenesis, and Diagnosis." *Expert Review of Respiratory Medicine*, 2017, pp. 1-17, doi:10.1080/17476348.2017.1312346.

Olson, Amy L., et al. "The Epidemiology of Idiopathic Pulmonary Fibrosis and Interstitial Lung Diseases at Risk of a Progressive-Fibrosing Phenotype." *European Respiratory Review*, vol. 27, no. 150, 2018, p. 180077, doi:10.1183/16000617.0077-2018.

Raghu, Ganesh, et al. "An Official ATS/ERS/JRS/ALAT Statement: Idiopathic Pulmonary Fibrosis: Evidence-Based Guidelines for Diagnosis and Management." *American Journal of Respiratory and Critical Care Medicine*, vol. 183, no. 6, 2011, pp. 788-824, doi:10.1164/rccm.2009-040gl.

Raghu, Ganesh, et al. "Incidence and Prevalence of Idiopathic Pulmonary Fibrosis." *American Journal of Respiratory and Critical Care Medicine*, vol. 174, no. 7, 2006, pp. 810-816, doi:10.1164/rccm.200602-163oc.

In: Respiratory Ventilatory Strategies … ISBN: 978-1-53617-847-0
Editor: Antonio M. Esquinas © 2020 Nova Science Publishers, Inc.

Chapter 3

BASIC KEY ASPECTS OF PHYSIOLOGY OF IDIOPATHIC PULMONARY FIBROSIS

Gregorino Paone[1,*], Giulia De Rose[1] and Josuel Ora[2]
[1]Department of Cardiovascular, Respiratory, Nephrologic, Anesthesiologic, Geriatric Sciences Sapienza University of Rome, Rome, Italy
[2]2nd Division of Respiratory Medicine, University Hospital "Tor Vergata", Rome, Italy

ABSTRACT

In Idiopathic Pulmonary Fibrosis there is typically recognizable restrictive ventilatory pattern: in this pattern the static expiratory pressure – volume (P-V) curve of the lung is moved down and to the right compared with normal subjects. Lung recoil is increased over the entire range of the reduced inspiratory capacity and both vital capacity (VC) and total lung capacity (TLC) are reduced.

The causes of decreased lung compliance in ILD are multifactorial and involve leak of lung volume, decreased alveolar distensibility, alterations in the elastic properties and raised alveolar surface tension.

Lung diffusing capacity is nearly always reduced in subjects with IPF. DLCO decrease come out from parenchymal and vascular damages.

Pulmonary hypertension (PH) is usually associated with higher mortality in subjects with IPF.

The causes of pulmonary hypertension in IPF are still not known. Latest data offer a multifactorial etiology (e.g., primary lesions of vessels and vasoconstriction).

* Corresponding Author's E-mail: gregorino.paone@uniroma1.it.

PATHOGENESIS

Idiopathic Pulmonary Fibrosis (IPF) is a specific form of chronic, progressive fibrosing interstitial pneumonia of unknown cause, occurring in adults, limited to the lungs, and associated with the histopathologic and/or radiologic pattern of Usual Interstitial Pneumonia (UIP) [1]. Idiopathic pulmonary fibrosis (IPF) is one of the most commonly diagnosed interstitial lung diseases (ILDs) [2, 3].

IPF is very attractive to the lung physiologist because its clinical expression, which ranges from exertional dyspnea, occurring early in the disease, to end-stage respiratory failure, is directly related to alterations in lung physiology [4].

The trigger factors in the development of IPF are undetermined. It is very likely that the fibrotic and destructive changes twist the normal lung architecture and result in the high mortality and morbidity. Most information comes from analysis of the tissue acquired from pulmonary biopsies. In the lungs numerous risk factors have been recognized: smoke, viral infections, Gastroesophageal Reflux Disease (GERD), environmental and professional exposure. All those issues could be responsible for the multiple microinjuries damage of the parenchyma [5].

Lung fibrosis is determined by replacement of normal, compliant lung extracellular matrix, rich in elastin, with an unusual one rich in fibrillar collagen. Alveolar lesions obey the usual interstitial pneumonia pattern. The UIP pattern is described by: 1) spatial heterogeneity, like areas of normal lung alternate with lesions; 2) temporal heterogeneity, with the coexistent presence of fibrotic areas, mainly constituted of dense acellular collagen, and distinct lesions in lung tissue that seems then normal, named fibroblastic foci; 3) the presence of honeycomb lesions, abnormal dilated airspaces with fibrotic tissue walls, lined by an epithelium sharing the same characteristics of the airway.Tissue adjustments are moreover observed in other parts of the respiratory system. For example, expression of Ki67, a marker of cell proliferation, is detected in airway epithelial cells.

Selman and colleagues () suppose that UIP signifies a pattern of lung anomalous wound healing, described by the deficiency of satisfactory reepithelialization and aberrations in myofibroblast functioning [6]. The pathologic process of fibrosis is the effect of persevering makeover of the lung interstitium.

The alveolar epithelial cells (AEC) play a key role in the pathogenic of IPF. The AEC type I are squamous cells recovering the 90 – 95% of the alveolar surface and they make a thin layer trough which the gases can pass; otherwise the AEC type II are involved in repairing processes and in the production of Surfactant, a complex lipoprotein molecule [7].

The AEC exposition to risk factors may damage the epithelium causing an abnormal activation of these cells, loss of epithelium integrity and apoptosis.

The activated alveolar epithelial cells induce an antifibrinolytic environment in the alveolar spaces, enhancing wound clot formation.

Alveolar epithelial cells produce growth factors and stimulate migration and proliferation of fibroblasts and differentiation into myofibroblasts. Proposed hypothesis suggests that the fibroblastic foci are the main sites of ongoing injury and repair in UIP. These small aggregates of actively proliferating myofibroblasts and fibroblasts are localized within the interstitial space directly beneath the alveolar epithelium. They are frequently at the interface between dense-collagenized and normal-appearing lung. Subepithelial myofibroblasts and alveolar epithelial cells produce gelatinases that might enhance basement membrane disruption and allow fibroblast–myofibroblast migration. Angiogenic factors induce neovascularization. Either intra–alveolar and interstitial myofibroblasts release extracellular matrix proteins, principally collagens.

Therefore, these foci make up many microscopic sites of ongoing alveolar epithelial injury and their activation is associated with developing fibrosis.

A derangement between interstitial collagens and tissue inhibitors of metalloproteinases causes the continuous deposition of extracellular matrix, pathologic alterations that characterize the IPF alveolar microenvironment. Recently, it has been demonstrated that matrix metalloproteinases MMP1 and MMP7, both previously implicated in the pathogenesis of IPF, are significantly increased in plasma, serum, bronchoalveolar lavage fluid (BAL), and lung tissue of IPF patients. This may reflect that MMP1 and MMP7 are involved in tissue remodeling or contribute to fibrosis through recruitment of neutrophils, which release reactive oxygen species (ROS) and transforming growth factor–beta (TGF - β).

Increased plasma concentration of MMPs may, therefore, reflect increased extracellular matrix turnover and disease activity. Signal responsible for myofibroblast apoptosis seem to be absent or delayed in UIP, increasing cell survival. Myofibroblasts produce angiotensinogen, which, as angiotensin II, provokes alveolar epithelial cell death, further impairing reepithelialization.

The endoplasm reticulum (ER) stress is caused by unfolded and/or misfolded proteins accumulation. IPF patients have high level of ER stress marker like Binding Immunoglobulin Protein (BIP), ER degradation enhancing α- mannosidase I – like protein (EDEM) and X-box binding protein 1 (XBP – 1).

The accumulation of these proteins defines the activation of a repair mechanism called Proteostasis involving several systems as Unfolded Protein Response (UPR), Endoplasmic – reticulum – associated protein degradation (ERAD) and autophagy. The UPR system is the first to play a role in this process promoting the proteins folding or increasing their destruction. This system is regulated by sensors consist of trans membrane proteins [Protein Kinase RNA – like endoplasmic reticulum kinase (PERK), Activating Transcription Factor 6 (ATF6) and Iron Responsive Element (IRE)], usually inactive because linked to the chaperone BIP/GRP78. Increased levels of unfold proteins could cause the dissociation of BIP from the sensors determining the activation of repair mechanism.

PHYSIOPATHOLOGY

In IPF is typically recognizable a restrictive ventilatory pattern: the static expiratory pressure – volume (P-V) curve of the lung is moved down and to the right compared with normal subjects [8]. Lung recoil is amplified over the entire range of the reduced inspiratory capacity. Thus, the P-V relation of the lung is acquired along its volume axis, and both vital capacity (VC) and total lung capacity (TLC) are reduced. The procedure of decreased lung compliance in ILD are multifactorial and involves leak of lung volume, decreased alveolar distensibility, alterations in the elastic properties and raised alveolar surface tension. A reduction in lung volume is perhaps the most important explication for decreased static compliance. Gibson and Pride have analyzed patients with progressive IPF and reduced static lung compliance. They concluded that these phenomena can be mainly explained by the loss of functioning alveoli occurring heterogeneously throughout the lungs. These authors analyzed static expiratory P-V curves with the lung volume expressed as a percentage of the predicted TLC or as a percentage of the actual TLC. They saw that in many patients P-V curves were regularized when expressed as percentages of the current TLC. Then, it is important underline that decreased static lung compliance is determined by loss of functioning alveolar units. Though this is one of the significant factors, it is possible to search out further for other potential contributors to decreased lung compliance in IPF. These factors enclose: altered tissue elastic component, decreased alveolar size and surface tension addition because of not regular configuration or amounts of pulmonary surfactant.

It is clear that static lung volumes are usually reduced in IPF. VC is unevenly diminished, even if the reduction is not IPF specific and may happen in several diseases: obstructive lung diseases, inspiratory muscle failing, chest wall restriction and after lung resection. Decreased VC reflects insufficient functioning of the alveoli. In fact, the disease process causes obliteration of the alveolar units because of exudate, inflammatory material or edema.

Functional residual capacity (FRC) is reduced as well in IPF but usually less than VC and TLC. The FRC is determined by the equilibrium among the external chest wall recoil and in the inward elastic recoil. Since the reduction in gas volume is typically attended by increased lung tissue volume, FRC is usually preserved. Thus, intrapleural pressure (P_{Pl}) would be expected to be diminished at that volume. Conversely, lots of studies have shown that total thoracic gas volume is normal in association with a normal chest wall recoil pressure determining P_{pl} to be normal or actually increased at FRC. Standard chest wall configuration may be related to adaptive changes in diaphragmatic length in response to chronically diminished lung volumes.

The reduction in TLC is relatively lower than in VC. TLC is the equilibrium between inspiratory muscle vigor and the recoil of the lung and chest wall. TLC is reasonably well preserved in spite of reduced lung compliance due to inspiratory muscles mechanical advantage and the normal chest wall recoil pressure. In case of other concomitant diseases, like small airways disease with air trapping, TLC can be increased toward normal values.

Residual Volume (RV) is usually 80% predicted normal in IPF, and the RV/TLC ratio is often increased. The preservation of RV appears to be for the presence of slightly ventilated cystic air space that concur to lung volumes measured by body plethysmography and the coexistence of small airways disease as part of the disease process or as a result of damage from smoking.

Deterioration of lung function over time depends on different factors, including the nature of the basic disease, host factors, and therapy reaction. In IPF the static lung volumes worsening is generally gradual: some patients might have acute exacerbations with a fast and sudden downhill of FVC. The clinical deterioration often correlates with worsening radiographic appearance.

Airway function is generally well preserved;spirometric measurements are typically regular. or slightly atypical. Examination of the highest expiratory flow–volume loop shows that although peak expiratory flows may be reduced in absolute terms, flow rated are consistently increased at a given volume compared to normal. This behavior is explained by the increased driving pressure for expiratory flow as a result of increased lung recoil pressures at volumes above FRC and by attendant preservation of static airway dimensions. Clinical suspicion of small airway dysfunction arises if, for example, $FEF^{25\text{-}75}$ is reduced or if the maximal expiratory flow curve is oriented concave to the horizontal volume axis. Several studies have shown that plethysmographic measurements of total airway conductance are usually in the normal range even in the presence of documented pathologic involvement of the small airways. This suggests that tests of total airway resistance are not sufficiently sensitive to detect increased resistance in small airways where conditions of laminar flow prevail.

Other exams to estimate small airways dysfunction in ILD include isovolume pressure – flow measurements, the ratio of dynamic to static compliance capacities and closing volume.

Lung diffusing capacity is nearly always reduced in subjects with IPF. The DLCO is reduced in most of IPF patients at the time of initial evaluation, although several individuals had regular TLC and FVC. DLCO decrease come out from parenchymal and vascular damages. The latter being mostly dependent on the pulmonary capillary volume as reported in Roughton–Forster model, where gas diffusion across the alveolar wall hang on membrane conductance (DmCO) and vascular conductance.

DLCO is usually estimated by a single-breath exam where the patient inhales a gas mix including an insoluble, like helium (He) or methane (CH4), with carbon monoxide (CO). The volume where gases switch occurs [alveolar volume (VA)] and the transfer constant of carbon monoxide (KCO) are measured on the reduction of He/CH4 and carbon monoxide concentrations in exhaled breath. DLCO is calculated by multiplying

VA and KCO. Generally, DLCO considers the gas-exchanging function of the entire lungs, while KCO reflects gas exchange per unit of lung volume [9]. Reference values for DLCO, VA and KCO were achieved in healthy patients at full lung inflation. When the lungs are inflated below TLC (i.e., low VA), DLCO slightly decreases while KCO increases. The increase in KCO at low lung volume in normal individuals is due to the unfolding of alveolar walls resulting in increased mass of gas-exchanging tissue per unit of volume.

Both VA and KCO are reduced in IPF. Of note, KCO is in the usual range in up to 30% of patients with IPF, especially in those with moderately reduced DLCO. It is important not to distort this finding as being indicative of a preservation of gas exchange units; indeed, it can be supposed that full lung inflation might not be attainable in IPF. In normal patients, KCO rises at low lung volumes. Then predicted values are insufficient to interpret it in patients with restrictive disease. On the other hand, the spatial heterogeneity of damage in IPF may influence KCO. So, a normal KCO value in IPF patients does not mean that pulmonary gas exchange is normal. DLCO correlates better than KCO with exertional growth in PaO_2. DLCO and KCO are both tightly correlate with the extension of disease as seen by scoring of computed tomography scans. Supporting the significance of DLCO to the clinical evaluation of IPF, DLCO is highly correlated both with dyspnea and survival. It remains unclear which changes in the alveolar–capillary membrane or in the lung circulation are the predominant gear of DLCO cut in IPF. At the opposite, KCO is correlated both with diminished oxygen diffusion and with alveolar ventilation (V′A)/Q′ mismatch, as shown by the multiple inert gas elimination test (MIGET). Concurrent carbon monoxide (CO) and nitric oxide (NO) diffusion measurements can aid to analyze what extent alterations in membrane take part in DLCO reductions [10, 11]. NO reacts nearly directly with haemoglobin, so the diffusing capacity of the lung for nitric oxide (DLNO) is independent of vascular conductance and is equivalent to the conductance of the alveolar–capillary membrane to nitric oxide (DmNO). Because DmNO/DmCO is setted, both DmCO and vascular conductance can be calculated with the DLCO/DLNO technique. Several studies demonstrate severe and analogous decreases in both membrane conductance and lung capillary volume, showing that alterations in both membranes contribute to the worsening of gas diffusion in IPF.

The specific arterial blood gas abnormalities in ILD are resting hypoxemia and rise alveolar – arterial oxygen tension gradient. Arterial CO_2 tension ($PaCO_2$) is usually in the normal range but may be decreased at rest in a number of patients due to alveolar hyperventilation. Arterial pH is typically normal. An increased $PaCO_2$ is clearly uncommon except in the terminal stage of the disease; airway function is relatively saved; eucapnia is guaranteed by raised minute ventilation even in the presence of gas exchange mismatch at the interface between alveoli and capillary.

Damaged gas diffusion from the alveolus to the capillary may result from either an anomaly of membrane or a decrease in pulmonary capillary blood volume. Some authors experimentally split membrane and blood components establishing that their relative contribution to lung diffusion can vary but the membrane conductance anomalies frequently predominate in ILD. These membrane abnormalities have been demonstrated, from morphometric analysis of lung biopsy specimens, not to be due to increased membrane thickness and to reduced alveolar surface area.

The pathologic process commonly has a rambling distribution throughout the lungs. The result is a substantial regional variation in lung compliance and an unusual distribution of ventilation time. Recently, a lot of inert gas removal tests have validated heterogeneity of ventilation – perfusion (V/Q) distribution. An abnormal V/Q ratio has been proved to resting hypoxemia. Wagner and colleagues handling multiple inert gas elimination techniques, showed that the distribution of V/Q relationship was bimodal; the majority of alveolar units have usually preserved V/Q ratios (ie, V/Q ratio = 1.0) and the other units (9% of total) indicate markedly reduced ventilation (V/Q ratio < 0.1). These tests have demonstrated that arterial hypoxemia at rest in patients with ILD could be presented on the basis of V/Q derangements.

Several studies demonstrate that intrapulmonary right – to – left shunting concurs minimally to resting arterial hypoxemia. Though, shunts are usually linked to one more of the following: 1) the anastomosis among pulmonary and bronchial circulation, 2) pulmonary hypertension 3) development of right – to – left intracardiac shunts accompanied by sever pulmonary hypertension with right ventricular hypertrophy.

Pulmonary hypertension (PH) is usually associated with higher mortality in subjects with IPF [12]. Diagnosis of PH is based upon clinical evaluation, reduction in diffusing capacity, severe hypoxemia or exercise – induced oxygen desaturation, echocardiography findings or the presence of biomarkers, like B-type natriuretic peptide (BNP) [13].

It is important to underline that the evaluation of pulmonary artery systolic pressures trough echocardiographic exam does not exactly correlate with right heart catheterization, considered the gold standard for hemodynamic estimation of pulmonary circulation. Therefore, in every patient with evidence of IPF identified by noninvasive investigations should be performed the right heart catheterization. PH rarely occurs at rest in patients with early IPF and it can be expected when the VC is less than 50% of predicted or the DLCO get down below 45% of predicted. Nevertheless, PH during exercise is usual even during the early stages. Auscultatory findings consistent with pulmonary hypertension are attendant in more than 70% of subjects with advanced IPF. The pulmonary arterial pressure at rest ranges among 23 and 28 mmHg and rarely overtake 40 mmHg and a pressure at rest higher than 30 mmHg is associated with a poor prognosis. Particularly, patient with emphysema appear prone to the develop severe pulmonary hypertension resulting in a much higher mortality matched with those without emphysema [14].

The causes of pulmonary hypertension in IPF are still unknown. (3) Latest data offer a multifactorial etiology: 1) primary lesions of pulmonary vessels (e.g., vasculitis); 2) compression and destruction of pulmonary vessels by the interstitial process; 3) vasoconstriction of vessels mediated by hypoxia, acidosis and autacoids; 4) pulmonary blood volume, pulmonary arterial compliance and left ventricular function. It has been demonstrated that oxygen therapy at rest and during exercise gets better pulmonary hemodynamics and improves exercise capacity and prognosis as well. However, little data exist on the value of vasodilator therapy in the treatment of pulmonary hypertension in the ILDs.

Obstructive sleep apnea is common in IPF patients even if, in most cases, may be underestimated [15]. It has been shown that IPF patients, particularly those with a daytime $Sa0_2$ of less than 90% and/or a story of snoring, develop sleep disorders. These patients present other characteristic such as: reduced rapid eye movement (REM) sleep, lighter and more fragmented sleep and hypoxemia during REM sleep. When there is a clinical worsening with disease progression, linear densities and reticulation become more extensive and eventually result in a honeycombed appearance. Pleural involvement is very unusual in IPF; thus, its presence may indicate other diagnosis: mitral valve disease, collagen vascular disease (especially rheumatoid arthritis or systemic lupus erythematosus), asbestosis, congestive heart failure, drug induced lung disease, infections or lymphangitic carcinosis.

References

[1] Schwarz, M. I., King, T. E. 2011. "*Interstitial Lung Disease,* 5th edition". People's Medical Publishing House – USA, Shelton, Connecticut.

[2] Raghu, G., Collard, H. R., Egan, J. J. et al. 2011. "An official ATS/ERS/JRS/ALAT statement: idiopathic pulmonary fibrosis: evidence-based guidelines for diagnosis and management". *American Journal of Respiratory and Critical Care Medicine,* 183: 788 - 824. doi: 10.1164/rccm.2009-040GL.

[3] Faverio, P., De Giacomi, F., Bonaiti, G. et al. 2019. "Management of Chronic Respiratory Failure in Interstitial Lung Diseases: Overview and Clinical Insights". *International Journal of Medical Sciences,* 16(7):967 - 980. doi: 10.7150/ijms.32752.

[4] Plantier, L., Cazes, A., Dinh – Xuan, A. T. et al. 2018. "Physiology of the lung in idiopathic pulmonary fibrosis". *The European Respiratory Review,* 27:170062. doi: 10.1183/16000617.0062-2017.

[5] Raghu, G., Ley, B., Brown, K. K. et al. 2019. "Risk factors for disease progression in idiopathic pulmonary fibrosis". *Thorax,* doi: 10.1136/thoraxjnl-2019-213620.

[6] Selman, M., Pardo, A. 2019. "The leading role of epithelial cells in the pathogenesis of idiopathic pulmonary fibrosis". *Cell Signal,* 66:109482. doi: 10.1016/j.cellsign.2019.109482.

[7] Sgalla, G., Iovene, B., Calvello, M. et al. 2018 "Idiopathic pulmonary fibrosis: pathogenesis and management". *Respiratory Research,* 22; 19(1):32. doi: 10.1186/s12931-018-0730-2.

[8] Sansores, R. H., Ramirez – Venegas, A., Pérez – Padilla, R. et al. 1996. "Correlation between pulmonary fibrosis and the lung pressure–volume curve". *Lung,* 174: 315 - 323. doi: 10.1007/bf00176190.

[9] Johnson, D. C. 2000. "Importance of appropriately adjusting carbon monoxide diffusing capacity (DLCO) and carbon monoxide transfer coefficient (KCO) for alveolar volume. *Respiratory Medicine,* 94(1): 28 - 37. doi: 10.1053/med.1999.0740.

[10] Barisione, G., Brusasco, C., Garlaschi, A. et al. 2016. "Lung diffusing capacity for nitric oxide as a marker of fibrotic changes in idiopathic interstitial pneumonias". *Journal of Applied Physiology,* 120: 1029 - 1038. doi: 10.1152/japplphysiol.00964.2015.

[11] Borland, C., Hughes, J. M. B., Guénard, H. 2017. "The blood transfer conductance for CO and NO. Review article". *Respiratory Physiology and Neurobiology,* 241:53 - 57. doi: 10.1016/j.resp.2017.02.010.

[12] Nathan, S. D., Shlobin, O. A., Ahmad, S. et al. 2007. "Pulmonary hypertension and pulmonary function testing in idiopathic pulmonary fibrosis". *Chest,* 131: 657 - 663. doi: 10.1378/chest.06-2485.

[13] Nathan, S. D., Barbera, J. A., Gaine, S. P. et al. 2019. "Pulmonary hypertension in chronic lung disease and hypoxia". *European Respiratory Journal,* 24; 53(1). doi:10.1183/13993003.01914-2018.

[14] Cottin, V., Hansell, D. M., Sverzellati, N. et al. 2017. Effect of emphysema extent on serial lung function in patients with idiopathic pulmonary fibrosis. *American Journal of Respiratory and Critical Care Medicine,* 196:1162 - 1171. doi: 10.1164/rccm.201612-2492OC.

[15] Mermigkis, C., Boulokaki, I., Schiza, S. E. et al. 2017. "Sleep as a New Target for Improving Outcomes in Idiopathic Pulmonary Fibrosis". *Chest,* 152(6):1327 - 1338. doi:10.1016/j.chest.2017.07.019.

In: Respiratory Ventilatory Strategies …
Editor: Antonio M. Esquinas
ISBN: 978-1-53617-847-0
© 2020 Nova Science Publishers, Inc.

Chapter 4

IMMUNITY, INFLAMMATION AND LUNG FIBROSIS

Thomas Planté-Bordeneuve, MD and Antoine Froidure, MD, PhD
Pneumology department, Cliniques universitaires Saint-Luc, Bruxelles
Université catholique de Louvain, Belgium

ABSTRACT

The role of the immune system in idiopathic pulmonary fibrosis (IPF) pathogenesis has been debated, with seemingly contradictory results between promising experimental data and disappointing clinical trials. As the understanding of the paramount role of the epithelium in the disease arose, the concept that immunity and inflammation influence rather than drive fibrosis developed. Immune cells involved in both innate and adaptive immunity have been implicated in experimental fibrosis development and display alterations in idiopathic pulmonary fibrosis, shaping a pro-fibrotic environment. Accordingly, the levels of several cytokines with a pro-fibrotic potential, such as IL-4, IL-13, IL-1β, TNF-α and IL-17A are elevated in IPF patients. Additionally, the interplay with cellular stress components such as danger associated molecular patterns and infectious alarm signals under the form of pathogen associated molecular patterns is an area of ongoing investigation. Finally, recent advances in sequencing techniques have unraveled a potential role for viruses and bacteria.

INTRODUCTION

The role of inflammation in the pathogenesis of idiopathic pulmonary fibrosis (IPF) has been a matter of debate for over 50 years. The observations that inflammatory cell counts were increased in the broncho-alveolar lavage (BAL) of patients and influenced fibroblast behavior led to the hypothesis that alveolitis preceded the fibrotic stage of the disease and that anti-inflammatory therapies could alter its relentless course. Based on this assumption, corticosteroids, later combined with other drugs, formed the cornerstone of IPF treatment for several years until almost a decade ago, when our understanding of the place and harmfulness of inflammation was questioned by the failure of several trials evaluating immune modulation. In the aftermath of these results, our current understanding of the place of inflammation and immunity in IPF emerged, in which they would act as an influencing force on the fibrotic process rather than be at its origin [1]. In this chapter, we propose to review the evidence linking the immune system, inflammation and IPF in the light of these recent concepts.

Immune Cells in IPF

Although IPF is an almost purely fibrotic disease, there is evidence of diffuse lung infiltration by immune cells, leading to question their putative role in the fibrotic process. Experimental evidence suggests a role for both innate immunity, with the bulk of data pointing towards monocytes, neutrophils and macrophages, and adaptive immunity, more specifically T-lymphocytes, in lung fibrosis.

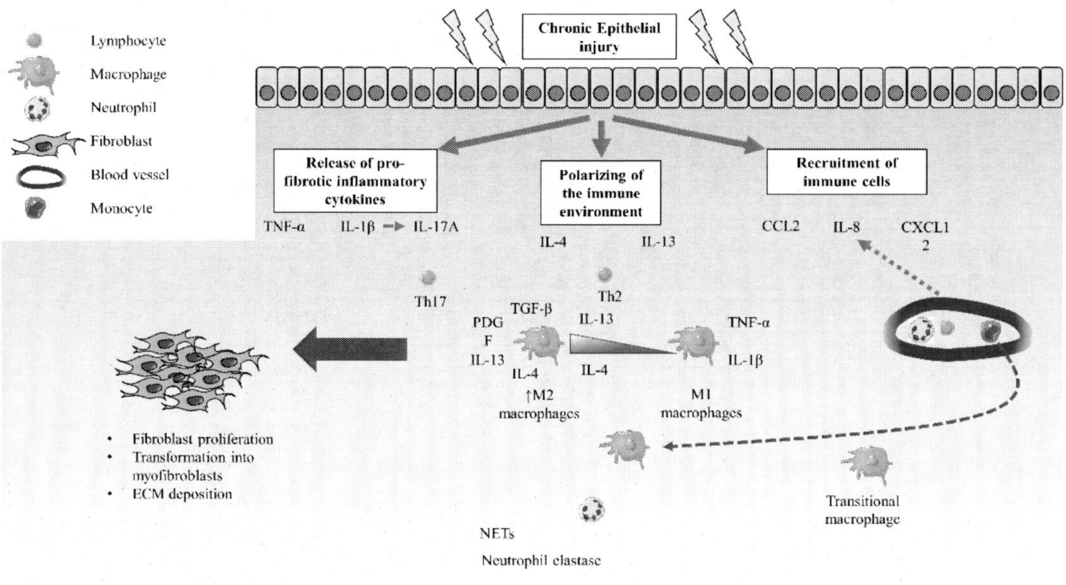

Figure 1. Overview of inflammatory and immune mechanisms at stake in lung fibrosis. Chronic epithelial lung injury affect epithelial cells that release pro-fibrotic and polarizing cytokines, recruit immune cells and ultimately favor lung fibrosis.

Macrophages

Lung macrophages are part of a complex habitat, at the interface between environment and host and fulfill a wide array of functions, including surfactant homeostasis, clearance of apoptotic cells and inflammatory modulation. Under normal conditions, these cells can be divided into two distinct groups, with different location, ontology, cell markers and function. Alveolar macrophages (AM) are a self-renewing population arising from fetal precursors that may reside both in alveoli and in the airways. Their role at the forefront of the mucosa demands a tight regulation of inflammatory mechanisms, as frequent exposure to benign stimuli occurs. For a long time, interstitial macrophages (IM), embedded within the lung tissue, were thought to only represent a transitional state between circulating monocytes and AM, but more recent data has highlighted their distinctiveness as a population. They seem to have a more immunomodulating role, with the expression of the anti-inflammatory IL-10 and alteration of dendritic cell maturation and migration [2].

To exert their functions, macrophages can polarize into different subsets. Although historically, they have been divided into two subtypes, macrophage polarization should be seen as a reversible continuum rather than a definitive dichotomic classification. Briefly, M1 or classically activated macrophages are induced by LPS, IFN-γ and TNFα, produce pro-inflammatory cytokines such as IL-1β, TNF-α, IL-12, IL-23, promote Th1 response and display enhanced pathogenicidal properties. M2 macrophages on the other hand are induced by TGF-β, IL-4 and IL-13 and are able to secrete pro-fibrotic cytokines such as TGF-β and PDGF, promoting tissue repair, immunomodulation and parasite containment [3].

In IPF, macrophages can be found in the vicinity of myofibroblasts, express TGF-β and are skewed towards an M2 type [4, 5]. They interact with fibroblasts promoting their growth and collagen deposition laying the basis of their pro-fibrotic actions [1]. Interestingly, the macrophage population is altered in the disease with the expansion of a distinct SPP1^{high} population in diseased individuals [6, 7]. Additional data regarding the pro-fibrotic potential of macrophages has been gathered from experimental studies: Mirroring what happens in humans, macrophages produce TGF-β [1], M2 macrophages in bleomycin treated rodents are increased and are able to influence fibroblast behavior [5]. Illustrating the important role of lung macrophages in fibrosis, depletion of those cells decreases collagen deposition [5] while specific deletion of TGF in myeloid cells was similarly protective *in vivo.* Aside from TGF-production, macrophages are also capable of secreting a wide array of compounds modulating their environment such as CCL18. This chemokine is increased in IPF patients and has been linked with M2 skewing of macrophages. Interestingly, fibroblasts interactions with the ECM promoted CCL18 secretion by macrophages, further enhancing collagen deposition by fibroblast and forming a feed-forwards loop [8].

Monocytes

Monocytes can be divided into classical monocytes ($CD14^{high}$ $CD16^{-}$), intermediate monocytes ($CD14^{+}CD16^{+}$) and non-classical monocytes ($CD14^{+}CD16^{++}$). Although serum monocytes count does not seem to vary over time, higher levels were recently shown to be prognostic of poor outcome in IPF patients [9]. When lung injury occurs, macrophages, monocytes and other immune cells can be recruited to the lung by several chemokines, including CCL2. CCL2 is implicated in fibrosis as it is elevated in the BAL as well as endothelial cells of IPF patients and modulation experiments in $CCR2^{-/-}$ (the receptors for this cytokines) animals have shown a protective effect from the mutation [8].

If lung injury is sufficiently important, local population of macrophages will be replaced by recruited circulating monocytes. Differentiation of monocytes to alveolar macrophages is linked with a pro-fibrotic transitional state, driving experimental lung fibrosis [10]. Single-cell RNA sequencing has allowed for a further identification into this monocyte-macrophage differentiation process and complementary studies localized these transitional cells in the proximity of fibroblasts [11].

Neutrophils

Neutrophils are among the first recruited cells at the site of injury, where they assist in the removal of pathologic material. Recruitment occurs through several chemokines, of which IL-8 (CXCL8) is the most important. In lung fibrosis patients, concentrations of this compound have been shown to be elevated both in BAL, sputum and serum correlating to some extent with lung functional parameters [8]. Data regarding the prognostic value of BAL neutrophilia is more mitigated with contradictory reports and high neutrophil counts have also been observed in several other interstitial pneumonia's thus seemingly more reflective of a specific fibrosis extensiveness than an IPF specific mechanism.

Neutrophils in IPF are activated as patients display higher concentrations of the serine protease neutrophil elastase (NE) in BAL and serum. NE seems capable of modulating fibrosis as $NE^{-/-}$ mice are protected from fibrosis in several experimental models and rodents treated with the NE inhibitor *Sivelestat* display lower levels of collagen deposition than controls [1]. NE seems to exert its pro-fibrotic actions by on the one hand increasing TGF-β activation and on the other hand inducing fibroblast proliferation and differentiation to myofibroblasts in a TGF-independent manner [12].

Next to NE, neutrophils are also capable of releasing networks of extracellular fibers of chromatin covered with antimicrobial proteins called neutrophil extracellular traps (NETs) which are involved in innate defense mechanisms. The exact role of those structures has yet to be determined in IPF, but experimental data supports the implication of both their DNA/histone structure and embedded proteins in fibrotic processes. Indeed, inhibition of NET formation alleviates cardiac fibrosis and NETosis induces primary lung fibroblast proliferation and myofibroblast differentiation while the IL-17 present within NETs has been linked with mesenchymal proliferation.

Despite this data suggesting a pro-fibrotic potential for neutrophils, IPF tissue is not characterized by neutrophilic influx and the role of these acute-injury components is unclear.

Lymphocytes

T-Lymphocytes are among the best studied immune cells in IPF and can be grossly divided into $CD4^+$ helper cells and $CD8^+$ cytotoxic cells. Typically, IPF biopsies can show a lymphocytic infiltrate, consisting of both types of cells. The importance of this infiltration seems to vary over time as histologic studies have shown an increase in lymphocyte aggregates over time. The role of T-cells in lung fibrosis is further supported by modulating experiments where athymic (thus lacking functional T-cells) and T-cell depleted animals were protected from lung fibrosis implying a pro-fibrotic role of (some) lymphocyte populations. Analysis of peripheral blood monocyte gene expression profile revealed that a decrease in several genes associated with costimulatory signals during T cell activation, including CD28 and ICOS, were associated with shorter transplant free survival [13]. Moreover, CD28 and ICOS expression was found to be a negative prognostic marker, while injection of $CD28^{null}$ lymphocytes in mice triggered the development of lung fibrosis [14].

The Inflammatory Environment in IPF

IPF Is Skewed Towards a Type 2 Inflammatory Profile

Experimental and human data link type 2 immunity and fibrotic processes while Th1 environments are seen as anti-fibrotic. Research conducted in lung fibrosis suggest similar influences as overexpression of GATA3, a transcription factor implicated in Th2 differentiation induces lung fibrosis in an experimental model [15]. Additionally, deletion of IL-4 and IL-13, two typical type 2 cytokines, in $IL\text{-}4^{-/-}$ and $IL\text{-}13^{-/-}$ animals, protected from bleomycin induced collagen deposition while treatment of fibroblasts with either cytokine promotes myofibroblast transformation [16]. Further mechanistic evaluation have identified IL-13 as the principal driver of these properties. IL-13 promotes fibrosis by enhancing TGF-β production by macrophages and epithelial cells, increasing TGF-β activation, and by directly acting on myofibroblast differentiation. Additional mechanisms have been evoked but their implication in pulmonary pathology is unclear. In IPF, concentrations of IL-4 and IL-13 are elevated in the BAL, suggesting activation of this type 2 axis. Following promising results in animal models, IL-13 and combined IL-4/IL-13 blockade was evaluated in IPF patients. Unfortunately, anti-IL-13 antibodies tralokinumab and lebrikizumab as well as SAR156597, inhibiting IL-4 and IL-13 have returned disappointing results, failing to meet their primary endpoints.

Conversely, type 1 inflammation seems to be repressed in IPF. One of the prototypical type 1 cytokines, interferon-γ (IFN-γ), possesses anti-fibrotic qualities since it impairs downstream TGF-β signaling by interfering with SMADs, reducing ECM deposition by TGF-exposed fibroblasts. Supporting this antifibrotic role, mice treated with IFN-γ display reduced TGF-β and collagen mRNA as well as diminished fibrosis, suggesting an additional upstream effect of the molecule. Congruently, IPF patients have a relative deficit in this cytokine, strengthening this Th2/Th1 imbalance concept.

Several therapeutic strategies have been designed to interfere with this skewed environment, either through inhibition of IL-4 and/or IL-13 or by substitution of IFN-γ. Despite promising results in murine models, trials evaluating both approaches have failed to meet their primary endpoints, relativizing this polarized view.

Pro-Inflammatory Cytokines in IPF

Aside from the aforementioned pathways, pro-inflammatory cytokines seem to play a role in lung fibrosis by shaping the environment, inducing apoptosis and triggering a cascade of events that will eventually lead to fibrosis.

IL-1β

Pro-IL-1β can be cleaved to IL-1β by inflammasome-dependent and -independent pathways, resulting in active secretion or passive release by dying cells of the cytokine in the surrounding milieu. Remarkably, the levels of this pro-inflammatory compound are elevated in the BAL of IPF patients [17], questioning its role in fibrotic diseases. The effects of IL-1β on the fibrotic process are seemingly contradictory. Indeed, adding this cytokine impairs fibroblast to myofibroblast transformation in cell cultures while overexpression in a rodent model induces lung fibrosis. Moreover, overexpression of this pro-inflammatory cytokine was associated with marked upregulation of PDGF and TGF, two typical fibrotic cytokines, as well as accumulation of myofibroblasts. Based on these observations, one could formulate the hypothesis that IL-1β exerts pro-fibrotic actions through its downstream cascade rather than by acting directly on mesenchymal cells. This was subsequently confirmed when IL-1β-mediated fibrosis was shown to be dependent on IL-17A [17].

TNF-α

The production of TNF-α has been linked to several cell types, including macrophages, lymphocytes and epithelial cells. The influence of this cytokine on the fibrotic process is complex with seemingly antagonistic reported effects. Indeed, it can favor a pro-fibrotic environment by stabilizing TGF-β mRNA, increasing TGF-β synthesis and PDGF transcription by fibroblasts as well as promoting EMT of cells of both bronchial and alveolar origin. Meanwhile, it is also capable of enhancing fibroblast apoptosis, decreasing fibroblast proliferation and reversing macrophage polarization from M2 to M1. *In vivo* observations reveal its complex role, as on the one hand TNF overexpression resulted in the development of lung fibrosis while on the other hand, TNF knock-out experiments have yielded more mitigated results, with some studies reporting reduced lung fibrosis and others documenting a protective effect [4, 16]. Remarkably, TNF-α treatment of bleomycin-stimulated mice enhanced fibrosis resorption possibly through reversal of M2 polarization and/or increased apoptotic signaling [4]. In addition to these experimental data, IPF patients present higher concentration of the cytokine than controls. Given the initial body of evidence suggesting a pro-fibrotic role, modulation with anti-TNF therapies was undertaken, alleviating lung fibrosis in murine models and suggesting a therapeutic potential for anti-TNF-α treatments. Etanercept, a recombinant soluble TNF-receptor capable of binding and neutralizing human TNF has been evaluated in IPF but failed to demonstrate its efficacy versus placebo.

IL-17: A New Player in the Field?

The IL-17 cytokine family consists of 6 different members, IL-17A-F, involved in host defense mechanisms, epithelial integrity and wound healing. IL-17A, the best described agent and the focus of this paragraph, has been implicated in several auto-immune diseases, perpetuating inflammation. Initially, IL-17A was shown to originate from a distinct lineage of effector $CD4^{+}$T-cells named Th17 cells, but later researches identified Tc17, γδ and natural killer T-cells, group 3 innate lymphoid cells and, more controversially, neutrophils, as alternative sources. Next to its inflammatory properties, IL-17A can influence fibrotic processes. Indeed, it is able to impact fibroblasts behavior, increasing their proliferation, myofibroblast differentiation and ECM synthesis while contributing to epithelial EMT [1, 12]. *In vivo*, $IL\text{-}17^{-/-}$ and anti-IL-17 treated animals are protected from lung and recombinant Il-17A administration induces collagen deposition

[17, 18]. Additionally, IL-17 influences ECM turn-over by inhibiting autophagy associated collagen resorption in a TGF-β independent manner [18]. The mechanisms underlying exaggerated IL-17 secretion are currently an area of investigation but epithelial injury seems to result in (a) secretion of IL-1β subsequently increasing IL-23 levels and (b) IL-6 production, consecutively promoting IL-17. Although experimental evidence points towards a role for IL-17 and IL-17 levels are elevated in the BAL and tissue of patients [17], the exact applicability of these findings to human IPF remains to be established and until then modulation of IL-17 in this disease seems precocious.

DAMPs and PAMPs

Damage associated molecular patterns (DAMPs) are components released upon cellular stress or tissue injury which act as "danger signals" leading to the activation of inflammatory pathways and the promotion of damaged structures clearance. Pathogen associated molecular patterns (PAMPs) on the other hand, are products of viruses or bacteria that are recognized by the organism. They both signal through pattern recognition receptors (PRR), such as Toll-like receptors (TLR), found on epithelial, mesenchymal and immune cells which mediate the inflammatory response elicited upon ligand binding.

DAMPs

The high mobility group box 1 (HMGB1) protein, extracellular ATP (eATP) and uric acid all act as DAMPs upon release by necrotic or damaged cells or secretion by immune cells [19]. These mediators all display elevated levels in the BAL of IPF patients compared to controls. Evaluation in bleomycin treated mice similarly show augmented concentrations in the BAL [19] while inhibition through drugs, genetic constructs or antibodies resulted in lower collagen deposition, implying a role in fibrosis. The underlying mechanisms are divergent, but one common element seems the production of IL-1β. Aside from this common pathway, some DAMPs seem capable of influencing fibrosis directly as, for example, HMGB1 stimulates proliferation of human fibroblasts.

PAMPs and Pattern Recognition Receptors

Several polymorphisms have implicated PRR and more specifically TLR in the pathogenesis of IPF. Indeed, single nucleotide polymorphisms (SNPs) in the gene coding for TOLLIP, an inhibitory protein of downstream TLR2/4 signaling, have been associated with IPF and a TLR3 polymorphism was associated with increased mortality [1]. Next to this genetic evidence, the physiological impact of TLR on the fibrotic process is variable, depending on the ligand and the type of receptor. Illustrating this, TLR4$^{-/-}$ mice display an enhanced susceptibility to bleomycin lung injury linked to altered signaling by hyaluronan DAMPs, causing increased alveolar injury and impaired AEC2 renewal . TLR9, a PRR recognizing unmethylated CpG DNA present in virus, bacteria and mitochondria, is increased in the lung tissue of IPF patients and its expression profile distinguishes rapid from slow IPF progressors. Treatment of fibroblast or monocytes with CpG promoted *in vitro* transformation to myofibroblasts and fibrocytes respectively. Even though TLR9 seemed to have pro-fibrotic actions, TLR9$^{-/-}$ mice develop more lung fibrosis, suggesting additional roles for this receptor [20].

VIRUSES

A link between IPF and viral infections has been suggested more than 30 years ago and several indirect arguments point towards a possible relationship. Although reports have been published regarding associations with hepatitis C virus, adenovirus and Torque-Teno virus, conclusive data is lacking and most of the attention has been drawn towards herpes viruses [21]. These double stranded DNA viruses replicate in the host cell nucleus and can induce latent infections, remaining quiescent for several years before reactivating. IPF patients have been reported to have higher IgG titers against EBV, CMV and HSV-1 suggesting a potential role for latent viral infection. IPF is a disease affecting primarily aged patients, possibly leaving them more vulnerable to viral infections due to mechanisms of immunosenescence or impaired ER-stress response. Contrarily to the prior observations in younger individuals, γHV-68 infection by itself was sufficient to induce lung fibrosis in aged mice. Moreover, γHV-68 exposed aged fibroblasts produced more TGF-β than uninfected counterparts along with increased responsiveness to this cytokine, resulting in augmented α-SMA and collagen production. The use of cidofovir, an antiviral drug, reduced lung fibrosis in γHV-68 infected mice, prompting evaluation in human subjects. Incidental data regarding this drug has shown that a select group of patients with prior reported EBV contact could benefit from ganciclovir treatment. Although there seems to exist a relationship between viral infections and IPF, a definite causal link is currently lacking, and further studies are needed.

The Role of Bacteria

High throughput bacterial sequencing has allowed the identification of a diversified bacterial flora in healthy human lungs, shattering the belief that this was a sterile compartment. IPF patients display an increased bacterial burden, decreased diversity compared to controls. Meanwhile, a higher bacterial charge was predictive of a worse survival in fibrotic patients [22]. Microbiome composition is able to alter host processes, as decreased bacterial diversity was associated with the presence of pro-inflammatory cytokine while certain *Streptococcus* and *Staphylococcus* operational taxonomic units (OTU) influenced disease progression [22]. Experimental data has further highlighted the role of the microbiome since bleomycin treated germ-free mice display increased survival and decreased fibrosis while inoculation of S*treptococcus pneumoniae* exacerbates collagen deposition [22]. Inoculation of specific bacterial species increases fibrogenesis in a microbiome-depleted bleomycin model underlining the effect of flora imbalance. The mechanisms underlying these observations are currently an area of active investigation, but increased synthesis of IL-17B by alveolar macrophages triggering a pro-inflammatory and pro-fibrotic cascade has been implicated. Since bacterial load and diversity seem to be altered in IPF, antibiotic treatment seems promising at first glance. Indeed, treatment with amoxycilline or clarithromycine is able to ablate the augmented collagen deposition observed after Streptococcus pneumoniae infection in a murine model. Only one trial, evaluating co-trimoxazole prophylaxis in IIP patients (of which 89% had IPF), has been conducted to this day in humans, with mitigated results as it is weakened by a high drop-out rate due to adverse events, reporting only a possible survival benefit in the per protocol analysis [22]. Further studies assessing the exact impact of antibiotic prophylaxis in IPF are under way and results are expected in 2019.

Next to these chronic interactions, IPF patients can experience acute infectious episodes such as pneumonia or bronchitis, associated with a high mortality. Gram negative bacteria seem to be more present in cultures from IPF patients suffering from respiratory infections than in the general population with H. influenzae, P. aeruginosa and K. Pneumonia reported as the main infectious agents.

Acute Exacerbations

The disease course of IPF patients can be complicated by acute, non-cardiac respiratory deterioration events corresponding to acute exacerbations (AE). The incidence of this complication is estimated to be 4 per 100 patient years, although this is probably an underestimation as a new, more liberal, definition of AE has recently been proposed and this proportion rose to 20 per 100 patient years when suspected events were considered [23]. Up to 46% of patient's death in IPF can be attributed to AE and median survival after such an episode is 3 to 4 months. The trigger can be diverse but encompasses episodes of physiological stress, such as surgery, infections and endoscopic procedures which will cause respiratory deterioration with new onset zones of ground glass or consolidation on chest-CT and diffuse alveolar damage on biopsy [23].

The exact cascade of events provoking AE is currently unknown and it is unclear whether this process reflects an intrinsic acceleration of the disease or the influence of external factors such as subclinical infection. Several elements plead in favor of an infectious origin, as (1) exacerbations are more frequent during winter and spring months, (2) immune suppression is a risk factor for AE and (3) acute infectious events share a similar prognosis to AE where the trigger remains unknown [23]. The presence of viruses in AE patients has been reported but their causal role remains to be established. The BAL of those patients is characterized by a relative increase in neutrophils, along with higher concentrations of pro-inflammatory and M2 polarizing cyto/chemokines [1]. Conversely, genetic evaluation of AE patients showed no important upregulation of inflammatory pathways compared to stable IPF controls with surprisingly close genetic signatures [24], mitigating the strength of an infectious hypothesis. Historically, the cornerstone of treatment has been corticosteroids, although data supporting their use is scant. Multiple reports of additional therapies have been published but well-conducted randomized controlled trials are direly needed.

Conclusion

The failure of immunosuppressive treatments in IPF led to the assumption that it was a "purely" fibrotic disease. However, strong evidence supports that IPF development is underlined by the activation and recruitment of several immune cell subsets. Those cells undergo differentiation under the influence of inflammatory cytokines. Those mechanisms amplify one another, participating to disease progression. A key open question for the future is the precise role of lung microbiota and its potential as a treatment target. Whether some antibiotic and/or anti-inflammatory drugs might be useful to prevent and cure exacerbations is still undetermined.

References

[1] Desai O, Winkler J, Minasyan M, Herzog EL. The Role of Immune and Inflammatory Cells in Idiopathic Pulmonary Fibrosis. *Frontiers in Medicine.* 2018;5:43.

[2] Schyns J, Bureau F, Marichal T. Lung Interstitial Macrophages: Past, Present, and Future. *Journal of immunology research*. 2018;2018:5160794-.

[3] Zhang L, Wang Y, Wu G, Xiong W, Gu W, Wang C-Y. Macrophages: friend or foe in idiopathic pulmonary fibrosis? *Respiratory Research*. 2018;19(1):170.

[4] Byrne AJ, Maher TM, Lloyd CM. Pulmonary Macrophages: A New Therapeutic Pathway in Fibrosing Lung Disease? *Trends in molecular medicine*. 2016;22(4):303-16.

[5] Gibbons MA, MacKinnon AC, Ramachandran P, Dhaliwal K, Duffin R, Phythian-Adams AT, et al. Ly6Chi monocytes direct alternatively activated profibrotic macrophage regulation of lung fibrosis. *Am J Respir Crit Care Med*. 2011;184(5): 569-81.

[6] Morse C, Tabib T, Sembrat J, Buschur K, Bittar HT, Valenzi E, et al. Proliferating SPP1/MERTK-expressing macrophages in idiopathic pulmonary fibrosis. *European Respiratory Journal*. 2019:1802441.

[7] Reyfman PA, Walter JM, Joshi N, Anekalla KR, McQuattie-Pimentel AC, Chiu S, et al. Single-Cell Transcriptomic Analysis of Human Lung Provides Insights into the Pathobiology of Pulmonary Fibrosis. *Am J Respir Crit Care Med*. 2018.

[8] Heukels P, Moor CC, von der Thusen JH, Wijsenbeek MS, Kool M. Inflammation and immunity in IPF pathogenesis and treatment. *Respir Med*. 2019;147:79-91.

[9] Scott MKD, Quinn K, Li Q, Carroll R, Warsinske H, Vallania F, et al. Increased monocyte count as a cellular biomarker for poor outcomes in fibrotic diseases: a retrospective, multicentre cohort study. *The Lancet Respiratory Medicine*. 2019;7(6):497-508.

[10] Misharin AV, Morales-Nebreda L, Reyfman PA, Cuda CM, Walter JM, McQuattie-Pimentel AC, et al. Monocyte-derived alveolar macrophages drive lung fibrosis and persist in the lung over the life span. *The Journal of Experimental Medicine*. 2017;214(8):2387.

[11] Aran D, Looney AP, Liu L, Wu E, Fong V, Hsu A, et al. Reference-based analysis of lung single-cell sequencing reveals a transitional profibrotic macrophage. *Nature Immunology*. 2019;20(2):163-72.

[12] Kolahian S, Fernandez IE, Eickelberg O, Hartl D. Immune Mechanisms in Pulmonary Fibrosis. *American Journal of Respiratory Cell and Molecular Biology*. 2016;55(3):309-22.

[13] Herazo-Maya JD, Noth I, Duncan SR, Kim S, Ma S-F, Tseng GC, et al. Peripheral Blood Mononuclear Cell Gene Expression Profiles Predict Poor Outcome in Idiopathic Pulmonary Fibrosis. *Science Translational Medicine*. 2013;5(205): 205ra136.

[14] Habiel DM, Espindola MS, Kitson C, Azzara AV, Coelho AL, Stripp B, et al. Characterization of CD28(null) T cells in idiopathic pulmonary fibrosis. *Mucosal Immunol*. 2019;12(1):212-22.

[15] Kimura T, Ishii Y, Yoh K, Morishima Y, Iizuka T, Kiwamoto T, et al. Overexpression of the transcription factor GATA-3 enhances the development of pulmonary fibrosis. *Am J Pathol.* 2006;169(1):96-104.

[16] Wynn TA. Integrating mechanisms of pulmonary fibrosis. *The Journal of Experimental Medicine*. 2011;208(7):1339.

[17] Wilson MS, Madala SK, Ramalingam TR, Gochuico BR, Rosas IO, Cheever AW, et al. Bleomycin and IL-1beta-mediated pulmonary fibrosis is IL-17A dependent. *J Exp Med.* 2010;207(3):535-52.

[18] Mi S, Li Z, Yang HZ, Liu H, Wang JP, Ma YG, et al. Blocking IL-17A promotes the resolution of pulmonary inflammation and fibrosis via TGF-beta1-dependent and -independent mechanisms. *Journal of immunology*. 2011;187(6):3003-14.

[19] Ellson CD, Dunmore R, Hogaboam CM, Sleeman MA, Murray LA. Danger-Associated Molecular Patterns and Danger Signals in Idiopathic Pulmonary Fibrosis. *American Journal of Respiratory Cell and Molecular Biology*. 2014;51(2):163-8.

[20] . Luckhardt TR, Coomes SM, Trujillo G, Stoolman JS, Vannella KM, Bhan U, et al. TLR9-induced interferon β is associated with protection from gammaherpesvirus-induced exacerbation of lung fibrosis. *Fibrogenesis & tissue repair*. 2011;4:18-.

[21] Moore BB, Moore TA. Viruses in Idiopathic Pulmonary Fibrosis. Etiology and Exacerbation. *Ann Am Thorac Soc*. 2015;12 Suppl 2:S186-92.

[22] Warheit-Niemi HI, Hult EM, Moore BB. A pathologic two-way street: how innate immunity impacts lung fibrosis and fibrosis impacts lung immunity. *Clinical & Translational Immunology*. 2019;8(6):e1065.

[23] Collard HR, Ryerson CJ, Corte TJ, Jenkins G, Kondoh Y, Lederer DJ, et al. Acute Exacerbation of Idiopathic Pulmonary Fibrosis. An International Working Group Report. *Am J Respir Crit Care Med*. 2016;194(3):265-75.

[24] Konishi K, Gibson KF, Lindell KO, Richards TJ, Zhang Y, Dhir R, et al. Gene expression profiles of acute exacerbations of idiopathic pulmonary fibrosis. *Am J Respir Crit Care Med*. 2009;180(2):167-75.

In: Respiratory Ventilatory Strategies ...
Editor: Antonio M. Esquinas ISBN: 978-1-53617-847-0
© 2020 Nova Science Publishers, Inc.

Chapter 5

EXTRAPULMONARY ALTERATIONS IN IDIOPATIC PULMONARY FIBROSIS

Francisco V. Lima[1,*], PT, MSc
and Carlos H. G. Uchôa[2,†], PT, PhD
[1]Department of Physical Therapy, University of Brasilia, Brasilia, Brazil
Cancer Institute of São Paulo, University of São Paulo, São Paulo, Brazil
[2]Department of Physical Therapy, Nove de Julho University, São Paulo, Brazil

ABSTRACT

Idiopathic pulmonary fibrosis is a noninfectious chronic disease of unknown cause of progressive and often fatal character, which has as its most striking feature the reduction in the ability to perform gas exchange. Although this disease is known to be limited to the respiratory system, patients with IPF are often affected by various alterations in other systems, such as the nervous system, cardiovascular system and skeletal muscular system, which may be determinant in the prognosis of these patients.

Keywords: idiopathic pulmonary fibrosis, comorbidities, risk factors

INTRODUCTION

Idiopathic pulmonary fibrosis (IPF) is a severe inflammatory disorder, with an almost invariably poor prognosis, defined as an specific form of chronic, progressive, fibrosing

* Corresponding Author's E-mail: limasvaldez03@gmail.com.
† Corresponding Author's E-mail: carloshgu@hotmail.com.

interstitial pneumonia with a steady worsening of respiratory symptoms, and decline of pulmonary function, which may lead to death [1, 2]. It is associated with increasing cough and dyspnea and impaired quality of life (QoL). IPF affects average of 3 million people worldwide. The incidence increases dramatically in patients over 65 years and the estimated prevalence is as high as 400 cases per 100.000 people [3]. Most studies report a slight male predominance. However, whether this finding reflects a biological susceptibility or results from behavioral and environmental factors is unclear [4, 5].

Currently the comprehensive understanding of IPF pathogenesis remains misleading. Several environmental and microbial exposures have been proposed as playing roles in IPF pathobiology that might be far from collateral, making the concept of "idiopathic" less used [6]. Individual genetic and epigenetic factors remain the most important aspect for the development of the fibrotic process, although the contribution of the variants so far identified, or their interaction with the presumed external factors has yet to be clarified. In this context of genetic susceptibility, the repeated micro-injury of the alveolar epithelium has been recognized as the first driver of an altered repair process where several lung cells develop poor deportment, leading to the development and sustainment of the fibrotic process [7, 8].

Several risk factors have been associated to IPF such as tobacco smoke, male gender, advanced age, environmental exposures. Moreover, among the various comorbidities present in these individuals we can mention pulmonary hypertension (PH), Chronic obstructive pulmonary disease (COPD), pulmonary emphysema, lung cancer and Obstructive Sleep Apnoea (OSA). Prompt treatment and identification of comorbidities may have a clinically significant impact on overall outcome that is meaningful for patients with IPF [9, 10].

Main Extrapulmonary Alterations in Patients with Idiopatic Pulmonary Fibrosis

Specific comorbid conditions that may be present in patients with IPF are important for the treatment, as prompt identification and treatment of comorbid conditions may also have a clinically significant impact on overall outcomes in patients with IPF. Respiratory comorbidities, including COPD, Pulmonary hypertension (PH) and Obstructive Sleep Apnea (OSA), have been common in many studies, although estimates varied widely depending on the source population. Non-respiratory comorbidities such as sleep disorders, cardiovascular and muscle alterations were also highly prevalent in this population of patients [11].

Sleep related breathing disorders (SRBD) in patients with IPF, especially OSA, are very common [12]. Studies show that the incidence is 59% and 90% of individuals. [13].

The two main components thought to emphasize the pathogenesis of OSA are increased upper airway collapsibility and instability of the ventilatory control system. Another important factor is that REM-related sleep disordered breathing is associated with changes in sleep structure, reduced quality of life (QOL), and increased risk of mortality. On the other hand, in patients with IPF, OSA is a predominant disorder, usually moderate to severe [14]. In other chronic lung diseases (COPD, obesity hypoventilation syndrome), OSA overlap is an important factor that worsens sleep quality, QOL, gas exchange, increased exacerbations, and mortality. This is thought to be due to increased intrinsic elastic load of the respiratory muscles and stimulation of peripheral mechanoreceptors [14].

Patients with IPF have changes in sleep architecture, including decreased sleep efficiency, slow-wave sleep and rapid eye movement (REM) sleep, and increased sleep fragmentation. In addition, sleep-related hypoventilation during the vulnerable period of REM and OSA sleep is frequent but generally remains underdiagnosed. These SRBD in IPF are associated with changes in sleep structure, reduced QOL, and increased risk of mortality [15].

Following diagnosis of OSA these patients should be referred to experienced centers capable of managing an effective therapy with Continuous Positive Airway Pressure (CPAP) and able to overcome interfering clinical problems (especially cough, claustrophobia, insomnia, and low adherence to use) [14].

Cardiovascular Alterations in IPF Patients

Cardiovascular comorbidities in individuals with IPF have been considered an important source of studies in this patient population. In a previous study, Sprunger et al. used a database from the National Center for Health Statistics in the USA over a period of 1988 to 2007 to determine the risk of individuals with IPF presenting with Venous Thromboembolism (VTE). The authors demonstrated that the diagnosis of VTE was present in approximately 2% of patients with IPFIPF who died in this period, the equivalent in a prevalence of 34% higher than in patients without this diagnosis, as well as 44% higher than in individuals with COPD and 54% higher than individuals who died due to lung cancer. These data place the IPF as an important risk factor for the involvement of these patients by VTE, especially in women over 65 years and men in any age group [15]. Additionally, a study by Dalleywater et al. investigating the risk of VTE in individuals with IPF through a longitudinal UK database of electronic primary care records, demonstrated that the VTE rate was twice as high as that of a group of properly matched healthy individuals (Crude rate per 1000 person-years and 95% CI: 4.3 (3.0-6.0) vs 2.2 (1.8-2.7), IPF and healthy, respectively) [16]. These findings provide further evidence that IPF increases the risk of VTE and confirm the strong association between

IPF and venous thromboembolism previously reported by Sprunger et al., due to a prothrombotic state present in these patients. More recently, to investigate the prevalence of venous thromboembolic events in hospitalized IPF patients, Farghaly and El-Abdin retrospectively analyzed data from 629 patients diagnosed with IPF from an interstitial lung disease (ILD) database from 2007 to 2013. The authors found a significantly higher risk for VTE in patients with IPF when compared to patients diagnosed with COPD (OR: 1.9; 95% CI: 1.039-3.530; $p = 0.035$). In addition, female individuals (OR: 2,871 [1,276-6,456], $p = 0.008$) and non-smokers (OR: 2,744 [1,219-6,177], $p = 0.011$) also had a significantly higher risk of VTE in relation to individuals with same-sex COPD and non-smokers [17]. The main mechanisms involved in the association between VTE and IPF are procoagulant abnormalities such as elevated levels of C protein, reduced thrombomodulin and presence of TF antigens (markers of active extrinsic coagulation pathways) in the respiratory system of patients with IPF. Furthermore, reduced mobility with venous stasis may also be involved as mechanisms that may potentiate procoagulant and antifibrinolytic effects in this population, increasing predisposition to VET in these patients [18] (Table 1).

The relationship between IPF and Coronary Artery Disease (CAD) has been previously reported in the literature. According to a recent review by Agrawal et al. reported as main mechanisms responsible for CAD in these patients increased serum levels of interleukins (mainly IL-4 and IL-8), cytokines (mainly tumor necrosis factor [TNF-α]), circulating immune complexes and development of fibrosis in extrapulmonary organs like the mediastinum. These mechanisms may be determinant in extrapulmonary fibroproliferative process and increased cardiac atherogenesis in this patient population (Table 1). Overall, the prevalence of CAD in patients with IPF ranges from 28.6% to 65.8% in the literature. These prevalence values are significantly higher when compared to COPD patients with values ranging from 9.8% to 46.1%. Regarding the risk of CAD in patients with IPF, the odds ratio ranges from 1.53 (95% CI: 1.15 to 2.03) to 2.18 (95% CI: 1.17 to 4.06) when compared to healthy subjects and patients with non-fibrotic pulmonary disease, respectively. The presence of CAD in patients with IPF and other comorbidities such as hypoxia and pulmonary hypertension are important factors related to the onset of cardiac arrhythmias in these patients. Changes such as increased sympathetic autonomic system activity, increased right ventricular afterload, and development of heart failures are mechanisms responsible for the appearance of various atrial arrhythmias in patients with IPF (Table 1). In addition, atrial arrhythmias are complications frequently present in the postoperative period of lung transplantation, where the presence of IPF has been an important risk factor for the onset of atrial fibrillation (OR: 2.3; 95%CI: 1.1 to 4.8; $p = 0.03$), atrial flutter (OR: 2.94; 95%CI: 1.31-6.62; $p = 0.009$) and supraventricular arrhythmias (OR: 1.98; 95%CI: 1.15 to 3.40; $p = 0.013$) [19].

Table 1. Summary of main action mechanisms related to extrapulmonary alterations

Extrapulmonary alteration	Main mechanism
Sleep Disorders	Sleep architecture, Breathing pattern during sleep, Sleep related hypoventilation in REM, Nocturnal hypoxemia, hypoxic pulmonary vasoconstriction
Venous Thromboembolism	Procoagulant State (elevated levels of protein C and reduced thrombomodulin and presence of TF antigens); reduced mobility (procoagulant and antifibrinolytic effects)
Coronary Artery Disease	Increase of interleukins (mainly IL-4 and IL-8), cytokines (mainly tumor necrosis factor [TNF-α]), circulating immune complexes
Cardiac arrhythmias	Increased sympathetic autonomic system activity, increased right ventricular afterload, and development of heart failures
Pulmonary hypertension and Right Heart Failure	Hypoxia-related pulmonary vasculopathy; reduced flow due to arterial thrombosis
Muscle disfunction	Chronic hypoxaemia, inflammatory and oxidative stress, corticosteroid use, physical inactivity and malnutrition

Legends: TF: Tissue Factor; IL: interleukins; TNF: Tumor necrosis factor.

Another important cardiovascular alteration in patients with IPF is pulmonary hypertension (PH) and consequent Right Heart Failure (RHF). According to Agrawal et al., despite its low prevalence in patients with moderate IPF (approximately 5%), in patients with severe IPF, PH may be present in 10% to 32% of these patients [19]. However, previous systematic review of Raghu et al. with the inclusion of 126 studies and 42 studies reporting prevalence of PH in these patients, there was a wide range from 3% to 86%, with a trend of 30% and 50% between studies about PH prevalence. The main factor associated with PH in these patients is hypoxia-related pulmonary vasculopathy. This alteration is responsible for several changes in the pulmonary vasculature such as hypertrophy, collagen deposition in small pulmonary arteries and vascular remodeling resulting from inflammatory process. In addition, increased pulmonary arterial pressure may also be associated with reduced flow due to arterial thrombosis (Table 1). These modifications are responsible for increased pulmonary vascular resistance with elevation of pulmonary arterial pressure levels above 25 mmHg at rest, considered gold standard for pulmonary hypertension definition [20].

Muscle Alterations in IPF Patients

Skeletal muscle dysfunction and exercise intolerance have been widely discussed in the literature in patients with chronic lung diseases such as COPD, but less frequently in patients with IPF. In a recent investigation comparing upper and lower limb skeletal muscle strength in 38 men diagnosed with IPF with an average age of 70 years, Nolan et al. demonstrated a preference for lower limb strength reduction over upper limb strength with isometric quadriceps maximum voluntary contraction (QMVC%pred) significantly lower than Handgrip (HG%pred). Additionally, the authors also demonstrated that QMVC%pred was independently associated with reduced exercise tolerance, measured in this study by incremental shuttle walk [21]. Moreover, Nishiyama et al. and Watanabe et al. have shown a quadriceps muscle strength reduction ranging from 65% to 82% of the predicted value, reinforcing the mechanism of exercise performance reduction due to lower limb muscle dysfunction [22, 23]. Reinforcing the findings previously described above, Mendes et al. investigating 26 individuals with interstitial lung disease (50% of patients with IPF) compared with a control group of healthy subjects demonstrated a significant reduction in the cross-sectional area (CSA) of rectus femoris (7.6 ± 2.1 vs 9.4 ± 2.4 cm^2; p = 0.03) and lower strength of knee extensors (119 ± 35 vs 147 ± 39 Nm; p = 0.02) and plantar flexors (37 ± 19 vs 50 ± 15 Nm; p = 0.02). The authors failed to demonstrate statistically significant difference between groups in upper limb strength [24]. Furthermore, Guler et al. have shown an association between disease severity and handgrip reduction in muscle strength in 115 ILD patients (40 IPF patients) regardless of body composition in male patients, but not showing the same results in women that were included in the study [25].

According to a previous review by Panagiotou et al., The main mechanisms involved in muscle fatigue in these patients are related to chronic hypoxaemia, inflammatory and oxidative stress, corticosteroid use, physical inactivity and malnutrition. Secondly, the authors related evidence of an inflammatory process and oxidative stress that result in an imbalance between degradation and resynthesis of skeletal muscle proteins resulting from systemic transmission in a reduction of skeletal muscle trophism. Additionally, Panagiotou et al. related evidences of a reverse relationship between doses of oral corticosteroids and muscular strenght of quadriceps, reinforcing the clinical relevance of steroid myopathy in these patients, results of increased oxidative stress and mitochondrial dysfunction. Finally, a reduction in the level of physical activity in these patients is a major alteration, not a mechanism for negative feedback on the ability to exercise or exercise symptoms. A muscular atrophy due to disuse has been attributed to this population of patients a decrease in protein content, fiber diameter, force production, and fatigue resistance [26] (Table 1).

References

[1] Raghu G, Collard H R, Egan J J, et al. An official ATS/ERS/JRS/ALAT statement: idiopathic pulmonary fibrosis: evidence-based guidelines for diagnosis and management. *Am. J. Respir. Crit. Care Med.* 2011; 183: 788-824.

[2] Raghu G, Remy-Jardin M, Myers J L, et al. Diagnosis of idiopathic pulmonary fibrosis. An official ATS/ERS/JRS/ALAT clinical practice guideline. *Am. J. Respir. Crit. Care Med.* 2018; 198: e44-e68.

[3] Nalysnyk L, Cid-Ruzafa J, Rotella P, Esser D, Incidence and prevalence of idiopathic pulmonary fibrosis: review of the literature. *Eur. Respir. Rev*. 2012 Dec 1;21(126):355-61.

[4] Richeldi L, Collard H R, Mark G J, Idiopathic pulmonary fibrosis. *Lancet* 2017;389: 1941-52.

[5] Raghu, G, et al. *Idiopathic pulmonary fibrosis in US Medicare beneficiaries aged 65 years and older: incidence, prevalence, and survival*, 2001-2011.

[6] Balestro E, Cocconcelli E, Tinè M, Biondini D, Faccioli E, Saetta M, Rea F, Idiopathic Pulmonary Fibrosis and Lung Transplantation: When it is Feasible. *Medicina* (Kaunas). 2019 Oct 19;55(10). pi: E702.

[7] American Thoracic Society. Idiopathic pulmonaryfibrosis: diagnosis and treatment. International consensus statement. American Thoracic Society (ATS), and the European Respiratory Society (ERS). *Am. J. Respir. Crit. Care Med.* 2000;161: 646-64.

[8] Mogulkoc, N, et al. Pulmonary Function in Idiopathic Pulmonary Fibrosis and Referral for Lung Transplantation. *Am. J. Respir. Crit. Care Med.* 164, 103-108 (2001).

[9] Martinez, F J, Collard, H R, Pardo, A, Raghu, G, Richeldi, L, Selman, M, Wells, A U, (2017). *Idiopathic pulmonary fibrosis. Nature Reviews Disease Primers*, 3, 17074. doi:10.1038/nrdp.2017.74.

[10] Fernandez, I E, Heinzelmann, K, Verleden, S & Eickelberg, O, Characteristic Patterns in the Fibrotic Lung. Comparing Idiopathic Pulmonary Fibrosis with Chronic Lung Allograft Dysfunction. *Ann. Am. Thorac. Soc.* 12, S34-S41 (2015).

[11] Raghu G, Amatto V C, Behr J, Stowasser S, Comorbidities in idiopathic pulmonar fibrosis patients: a systematic literature review. *Eur. Respir. J.* 2015. Oct;46(4):1113-30.

[12] A Pihtili, Z Bingol, E Kiyan, C Cuhadaroglu, H Issever, Z Gulbaran. Obstructive sleep apnea is common in patients with interstitial lung disease. *Sleep Breath*, 17 (2013), pp. 1281-1288.

[13] Mermigkis C, Chapman J, Golish J, Mermigkis D, Budur K, Kopanakis A, Polychronopoulos V, Burgess R, Foldvary-Schaefer N, Sleep-related breathing disorders in patients with idiopathic pulmonary fibrosis. *Lung*. 2007 May-Jun;185(3):173-8. Epub 2007 Apr 10.

[14] Milioli G, Bosi M, Poletti V, Tomassetti S, Grassi A, Riccardi S, Terzano M G, Parrino L, Sleep and respiratory sleep disorders in idiopathic pulmonary fibrosis. *Sleep Med. Rev*. 2016 Apr; 26:57-63.

[15] Perez-Padilla R, West P, Lertzman M, Kryger M H, Breathing during sleep in patients with interstitial lung disease. *Am. Rev. Respir. Dis.* 1985; 132:224e9.

[16] Sprunger D B, Olson A L, Huie T J, Fernandez-Perez E R, Fischer A, Solomon J J, Brown K K, Swigris J J, Pulmonary fibrosis is associated with an elevated risk of thromboembolic disease. *Eur. Respir. J.* 2012 Jan; 39(1):125-32.

[17] Shereen Farghaly, and Ashraf Z, El-Abdin. Pulmonary fibrosis as a risk factor for thromboembolic disease. *Egypt. J. Broncho* 2015 9:160-164.

[18] Paloma Millan-Billi, Candela Serra, Ana Alonso Leon, Diego Castillo. Comorbidities, Complications and Non-Pharmacologic Treatment in Idiopathic Pulmonary Fibrosis. *Med. Sci.* 2018, 6, 59; doi:10.3390/medsci6030059.

[19] Abhinav Agrawal, Isha Verma, Varun Shah, Abhishek Agarwal, Rutuja R Sikachi. Cardiac manifestations of idiopathic pulmonary fibrosis. *Intractable Rare Dis. Res.* 2016 May;5(2):70-5. doi: 10.5582/irdr.2016.01023.

[20] Ganesh Raghu, Valeria C, Amatto, Jürgen Behr, Susanne Stowasser. Comorbidities in idiopathic pulmonary fibrosis patients: a systematic literature review. *Eur. Respir. J.* 2015; 46: 1113-1130. doi: 10.1183/13993003.02316-2014.

[21] Claire M Nolan, Samantha S C Kon, Jane L Canavan, Sarah E Jones, Matthew Maddocks, Paul Cullinan, Toby M Maher, William D C, Man. Preferential lower limb muscle weakness in idiopathic pulmonary fibrosis: Effects on exercise capacity. *European Respiratory Journal* 2014 44: P4492.

[22] Nishiyama O, Taniguchi H, Kondoh Y, et al. Quadriceps weakness is related to exercise capacity in idiopathic pulmonary fibrosis. *Chest* 2005; 127: 2028-2033.

[23] Watanabe F, Taniguchi H, Sakamoto K, et al. Quadriceps weakness contributes to exercise capacity in nonspecific interstitial pneumonia. *Respir. Med.* 2013; 107: 622-628.

[24] Polyana Mendes, Lisa Wickerson, Denise Helm, Tania Janaudis-Ferreira, Dina Brooks, Lianne G. Singer, Sunita Mathur. Skeletal muscle atrophy in advanced interstitial lung disease. *Respirology*. 2015 Aug; 20(6):953-9. doi: 10.1111/resp.125 71.

[25] Sabina A Guler, Seo Am Hur, Scott A Lear, Pat G Camp, Christopher J Ryerson. Body composition, muscle function, and physical performance in fibrotic interstitial lung disease: a prospective cohort study. *Respir. Res.* 2019 Mar 12; 20(1): 56. doi: 10.1186/s12931-019-1019-9.

[26] Marios Panagiotou, Vlasis Polychronopoulos, Charlie Strange. Respiratory and lower limb muscle function in interstitial lung disease. *Chronic Respiratory Disease* 2016, Vol. 13(2) 162-172. doi: 10.1177/1479972315626014.

In: Respiratory Ventilatory Strategies …
Editor: Antonio M. Esquinas
ISBN: 978-1-53617-847-0
© 2020 Nova Science Publishers, Inc.

Chapter 6

EPITHELIAL DAMAGE AND REMODELING IN IDIOPATHIC PULMONARY FIBROSIS

Antoine Froidure, MD, PhD
Pneumology department, Cliniques universitaires Saint-Luc, Bruxelles,
Université catholique de Louvain, Louvain-la-Neuve, Belgium

ABSTRACT

Lung fibrosis is characterized by the progressive replacement of lung alveoli by a fibrotic scar tissue. The disease is considered as epithelial-derived: repeated lung injury or sustained inflammation leads to the destruction of alveolar epithelial cells, which reside at the forefront of the interface between lung and environment. This epithelial injury is followed by type 2 alveolar cell hyperplasia and dysfunction, along with the recapitulation of developmental pathways. Impaired cell differentiation is also a key characteristic of lung fibrosis, and the way the balance between epithelial repair and fibrosis is regulated still remains partially unexplained. Interestingly, epithelial remodeling and cell turnover provide opportunities for biomarkers. Finally, currently available drugs, as well as novel treatments, exert, at least partially, their function through epithelial cell regulation.

INTRODUCTION

Lung fibrosis is characterized by the progressive replacement of lung alveoli by a fibrotic scar tissue. The disease is now considered as epithelial-derived: In a predisposed patient, repeated lung injury or sustained inflammation leads to the destruction of alveolar epithelial cells, which reside at the forefront of the interface between lung and environment. Failure of wound healing leads to profound changes in lung architecture. In the present chapter, we will review the mechanisms underlying cell destruction and transformation in idiopathic pulmonary fibrosis. We will also consider data pointing to epithelial cells as potential disease drivers. In a second part of the chapter, we will review data regarding potential epithelial biomarkers and, finally, we will describe current evidence regarding the effect of current treatment options on epithelial differentiation.

Epithelial Cells as Primary Targets and Disease Drivers in Lung Fibrosis

The airways are covered by a pseudo-stratified epithelium that constitutes the first line of defense against external injury and microbes, acting both as a physical barrier and a key regulator of innate and adaptive immunity. At the alveolar level, the distal epithelium is composed by type 1 alveolar cell (AEC1), that constitute more than 90% of the alveolar surface area, and type 2 alveolar cells (AEC2), that have a cuboidal shape and display several functions including surfactant production and clearance of the alveolar fluid. Furthermore, AEC2 might play the role of local progenitor cells, based on data from preclinical models.

The way cell renewing and epithelial regeneration occurs in lungs still remains elusive. At this point, it is known that lung epithelium regenerates by the activation of regional lineage-restricted, facultative progenitor cells, namely (from proximal to distal airways) basal cells, club cells and broncho-alveolar stem cells. In conducting airways, $CK5^+$ basal cells that express p63 transcription factor represent the "niche" of progenitor cells. In contrast, experimental studies in mice implicated several populations of putative progenitor cells in the more distal lung [1], including AEC2 that are capable of self-renewing. To date, it remains uncertain to what extent all those recent findings apply to the human lung, although a recent work suggested a role for club cells in IPF progression [2].

As the epithelial layer stands at the forefront between lung parenchyma and the outer environment, chronic lung injury first results in the destruction of the alveolar epithelium. In normal state, repair mechanisms include stem cell recruitment, including AEC2 hyperplasia followed by transdifferentiation into AEC1. These mechanisms, among others, lead to the restauration of normal lung architecture. This normal repair phenomenon occurs following acute lung injury or pneumonitis for example.

However, lung fibrosis, and IPF in particular, is characterized by AEC2 dysfunction and senescence, putatively linked to genetic abnormalities affecting telomeres and surfactant proteins. Following chronic lung aggression (tobacco smoke, occupational dust, chronic viral infection and gastro-esophageal reflux), dysfunctional AEC2 no longer support epithelial regeneration but rather trigger several pathways leading to fibrosis.

Hyperplastic AEC2 secrete several cytokines and proteins that promote macrophage polarization towards a profibrotic "type 2" phenotype and trigger fibroblast recruitment and differentiation into myofibroblasts. The ectopic epithelium displays features of bronchial/bronchiolar epithelium [3]. An aberrant activation of developmental signaling pathways has also been observed in IPF [4], all of them promoting fibroblast recruitment and transformation into myofibroblasts. The reactivation of crucial embryonic pathways and networks in IPF, including WNT, SHH, TGF-β1 and FGF allows cells to transduce and integrate transcription factors, which then execute downstream target programs by modulating gene expression. For example, the activation of β-Catenin, GLI, SMAD2/3 and ETV TFs are respectively involved downstream of WNT (Wingless Integration), sonic hedgehog (SHH), TGF and FGF pathways during lung development and fibrosis [5]. Additional developmental transcription factors have been also described as participants to IPF pathogenesis, including members of the Forkhead family (FOXF1 [6], FOXO3 [7]) and The T-box (TBX) transcription factor (TBX4 [8]). Finally, epithelial to Mesenchyme transition (EMT) designates the transformation of a cell from an epithelial to a mesenchymal phenotype, with migration and proliferative properties. Transcription factors implicated in EMT are also upregulated in IPF (TWIST-1, SNAI1 and FOXM1 [9]).

The injured epithelium in fibrosis also activates several immune pathways, reviewed in chapter 3 of this book. Altogether, extracellular matrix production and lung remodeling ultimately lead to organ failure.

This model of epithelial-triggered fibrotic disease is supported by histological findings: Fibroblast foci, which are considered as the cardinal feature of fibrosis, are surrounded by a completely remodeled epithelium. Epithelial abnormalities comprise histological honeycombing, which are cysts bordered by hyperplastic AEC2 and areas of so-called bronchiolization, which consists of the development of an ectopic epithelium that displays characteristics of bronchi, within distal lung parenchyma.

CELL PLASTICITY IN LUNG FIBROSIS

The disruption of alveolar barrier and subsequent lung remodeling is linked to a failure of normal cell differentiation. In a recent study [10], Xu and colleagues performed single-cell transcriptome analysis of IPF and control lung slices. Their results demonstrate that IPF is characterized by several modifications of the genome of epithelial cells. IPF epithelial cells acquire both an abnormal differentiation program and an aberrant phenotype. Important changes are demonstrated in AEC2 but also in bronchial cells and progenitors, namely basal cells and goblet cells. The Authors also identify so-called indeterminate epithelial cells that display features of both AEC and AEC2. In line with their aberrant reprogramming, IPF epithelial cells express molecules that regulate myofibroblast activity and attract immune cells. This transcriptomic study also showed proofs of transforming growth factor (TGF)-β1 pathway activation within epithelial cells in IPF lungs.

The way balance between alveolar repair and lung fibrosis is regulated is yet to be explored. Nevertheless, Cao et al., [11] uncovered the existence of a hematopoietic-vascular niche composed that favours alveolar repair composed by capillary endothelial cells and macrophages interacting with one another. In an experimental model of fibrosis triggered by chronic injury (repeated instillations of bleomycin), this repair niche was inhibited and fibrosis was stimulated, further supporting the hypothesis that chronic lung injury is able to outrun normal lung repair mechanisms.

EPITHELIAL BIOMARKERS IN LUNG FIBROSIS

As epithelial remodeling and high cell turnover characterize lung fibrosis, several compounds are disseminated in the blood flow, hence offering perspectives for biomarkers that could predict disease progression or disease outcome. An ideal biomarker should be a proper surrogate for clinically meaningful endpoints, such as disease diagnosis and progression, mortality or prediction of key events (i.e., acute exacerbations of IPF). Ideally, a biomarker should also be modified by treatment, so that it could be used for the assessment of drug efficacy. In the complex field of interstitial lung diseases (ILD), a biomarker should be able to discriminate ILD subgroups (for instance separating IPF, a purely fibrotic disease, from chronic hypersensitivity pneumonitis, an inflammatory-driven fibrotic disease). In the following section, we will review recent key advances in the field of epithelial-derived biomarkers in IPF.

Krebs von den Lungen 6 (KL-6) or MUC-1 is a mucin protein secreted by type-2 alveolar cells. Several studies have demonstrated that elevated baseline KL-6 levels in patients' serum was predictive of unfavorable outcome in several interstitial lung diseases, including hypersensitivity pneumonia, non-specific interstitial pneumonia and IPF [12]. In another study by Ohshimo and colleagues [13], elevated baseline KL-6 levels predicted the onset of IPF-related acute exacerbations. Finally, a recent study reports a prognostic value of a combined measurement of KL-6 and calgranulin B, a calcium-binding inflammatory protein, in broncho-alveolar lavage (BAL) of IPF patients. Results show that a BAL concentration of both biomarkers above the 75th percentile is linked to poorer outcome.

Matrix metalloproteases (MMP) are enzymes that degrade extracellular matrix. There are 23 MMP identified in human, with several roles identified in human homeostasis and disease. The expression of several matrix metalloproteinases (MMP-1, MMP-3, MMP-7, MMP-9 and MMP-10) is increased during idiopathic pulmonary fibrosis, suggesting that they are putatively involved in the pathogenesis of the disease. The potential of MMP-1,

7 and MMP-10 as biomarkers of lung fibrosis was evaluated in several studies [14, 15]. The study by Rosa and colleagues showed that MMP-1 and MMP-7 were elevated in lung fibrosis microenvironment, reflected by their plasma concentration. The Authors did not find any elevation of MMP-1 and 7 in non-fibrotic lung diseases (sarcoidosis and chronic obstructive pulmonary disease). Moreover, elevated MMP-1 and MMP-7 were able to distinguish IPF from hypersensitivity pneumonitis. Sokai et al., demonstrated that both BAL and serum levels of MMP-7 and MMP-10 correlated to lung function (assessed by forced vital capacity and lung diffusion capacity), while only serum MMP-10 was linked to worsening of symptoms at six months and mortality [15].

A major leap forward was recently achieved thanks to the PROFILE (Prospective Observation of Fibrosis in the Lung Clinical Endpoints) study. PROFILE is a prospective longitudinal cohort of treatment-naïve idiopathic pulmonary fibrosis (IPF) patients. 106 patients and 50 age-matched controls were followed for up to 36 months and regularly assessed for clinical evaluation, lung function and serum biomarkers sampling an measurement. The investigators performed unbiased multiplex analysis for 123 biomarkers at different time points. The lung expression of potentially useful biomarkers was further assessed by immunostaining on lung biopsies from IPF patients that underwent a lung biopsy. Finally, findings were challenged in a validation cohort. Altogether, the analysis retained four epithelial biomarkers, namely surfactant protein-D, matrix metalloprotease 7 (MMP7), CA-19.9 and CA-125 [16]. The latter two were also confirmed as markers of epithelial damage in immunochemistry. Analysis of the replication cohort suggested that CA-19.9 and surfactant protein D serum concentration was higher in progressive patients as compared to stable patients. On a longitudinal point-of-view, a 3-months increase in CA-125 serum concentration was correlated to IPF-related mortality. Other biomarkers, related to collagen turnover, were also highlighted in the PROFILE study.

Unfortunately, at this point, none of the biomarkers has entered routine clinical practice, neither for diagnosis nor for follow-up of interstitial lung disease. Additional studies are warranted in order to confirm currently published results.

Effect of Antifibrotic Drugs and Stem Cell Therapy on IPF Epithelial Cells

Pirfenidone and nintedanib are both approved as treatment for IPF and are able to slow disease course. Pirfenidone is a pyridine with antifibrotic properties. Although its precise target is unknown, several effects on fibroblast migration, proliferation and survival have been demonstrated *in vitro* and *in vivo*. Interestingly, a recent transcriptomic study was performed on lung homogenates and primary fibroblasts from

IPF patients treated by pirfenidone as compared to naïve patients. The study led to the identification of multiple targets for the drug: The results suggest that pirfenidone displays multiple action not only on lung fibroblasts but also on other cell type including epithelial cells. This might explain the ability of the drug to control extracellular matrix production and deleterious inflammatory reactions [17]. The second drug that was approved as treatment for IPF, nintedanib, is a multiple tyrosine-kinase inhibitor. Although it mainly targets fibroblast homeostasis, recent *in vitro* experiments suggest that it has the ability to stabilize epithelial differentiation, similarly to pirfenidone [18].

Current available therapies only slow disease progression, without evidence of any effect on cell fate and differentiation per se. In this regard, much hope has been placed in mesenchymal stem cells as a potential way to restore alveolar epithelial integrity. Mesenchymal stem cells (MSC) are multipotent cells, defined by their ability to differentiate, their capacity to self-renew and their clonality. IPF is characterized by impaired wound healing, alveolar injuries and failure of re-epithelialization. Therefore, the idea emerged that treating patients with mesenchymal stem cells could restore a normal healing process and prevent fibrosis extension through inhibition of Wnt-30, TGF-β1 and FGF. In human disease, the first trial evaluating the safety and tolerability of MSC treatment in IPF was recently published. Glassberg and colleagues conducted a phase I study using allogeneic human mesenchymal stem cells in IPF patients (AETHER trial) [19]. Several studies indicate that stem cells exert their effect by regulating the transcription of pro-fibrotic pathways: Induced pluripotent stem cells inhibit fibroblast to myofibroblast differentiation and TGF-β1-dependent proliferation. Similarly, human bone marrow-derived stem cells are capable to promote regulatory T cell expansion and production of the anti-fibrotic molecule IP-10 [20]. Moreover, Dinh et al., have recently developed a method allowing lung spheroid cells isolation from transbronchial biopsies [21]. The authors were able to demonstrate angiogenic potential and lung distribution following cell transfer to athymic mice. This new method paves the way for future application in human, for example by preventing aberrant reprogramming of type 2 alveolar cells. Finally, Guo and colleagues have recently demonstrated that a careful reprogramming of AEC2 generated induced progenitor-like cells that dampen bleomycin-induced fibrosis when transferred to mice [22].

The clinical use of mesenchymal stem cell is still under consideration: While encouraging results were already obtained in systemic sclerosis-related interstitial lung disease [23], the use of MSC is currently evaluated in acute respiratory distress syndrome and chronic lung fibrosis.

Conclusion

Idiopathic pulmonary fibrosis is now considered as an epithelial-derived disease. Imapired chronic wound healing leads to aberrant epithelial cell reprogramming and fibroblast proliferation. As illustrated in this chapter, epithelial cells constitute thus both the first hit and the main drivers of the disease. The IPF epithelium is characterized by a profound architectural remodeling, the reactivation of several developmental pathway. Epithelial turnover is also illustrated by the identification of potential biomarkers, although they use in clinical practice is not yet validated. Finally, current antifibtotic drugs as well as emerging therapies exert their effect partly through an action on epithelial cells. Further untangling the mechanisms that underlie failure of normal alveolar repair might pave the way for a better management of idiopathic pulmonary fibrosis.

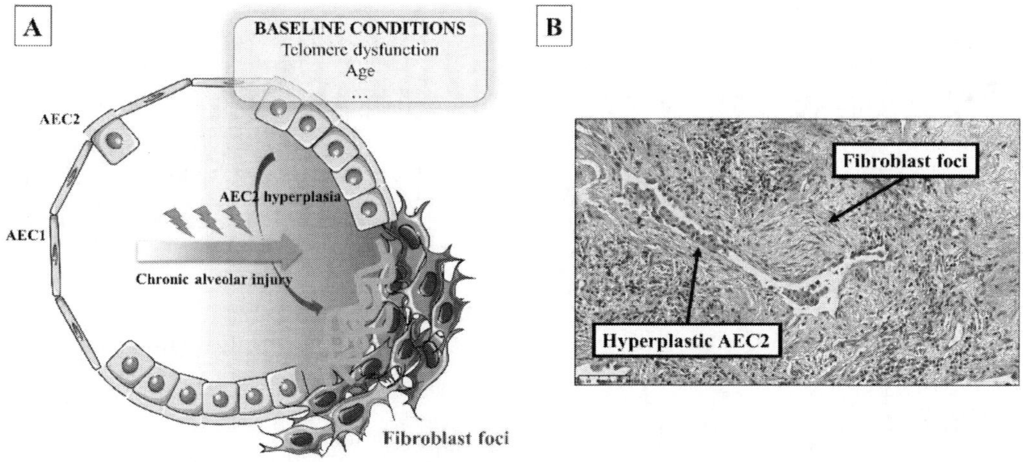

Figure 1. Panel A (left): Schematic view of aberrant alveolar repair, followed by type 2 alveolar cel hyperplasia and fibroblast recruitment. Panel B (right): Histological picture of an IPF patient illustrating close proximity between areas of epithelial cell hyperplasia and fibroblast foci (courtesy of Dr Delphine Hoton).

References

[1] Kotton D. N., Morrisey E. E. Lung regeneration: mechanisms, applications and emerging stem cell populations. *Nat Med.* 2014; 20(8):822-32.

[2] Fukumoto J., Soundararajan R., Leung J., Cox R., Mahendrasah S., Muthavarapu N., et al., The role of club cell phenoconversion and migration in idiopathic pulmonary fibrosis. *Aging* (Albany NY). 2016; 8(11):3091-109.

[3] Yang I. V., Coldren C. D., Leach S. M., Seibold M. A., Murphy E., Lin J., et al., Expression of cilium-associated genes defines novel molecular subtypes of idiopathic pulmonary fibrosis. *Thorax.* 2013; 68(12):1114-21.

[4] Selman M., Lopez-Otin C., Pardo A. Age-driven developmental drift in the pathogenesis of idiopathic pulmonary fibrosis. *Eur Respir J.* 2016.

[5] Chanda D., Kurundkar A., Rangarajan S., Locy M., Bernard K., Sharma N. S., et al., Developmental Reprogramming in Mesenchymal Stromal Cells of Human Subjects with Idiopathic Pulmonary Fibrosis. *Sci Rep.* 2016; 6:37445.

[6] Kalinichenko V. V., Lim L., Stolz D. B., Shin B., Rausa F. M., Clark J., et al., Defects in pulmonary vasculature and perinatal lung hemorrhage in mice heterozygous null for the Forkhead Box f1 transcription factor. *Dev Biol.* 2001; 235(2):489-506.

[7] Al-Tamari H. M., Dabral S., Schmall A., Sarvari P., Ruppert C., Paik J., et al., FoxO3 an important player in fibrogenesis and therapeutic target for idiopathic pulmonary fibrosis. *EMBO Mol Med.* 2017.

[8] Xie T., Liang J., Liu N., Huan C., Zhang Y., Liu W., et al., Transcription factor TBX4 regulates myofibroblast accumulation and lung fibrosis. *J Clin Invest.* 2016; 126(8):3063-79.

[9] Goossens S., Vandamme N., Van Vlierberghe P., Berx G. EMT transcription factors in cancer development re-evaluated: Beyond EMT and MET. *Biochim Biophys Acta.* 2017; 1868(2):584-91.

[10] Xu Y., Mizuno T., Sridharan A., Du Y., Guo M., Tang J., et al., Single-cell RNA sequencing identifies diverse roles of epithelial cells in idiopathic pulmonary fibrosis. *JCI Insight.* 2016; 1(20):e90558.

[11] Cao Z., Lis R., Ginsberg M., Chavez D., Shido K., Rabbany S. Y., et al., Targeting of the pulmonary capillary vascular niche promotes lung alveolar repair and ameliorates fibrosis. *Nat Med.* 2016; 22(2):154-62.

[12] Yokoyama A., Kondo K., Nakajima M., Matsushima T., Takahashi T., Nishimura M., et al., Prognostic value of circulating KL-6 in idiopathic pulmonary fibrosis. *Respirology.* 2006; 11(2):164-8.

[13] Ohshimo S., Ishikawa N., Horimasu Y., Hattori N., Hirohashi N., Tanigawa K., et al., Baseline KL-6 predicts increased risk for acute exacerbation of idiopathic pulmonary fibrosis. *Respir Med.* 2014; 108(7):1031-9.

[14] Rosas I. O., Richards T. J., Konishi K., Zhang Y., Gibson K., Lokshin A. E., et al., MMP1 and MMP7 as potential peripheral blood biomarkers in idiopathic pulmonary fibrosis. *PLoS Med.* 2008;5(4):e93.

[15] Sokai A., Handa T., Tanizawa K., Oga T., Uno K., Tsuruyama T., et al., Matrix metalloproteinase-10: a novel biomarker for idiopathic pulmonary fibrosis. *Respir Res.* 2015; 16:120.

[16] Maher T. M., Oballa E., Simpson J. K., Porte J., Habgood A., Fahy W. A., et al., An epithelial biomarker signature for idiopathic pulmonary fibrosis: an analysis from the multicentre Profile cohort study. *Lancet Respir Med*. 2017; 5(12):946-55.

[17] Kwapiszewska G., Gungl A., Wilhelm J., Marsh L. M., Thekkekara Puthenparampil H, Sinn K, et al., Transcriptome profiling reveals the complexity of pirfenidone effects in idiopathic pulmonary fibrosis. *Eur Respir J*. 2018; 52(5).

[18] Lehmann M., Buhl L., Alsafadi H. N., Klee S., Hermann S., Mutze K., et al., Differential effects of Nintedanib and Pirfenidone on lung alveolar epithelial cell function in *ex vivo* murine and human lung tissue cultures of pulmonary fibrosis. *Respir Res*. 2018; 19(1):175.

[19] Glassberg M. K., Minkiewicz J., Toonkel R. L., Simonet E. S., Rubio G. A., Difede D, et al., Allogeneic human mesenchymal stem cells in patients with idiopathic pulmonary fibrosis via intravenous delivery (AETHER): a phase I, safety, clinical trial. *Chest*. 2016.

[20] Liu M., Zeng X., Wang J., Fu Z., Wang J., Liu M., et al., Immunomodulation by mesenchymal stem cells in treating human autoimmune disease-associated lung fibrosis. *Stem Cell Res Ther*. 2016; 7(1):63.

[21] Dinh P. C., Cores J., Hensley M. T., Vandergriff A. C., Tang J., Allen T. A., et al., Derivation of therapeutic lung spheroid cells from minimally invasive transbronchial pulmonary biopsies. *Respir Res*. 2017; 18(1):132.

[22] Guo L., Karoubi G., Duchesneau P., Aoki F. G., Shutova M. V., Rogers I, et al., Interrupted reprogramming of alveolar type II cells induces progenitor-like cells that ameliorate pulmonary fibrosis. *NPJ Regen Med*. 2018; 3:14.

[23] Zhang H., Liang J., Tang X., Wang D., Feng X., Wang F., et al., Sustained benefit from combined plasmapheresis and allogeneic mesenchymal stem cells transplantation therapy in systemic sclerosis. *Arthritis Res Ther*. 2017; 19(1):165.

In: Respiratory Ventilatory Strategies …
Editor: Antonio M. Esquinas ISBN: 978-1-53617-847-0
© 2020 Nova Science Publishers, Inc.

Chapter 7

PULMONARY HYPERTENSION IN IDIOPATHIC PULMONARY FIBROSIS

Deniz Koksal**, MD
Department of Chest Diseases, Hacettepe University School of Medicine,
Ankara, Turkey

ABSTRACT

Pulmonary hypertension (PH) is commonly present in patients with idiopathic pulmonary fibrosis (IPF) and classified as group III PH due to chronic lung diseases and hypoxemia. PH should be suspected in patients with rapid clinical worsening, progressive exercise limitation and/or gas exchange abnormalities which are not deemed attributable to ventilatory impairment. Echocardiography and enlarged main pulmonary artery ratio are non-invasive modalities for screening PH. Right heart catheterization (RHC) is the gold standard test for the measurement of pulmonary artery pressure. It should be performed in patients in whom severe PH is suspected and the patient's management will likely be influenced by RHC results. Currently there is no specific therapy for IPF associated PH. Supplemental oxygen is prescribed for hypoxemic patients. PH targeted therapy is not typically indicated in IPF patients. It may be considered in patients with severe PH which cannot be explained with the underlying lung disease. These patients should be referred to specialized centers experienced in the management of PH for possible enrollment in clinical trials.

Keywords: idiopathic pulmonary fibrosis, pulmonary hypertension

---

* Corresponding Author's E-mail: dckoksal@gmail.com.

Introduction and Definitions

Idiopathic pulmonary fibrosis (IPF) is a chronic, progressive, fibrotic interstitial lung disease of unknown etiology. Pulmonary hypertension (PH) is commonly present in patients with IPF and classified as group III PH due to chronic lung diseases (CLD) and hypoxemia [1]. The prevalence of PH amongst IPF patients is dependent on the severity of IPF. In the early stages, it affects approximately 10% of the patients [2]. In the advanced stages it affects as much as 40% of the patients and is considered one of the principal predictors of mortality [3]. The focus of this chapter is to review the current understanding and management of PH associated with IPF.

PH has been arbitrarily defined as mean pulmonary arterial pressure (mPAP) $\geq$ 25 mmHg at rest, measured by right heart catheterization (RHC) since the 1st world symposium on PH (WSPH) in 1973 [4]. Recent data from normal subjects has shown that normal mPAP is 14.0 $\pm$ 3.3 mmHg and 2 standard deviations above this mean value suggests mPAP >20 mmHg as the upper limit of normal. However, abnormal elevation of mPAP is not sufficient to define pulmonary vascular disease, as elevation of mPAP can be due to an increase in cardiac output or pulmonary arterial wedge pressure. Thus, the 6th WSPH Task Force proposed to include pulmonary vascular resistance (PVR) $\geqslant$ 3 Wood Units (WU) in the definition of all forms of pre-capillary PH associated with mPAP > 20 mmHg [1].

Cor pulmonale is defined as a complication of PH and refers to PH induced altered structure and/or impaired function of the right ventricle that is associated with CLD and/or hypoxemia. It is characterized by elevations in PVR and in PAP, which cause increased right ventricular afterload and eventually to right ventricular failure in susceptible patients. The development of PH and subsequent cor pulmonale is clinically important since it is common and associated with increased morbidity and mortality [5].

PH Associated with IPF

Like other pulmonary disorders in Group III, PH is commonly seen in patients with IPF. Most of the IPF patients have mild to moderate PH, but PH may also be severe. A longitudinal study suggested that in patients with IPF, mPAP increases by around 1.8 mmHg per year, but rapid progression has been reported in advanced stage IPF patients [6]. In the current literature, most of the available data regarding PH associated with IPF comes from advanced IPF patients who had been evaluated for lung transplantation. In the retrospective analysis of 79 consecutive IPF patients who had undergone pre-transplantation RHC, an mPAP of $\geq$ 25 mmHg was present in 31.6% of the patients. Those patients with PH had a lower diffusion capacity for carbon monoxide, a lower 6 minute walking distance, were more likely to require supplemental oxygen therapy, and had an increased risk of mortality [7]. In another study, the lung transplant registry of USA (between January 1995 and June 2004) was analyzed and IPF patients who had undergone RHC were identified. This was the largest series of IPF patients evaluated for lung transplantation. Of the 3457 patients listed, 2525 (73%) had undergone RHC. PH (mPAP $\geq$ 25 mmHg) was present in 46.1% of these patients and 9% of patients had severe PH (mPAP $\geq$ 40 mmHg). Those patients with PH were 1.6 times more likely to die after being listed for lung transplantation compared to those without PH [8].

In IPF patients, there is a poor correlation between lung function parameters and the severity of PH. In a retrospective analysis of 118 IPF patients, in whom both pulmonary function tests and RHC were performed, 48 patients (40.7%) had PH. The authors examined the relationship between PH and pulmonary function tests including the percentage of predicted forced vital capacity (FVC%), total lung capacity (TLC%) and diffusing capacity for carbon monoxide (DLCO%). While there was no correlation between lung volumes and PH, there was a modest association with DLCO%. The prevalence of PH was two folds higher in patients with DLCO% < 30% compared to patients with DLCO% $\geq$ 30%. The authors concluded that there was a poor correlation between the measured pulmonary functions and PH, suggesting that factors other than fibrosis may play a role in the etiology of PH. However a decreased diffusing capacity might predict the presence of PH. The early detection of PH in patients with well-maintained pulmonary functions might have implications for the management and prognosis of IPF patients [9].

PATHOPHYSIOLOGY

IPF is associated with multiple pathological alterations involving most of the compartments of the pulmonary system. It not only affects the alveoli but also other regions, such as conducting airways and pulmonary vasculature. The distribution of lesions in IPF is heterogeneous. The alterations of alveolar-capillary membrane impair both the diffusion capacity and ventilation perfusion relationships in the lung, leading to reduced diffusing capacity, increased dead space ventilation, increased alveolar-arterial oxygen gradients and finally chronic arterial hypoxemia. Distinct vascular alterations are observed both in fibrotic areas and more preserved regions. The pulmonary arteries are thickened by intimal fibrosis and medial hypertrophy. Occlusion of pulmonary venules is frequent in relatively preserved areas [10].

PH is characterized by extensive vascular remodeling, enhanced proliferation of pulmonary artery smooth muscle cells leading to narrowing and obliteration of vessel lumen resulting in increased vascular tonus. The mechanisms underlying the development and progression of PH are not completely understood and appear to be multifactorial. It is likely that early vascular endothelial injury due to hypoxemia, and inflammation leads to endothelial dysfunction and subsequently to the development of structural vascular changes leading to an increase in PVR and subsequently in PAP. Loss of peripheral pulmonary vessels are also important for the onset of PH. The presence of PH in CLD is strongly associated with increased mortality. However it is not clear whether PH is the cause of this worse outcome or simply a marker of advanced lung disease.

In recent years, PH associated with IPF is suspected to be a specific phenotype of IPF. The traditional concept that hypoxic vasoconstriction and accumulation of scar tissue are mainly responsible for the development of PH in IPF, has been challenged. Recent studies suggest that the underlying pathobiology is much more complex, and includes a complicated interaction of epithelial cells, fibroblasts, and vascular cells. This interaction seems to be regulated by a large variety of angiogenesis promoters and inhibitors, as well as growth factors. Central components seem to be endothelial apoptosis and growth factor induced remodeling of pulmonary arterial wall [11].

DIAGNOSIS

Patients with IPF commonly present with the symptoms of progressive breathlessness with exertion and /or a persistent nonproductive cough. Since the symptom of exertional dyspnea is a common feature of both IPF and PH, there is a risk of underdiagnosing PH in IPF patients. Therefore PH should be suspected in patients with rapid clinical worsening, progressive exercise limitation and/or gas exchange abnormalities (extremely low diffusing capacity) which are not deemed attributable to ventilatory impairment [12].

Echocardiography is considered the best non-invasive modality as a screening tool for the diagnosis of PH. However, the ability to determine peak tricuspid regurgitation velocity to estimate the right ventricular systolic pressure is limited in IPF patients. Alternate echocardiographic measures such as right ventricular outflow tract diameter, tricuspid annular plane systolic excursion, and qualitative assessment of right chamber structure and function have been advocated [12, 13]. Enlarged main pulmonary artery (the ratio of main pulmonary artery/ aorta diameter > 1) on CT scan is also important to predict PH. Combining the echocardiographic measures with enlarged pulmonary artery ratio improves the accuracy of predicting PH [14].

RHC remains the gold standard test to measure PAP. However RHC should be performed in patients in whom severe PH is suspected and the patient's management will likely be influenced by RHC results, including referral for transplantation, inclusion in clinical trials or registries, treatment of unmasked left heart dysfunction, or compassionate use of therapy. Currently, there is no valid data to support the routine use of acute vasodilator testing in CLD associated PH [12].

In the 6th WSPH Task Force, PH is defined as PVR ⩾ 3 WU in the definition of all forms of pre-capillary PH associated with mPAP > 20 mmHg [1]. In the context of CLD associated PH the definition is adapted as [12, 15]:

1. CLD without PH (mPAP < 21 mmHg, or mPAP = 21-24 mmHg with PVR < 3 WU)
2. CLD with PH (mPAP = 21-24 mmHg with PVR ≥ 3 WU, or mPAP = 25-34 mmHg)
3. CLD with severe PH (mPAP ≥ 35 mmHg, or mPAP ≥ 25 mmHg with low cardiac index (< 2 L/min/m^2))

TREATMENT

Currently there is no specific therapy for IPF associated PH. Treatment of IPF should be optimized to reduce disease progression. As general measures, all patients should exercise as tolerated, receive routine vaccinations, be counselled against smoking and be treated with supportive measures including long term oxygen therapy and diuretics when indicated. Supplemental oxygen is prescribed for hypoxemic patients (at rest, during exercise or sleep) with the goal of maintaining a peripheral oxygen saturation higher than 90%. Diuretics are indicated in patients with fluid retention from PH related right heart failure.

PH targeted therapy is not typically indicated in IPF patients since it has no proven benefit and is associated with potential harm partially explained by vasodilatory effects of these agents that may exacerbate ventilation perfusion abnormalities and worsen gas exchange [15]. Safety and efficacy of PH targeted therapies have been evaluated in recent years. Riociguat and ambrisentan are both contraindicated. There is no evidence of benefit for other endothelin receptor antagonists. The very limited data on the use of sildenafil is conflicting. The evidence on prostanoid therapy is too limited for any current recommendation [12].

PH targeted therapies may be considered in patients with severe PH and mild to moderate lung disease in whom general measures have failed and a major component of PH is thought to be unrelated to the underlying lung disease. These patients should be referred to specialized centers experienced in the management of PH for possible enrollment in clinical trials.

REFERENCES

[1] Simonneau, G., Montani, D., Celermajer, D.S., Denton, C.P., Gatzoulis, M.A., Krowka, M., Williams, P.G., and Souza, R. (2019). "Haemodynamic definitions and updated clinical classification of pulmonary hypertension." *Eur. Respir. J.* 53: 1801913. (https://doi.org/10.1183/13993003.01913-2018)

[2] Klinger, James R. (2016). "Group III pulmonary hypertension: pulmonary hypertension associated with lung disease: epidemiology, pathophysiology, and treatments." *Cardiology Clinics* 34: 413-433.

[3] Collum, S.D., Amione-Guerra, J., Cruz-Solbes, A.S., DiFrancesco, A., Hernandez, A.M., Hanmandlu, A., Youker, K., Guha, A., and Karmouty-Quintana, H. (2017). "Pulmonary hypertension associated with idiopathic pulmonary fibrosis: Current and Future Perspectives." *Canadian Respir. J.* 2017: 1430350. (https://doi.org/10.1155/2017/1430350)

[4] Shuichi, Hatano and Toma Strasser. (1975). Primary pulmonary hypertension. *Report on a WHO Meeing.* Geneva, World Health Organization. https://apps.who.int/iris/handle/10665/39094, accessed June 30, 2019.

[5] Weitzenblum, E. (2003). "Chronic cor pulmonale." *Heart* 89: 225-230.

[6] Teramachi, R., Taniguchi, H., Kondoh, Y., Ando, M., Kimura, T., Kataoka, K., Suzuki, A., Furukawa, T., Sakamoto, K., and Hasegawa. Y. (2017). "Progression of mean pulmonary arterial pressure in idiopathic pulmonary fibrosis with mild to moderate restriction." *Respirology* 22: 986–990.

[7] Lettieri, C.J., Nathan, S.D., Barnett, S.D., Ahmad, S., and Shorr, A.F. (2006). "Prevalence and outcomes of pulmonary arterial hypertension in advanced idiopathic pulmonary fibrosis." *Chest* 129: 746-752.

[8] Shorr, A.F., Wainright, J.L., Cors, C.S., Lettieri, C.J., and Nathan, S.D. (2007). "Pulmonary hypertension in patients with pulmonary fibrosis awaiting lung transplant." *Eur. Respir. J.* 30; 715-721.

[9] Nathan, S.D., Shlobin, O.A., Ahmad, S., Urbanek, S., and Barnett, S.D. (2007). "Pulmonary hypertension and pulmonary function testing in idiopathic pulmonary fibrosis." *Chest* 131: 657-663.

[10] Colombat, M., Mal, H., Groussard, O., Capron, F., Thabut, G., Jebrak, G., Bruqiere, O., Dauriat, G., Castier, Y., Leseche, G., and Fournier, M. (2007). "Pulmonary vascular lesions in end-stage idiopathic pulmonary fibrosis: histopathologic study on lung explant specimens and correlations with pulmonary hemodynamics." *Hum. Pathol.* 38: 60-65.

[11] Farkas, L., Gauldie, J., Voelkel, N.F., and Kolb, M. (2011). "Pulmonary hypertension and idiopathic pulmonary fibrosis. A tale of angiogenesis, apoptosis, and growth factors." *Am. J. Respir. Cell Mol. Biol.* 45: 1-15.

[12] Nathan, S.D., Barbera, J.A., Gaine, S.P., Harari, S., Martinez, F.J., Olschewski, H., Olsson, K.M., Peacock, A.J., Pepke-Zaba, J., Provencher, S., Weissmann, N., and Seeger, W. (2019). "Pulmonary hypertension in chronic lung disease and hypoxia." *Eur. Respir. J.* 53: 1801914 (https://doi.org/10.1183/13993003.01914-2018)

[13] Nowak, J., Hudzik, B., Jastrzebski, D., Niedziela, J.T., Rozentryt, P., Wojarski, J., Ochman, M., Karolak, W., Zeglen, S., Gierlotka, M., and Gasior, M. (2018). "Pulmonary hypertension in advanced lung diseases: echocardiography as an important part of patient evaluation for lung transplantation." *Clin. Respi.r J.* 12:930-938.

[14] Alkukhun, L., Wang, X.F., Ahmed, M., Baumgartner, M., Budey, M., Dweik, R.A., and Tonelli, A.R. (2016). "Non-invasive screening for pulmonary hypertension in idiopathic pulmonary fibrosis." *Respir. Med.* 117:65-72.

[15] Seeger, W., Adir, Y., Barbera, J.A., Champion, H., Coghlan, J.G., Cottin, V., De Marco, T., Galie, N., Ghio, S., Gibbs, S., Martinez, F.J., Smigran, M.J., Simonneau, G., Wells, A.U., and Vachiery, J.L. (2013). "Pulmonary Hypertension in chronic lung diseases." *J. Am. Coll. Cardiol.* 62: D109-D116.

In: Respiratory Ventilatory Strategies …
Editor: Antonio M. Esquinas
ISBN: 978-1-53617-847-0
© 2020 Nova Science Publishers, Inc.

Chapter 8

BIOMARKERS IDIOPATHIC PULMONARY FIBROSIS AND LUNG FUNCTION

Dorina Esendagli*, MD, PhD
Department of Chest Diseases, Baskent University, Ankara, Turkey

ABSTRACT

Idiopathic pulmonary fibrosis (IPF) is a chronic, progressive and a form of interstitial pneumonia leading to fibrosis and loss of function of the lung. It is usually diagnosed in elderly population after excluding the known causes of interstitial lung diseases, the presence of the radiological findings and histopathology patterns of usual interstitial pneumonia (UIP). The fact that etiology is unknown makes it difficult to understand the complexity of the pathogenesis behind the disease, develop new treatment options, foresee the clinical outcome of different patients and the way they will respond to the available therapies. Taking in consideration the complexity of the disease the identification of biomarkers would help not only in determining the predisposition of patients for the disease, but also classify them according to the prognosis, choose the right treatment for specific groups and help in their follow-up. Many studies in the last 2 decades have been focused in identification of the ideal biomarker for IPF, but as a result of what these studies have shown it is yet unclear if any of the numerous potential biomarkers can be used in clinics.

Keywords: idiopathic pulmonary fibrosis, biomarkers, lung function

* Corresponding Author's E-mail: dr.dorina.de@gmail.com.

INTRODUCTION

IPF is usually diagnosed in elderly patients and has got a poor prognosis with an estimated average survival of 3-5 years, eventhough many patients might die within one year from diagnosis time. Guidelines for IPF diagnosis are used starting from 2011 yet there is a part of the patients who still needs an invasive procedure when the radiological findings are indeterminate and this might add a risk for this group of patients who are old and have many other comorbidities. This is one of the reasons which urges the usage of biological biomarkers that can be easily obtained in less invasive methods and low complication rates like for example blood or sputum. On the other hand the wide variety and heterogeneity of clinical outcome and the sudden episodes of acute exacerbations which worsen the prognosis and might be even fatal for the patients makes it difficult to foresee how the disease will progress and this is another reason which emphasis the need of biomarkers in this field. The current treatment approved for IPF is mainly composed of agents that try to slow down the fibrosis, but yet not enough to reverse the whole process and we still do not know who are exactly the specific patients that benefit from such treatment options. Biomarkers that are related to different steps of the pathophysiology of the disease might help not only in the elucidation of the mechanism of the disease but also lead to the development of new therapies and identification of patients' subsets that can benefit from them.

Biomarkers apart from being related to the mechanism of the diesease, prognosis and treatment response they should also be easily measured, specific, reproducible, cheap, highly sensitive and uniform even if they are measured in different populations of the world.

This chapter will summarize the research on biomarkers related to IPF according to different aspects of the underlying mechanisms of the diease, methods and ways of sampling and the latest approaches in the field.

GENE SIGNATURES IN IPF

Taking in consideration the complexity and heterogeneity of IPF disease various biomarkers have been shown in different studies with contradictory findings or have been found to be unable to differentiate among patients who undergo exacerbations and have a worse prognosis. This fact emphasis that a classification of the patients should be done from the start and that biomarkers might be specific for a certain group of patients. Wang et al., have examined the gene expression profiles in IPF patients and found that only a few number of genes are in common which are called as IPF core genes and that there is a high heterogeneity in patients genes which are not consistent with the clinical findings like forced vital capacity (FVC) or diffusing capacity of carbon monoxide (DLCO) results and cannot predict the acute exacerbations. They have identified six subtypes of IPF that reflect the severity of disease and decline in lung function by using transcriptional profiles on lung tissue from 131 patients with IPF and 12 patients without the disease as a control group. 55 genes were shown to be dysregulated in IPF patients and they were mainly involved in extracellular matrix, epithelial to mesenchymal cells cross-talk, calcium ion homeostasis and oxygen transport. Yet further studies are needed to validate the involvement of these genes in pathogenesis of the disease.

Biomarkers Involved in Pathogenesis of IPF

There are different pathways that are shown to have a role in pathogenesis of IPF like alveolar epithelial dysfunction as a result of an injury (viral or other type of infections, microaspirations, inhalation of hazardous agents like cigarette smoking) that leads to extracellular matrix remodeling and fibroproliferation and also an immune dysregulation that results in tissue destruction, unproper healing process and in progressive loss of function of the lung. Biomarkers related to these steps of pathogenesis have been studied mainly from peripheral blood because of easy sampling and low rate of complications.

Alveolar Epithelial Cell (AEC) Dysfunction

Surfactant proteins are lipoprotein complexes which are synthesized and secreted by type 2 alveolar epithelial cells. Despite reduction of intra-alveolar surface tension they are also involved in innate host defense against various infections. Among surfactant proteins SP-A and SP-D have been shown in many studies to be elevated in IPF especially in acute exacerbations, but also in other interstitial lung diseases (ILD). While SP-A has been shown to be higher in IPF rather than other ILDs thus might play role in diagnosis on the other hand SP-D high levels were related to prognosis and frequency of exacerbations.

Mutations in SP-A2 and SP-C can lead to a chronic endoplasmic reticulum (ER) stress and enhance the unfolded protein response in alveolar epithelial cells that ends with development of pulmonary fibrosis. This mechanism which is especially important for familial IPF patients has been investigated also in animal models that have shown the need for a second hit (e.g. any infection or hazardous agent for the lung) in some cases. On the other hand IPF and lung cancer also do co-exist in some patients and mutations in SP-A subgroups might be involved in this phenotype of IPF patients. Interestingly in 2 studies examining the levels of SP-A and SP-D in patients receiving any of the antifibrotic drugs there was shown no difference from the levels of patients taking placebo pills.

Krebs von den Lungen 6 (KL-6)/MUC1

KL-6 is a glycoprotein expressed on extracellular membrane of type 2 AEC and bronchiolar epithelial cells. KL-6 is increased in blood when alveolar epithelial cells are injured or proliferate and is not specific to IPF or lung since it also increases in other ILDs and can be released by other organs like breast or pancreas. High levels of KL-6 are especially measured in patients with acute exacerbations and levels higher than 1000 units are associated with low survival rates in IPF and other ILDs. High levels have been measured not only in blood but also in sputum and bronchoalveolar lavage (BAL) of IPF patients.

Interestingly no relationship between levels of KL-6 and treatment response was shown, suggesting that more research in the field is needed to determine the role of this biomarker in diagnosis and prognosis.

MUC5B

Mucins are glycoproteins that not only lubricate the respiratory system, but also play an important role as a part of innate immunity by neutralizing and inhibiting the penetration of infectious agents to the lung parenchyma. The MUC5B production is maintained by pseudostratified epithelium in distal airways. In 2011 a single nucleotide polymorphism (SNP) of MUC5B named as rs35705950 was detected which was shown to be associated with high MUC5B levels and development of IPF disease and was not related to other ILDs like scleroderma or sarcoidosis. MUC5B plays a role in predisposition of patients toward IPF, but studies have shown that it is related with a better prognosis in patients who are already diagnosed with the disease. Further studies are needed to elucidate the mechanism behind these findings and the importance of mucociliary clearance in pathogenesis of IPF.

Cleaved Cytokeratin 18 (cCK18)

cCK18 is a cytoskeletal protein in AECs. During apoptosis cytokeratin 18 is cleaved by caspases yielding cCK18. Serum levels of cCK18 were elevated in IPF patients and not in controls or other ILD patients. This biomarker was also detected by immunohistochemistry in lung tissues of IPF patients and not in the control normal lung tissues. cCK18 seems to be of a diagnostic value since no relationship was detected with the prognosis and clinical outcome.

Telomeres

Telomeres are non-coding nucleotide sequences located at the end of chromosomes which protect the DNA from degradation and shorten with age. Telomerases are enzymes that restore the telomere length. Shortening of telomeres in AEC cells of IPF patients leads to apoptosis or cell senescence and might explain why the disease is more common in elderly population.

Mutations in telomerase which lead to abnormal shortening of telomeres are reported especially in familial IPF patients (8-15%) and less in sporadic cases (only 3%). Other mutations of genes that are involved in telomere stabilization have been related with familial IPF. Analysis of telomere length in peripheral blood leucocytes have shown that short telomeres even when no mutation is present are associated with development of IPF both in sporadic and familial type and also helps in predicting the transplant-free survival in these patients.

Extracellular Matrix Remodeling and Fibrogenesis

As a result of alveolar epithelial injury like in wound healing the activation of profibrotic pathways, uncontrolled fibroblast proliferation and remodeling of extracellular matrix starts to occur. All these steps lead unfortunately to the tissue destruction and a defective architecture which results in progressive organ dysfunction and loss of lung function.

Matrix Metalloproteases (MMPs)

MMPs are zinc containing metallopeptidases that shape the extracellular matrix by degradation or activation of its components and also facilitate the cell migration process. MMPs are secreted by activated AECs and fibroblasts. They are expressed in normal conditions but their levels measured in either peripheral blood, BAL fluid or lung tissue were shown to be higher especially in wound healing process. There are various types of MMPs identified until nowadays but MMP1 and MMP7 are mainly the subtypes shown to be related with IPF and not other ILDs. MMP7 levels were shown to correlate inversely with the FVC and DLCO measures. MMP7 was also associated with disease progression and mortality which makes it a useful biomarker to be used not only in diagnosis but also in prognosis and survival of IPF patients. Despite the specificity and prognostic value this biomarker is yet not used in clinical practice because there is a lackage of standardization in protocols used in measurement of MMP levels and also the absence of a universal cut-off value.

MMP3 was also shown to have a role in pathogenesis of IPF and mouse models have shown that knocking out this gene protects mice from bleomycin induced lung fibrosis. MMP9 produced mainly by fibroblasts is upregulated in progressive disease and might have a role in prognosis and clinical outcome.

A recent study investigating MMP28 levels in IPF patients in two different cohorts (Mexico and Spain) showed that MMP28 was higher in IPF patients than in controls or patients with other ILDs and that a significant negative correlation of this biomarker with DLCO existed in both cohorts.

Collagen Synthesis Epitopes

Biomarkers related to collagen synthesis and tissue degradation have also been investigated especially in prediction of prognosis and therapeutic options in IPF. PRO-C3 and PRO-C6 which are neoepitopes measured in blood for collagen type 3 and 6 production were shown to be elevated in IPF patients when compared to normal populations and higher in the patients who had a progressive disease. These biomarkers did not correlate with the mortality rate.

Fibrocytes

Fibrocytes which are cells that express both hematopoietic and mesenchymal markers may differentiate into fibroblasts or myofibroblast and take role in ECM shaping. Activated AECs express CXCL12 chemokine which in turn recruits the circulating fibrocytes to the lung tissue. Even though studies have shown no correlation of fibrocytes with pulmonary function or radiological findings they were shown to be higher in IPF patients and especially show a peak in acute exacerbations which decreases after recovering. High levels of fibrocytes (>5%) are associated with a worse prognosis and survival rates.

Osteopontin (OPN)

OPN is a phosphorylated glycoprotein upregulated in inflammation and wound healing. It is located at AECs and macrophages and upregulates MMP7 in IPF patients. OPN enhances fibroblast proliferation and migration and is elevated in different ILDs. The cut-off value (>6 ng/ml) can be used to differentiate IPF from the other diseases. OPN seems to be only a diagnostic marker since studies have shown that the serum levels do not correlate with the disease progression.

Periostin

Periostin is a protein of ECM and plays a role in mesenchymal cell proliferation, wound healing and promotion of fibrotic processes in different organs including lungs. IPF patients have higher levels of periostin localized mainly in fibroblast loci and are related inversely with the lung function making it a potential prognostic marker. IL-13 which is secreted by bronchial epithelial cells promotes periostin production not only in asthma but also in IPF.

Lysyl Oxidase-Like (LOXL) Proteins

LOXL proteins play a role in collagen deposition and ECM homeostasis. LOXL2 and 3 subtypes enable fibroblast to myofibroblast trans-differentiation which is an important part of pathogenesis of IPF. LOXL levels are also related to disease prognosis and the overall survival.

Immune Dysregulation

Although immunosuppressive therapies are not effective in IPF treatment and lead to increased mortality in patients, the pathological examination of lung tissues in IPF have shown lymphoid aggregates and plasma cells which are present within fibrotic structure. Immune system even though not elucidated enough to explain the underlying mechanism seems to play an important role in different steps of pathophysiology of the disease. The way the immune system responds might be different as a result of an immune dysregulation thus making the immunosuppressive therapies approach fail.

Innate Immune System

Toll-Like Receptor 3 (TLR3)

Toll-like receptors are important components of innate immunity and play role in response to infection and injury. Studies have shown that a polymorphism of TLR3 named as L412F altered the cytokine production and dysregulated the fibroblasts production. In two different cohorts TLR3 polymorphism presence was associated with the disease progression and increased mortality in IPF patients.

Chemokines and Interleukins (IL-8, CCL18)

IL-8 which is a chemo-attractant for neutrophils was shown to be high in IPF patients serum and correlated negatively with DLCO, total lung capacity (TLC) and vital capacity (VC) parameters.

CC chemokine ligand 18 (CCL18) is secreted by antigen presenting cells mainly alveolar macrophages and induces the fibroblast production. CCL18 is elevated in different ILDs including IPF and antifibrotic treatments have been shown to reduce its production. CCL18 might be a prognostic biomarker in the future.

Defensins

Defensins are antimicrobial proteins that are secreted by neutrophils and epithelial cells. Alpha defensins were upregulated in IPF patients and especially in the ones who had acute exacerbations. They were related to the functional deterioration and impairment of DLCO.

YKL40

YKL40 is a chitinase-like protein expressed by bronchiolar epithelial cells and alveolar macrophages near fibrotic areas in IPF and is involved in injury and both acute and chronic inflammation. YKL40 levels were elevated both in serum and BAL samples of IPF patients and also in many other ILDs.

Adaptive Immune System

T Lymphocytes

T cells are the most common immune cells isolated from IPF patients lungs. Due to a continous stimulation CD28, which is a costimulatory protein, may be lost and $CD4+CD28^{null}$ cells are typical for a chronic immune activation. In some patients CD28 percentage was correlated with FVC and DLCO changes.

On the other hand regulatory T cells promote tolerance and prevent the autoimmune diseases. Tregs levels were low and abnormally functioning in IPF patients in both peripheral blood and BAL samples.

CXCL13

CXCL13 is a chemokine that enables homing of CXCR5 + B cells in lymphoid tissues. CXCL13 were elevated in IPF patients and were related with acute exacerbations, pulmonary hypertension and increased mortality.

Anti-Heat Shock Protein (HSP)-70 Antibodies

Autoantibodies especially IgG subtype that target HSP70 were detected in peripheral blood of IPF patients and were associated with progression of the disease and lower survival rates.

Adhesion Molecules and Growth Factors

Adhesion molecules like intracellular adhesion molecules (ICAM-1 and 2); insulin-like growth factor binding proteins (IGFBP-2) and vascular endothelial growth factor (VEGF) levels were also elevated in IPF patients. Their role in pathogenesis and the use in clinics needs further investigation. VEGF is even targeted by ninentanib, one of the anti-fibrotic drugs used in IPF and high FEGF levels were correlated with lower VC and survival rates. Whereas vimentin which is a protein expressed by mesenchymal cells and takes part in cytoskeletal structure is targeted by IgG autoantibodies in IPF patients. The higher the amount of these antibodies is in peripheral blood, the worse the lung function and prognosis will be.

OTHER POTENTIAL BIOMARKERS

Lung function parameters are used to monitor the disease activity and also used for the follow-up and response to the treatment for the IPF patients. Lately breath biomarkers have been studied if they can be used in diagnosis of IPF and their correlation with lung function tests to determine the different clinical groups and response to treatment. The concentration of NO at the level of alveolus (CalvNO) was the main biomarker found to be high in IPF patients and further study is needed to determine its potential role as a clinical biomarker.

Another way used in literature to define biomarkers is by examination of exosomes from the sputum of IPF patients. A negative correlation between miR-142-3p and DLCO was identified which suggests that miRNAs from sputum exosomes can be used as biomarkers to foresee the disease severity.

Another approach is to define biomarkers for IPF from samples other than lung or upper respiratory tract. Urine proteomics have identifed some proteins like MMP-7, human epididymis protein-4 (HE4) and urokinase plasminogen activator surface receptor (uPAR) to be different in IPF group when compared to the control.

Evaluation of oxidative stress biomarkers in different types of biological specimens of IPF patients has shown that some markers might be important, but unfortunately studies concerning the antioxidant treatments have shown no benefit in clinical improvement thus questioning the importance of this biomarkers in diagnosis, prognosis or treatment response.

Even microbiome isolated from IPF patients has been shown to be different from the normal lung. Higher bacterial content of *Streptococcus* and *Staphylococcus* species in BAL samples are related to a worse prognosis.

LIMITATIONS AND FUTURE DIRECTIONS

Many studies regarding the identification of potential biomarkers for IPF have been published and numerous markers have been shown to be important in the pathophysiology of the disease that might help in diagnosis, prognosis and treatment response for the patients. The studies are mainly performed in small groups of patients who belong to different populations, have used different ways of sampling and various kinds of biological specimens that have been measured by experimental protocols that differ from one group to another.

Regarding the fact that subgroups of patients exist and that clinical presentation is various in IPF this leads to the crucial need for the identification of not only a single biomarker but specific panels of markers which might help in patients follow-up and treatment decisions.

CONCLUSION

IPF is a complex disease with a clinical presentation that differs from one patient to another and the identification of subgroups according to the genetic background together with biological biomarkers would help for a better approach from the start concerning diagnosis and prognosis together with the expected treatment response in an individual basis. Many biomarkers have been identified which should further be studied for their validation in clinical usage and standardization between populations. A biomarker panel rather than a single one might provide information for the physicians and their correlation with clinical parameters like lung function tests would help in the treatment decisions during the follow-up.

REFERENCES

Drakopanagiotakis, F., Lukasz Wujak, Malgorzata Wygrecka, and P. Markart. "Biomarkers in idiopathic pulmonary fibrosis." *Matrix Biology* 68 (2018): 404-421.

Fois, A. G., Panagiotis Paliogiannis, Salvatore Sotgia, Arduino A. Mangoni, Elisabetta Zinellu, Pietro Pirina, Ciriaco Carru, and Angelo Zinellu. "Evaluation of oxidative stress biomarkers in idiopathic pulmonary fibrosis and therapeutic applications: a systematic review." *Respiratory research* 19, no. 1 (2018): 51.

Guiot, J., Catherine Moermans, Monique Henket, Jean-Louis Corhay, and Renaud Louis. "Blood biomarkers in idiopathic pulmonary fibrosis." *Lung* 195, no. 3 (2017): 273-280.

Hayton, C., Dayle Terrington, Andrew M. Wilson, Nazia Chaudhuri, Colm Leonard, and Stephen J. Fowler. "*Breath Biomarkers in Idiopathic Pulmonary Fibrosis: A Systematic Review.*" (2018): PA2921.

Ley, B., Kevin K. Brown, and Harold R. Collard. "Molecular biomarkers in idiopathic pulmonary fibrosis." *American Journal of Physiology-Lung Cellular and Molecular Physiology* 307, no. 9 (2014): L681-L691.

MMP28 is upregulated in idiopathic pulmonary fibrosis (IPF) epithelium and is a promising biomarker to distinguish IPF from non-IPF patients.

Njock, M. S., Julien Guiot, Monique A. Henket, Olivier Nivelles, Marc Thiry, Franck Dequiedt, Jean-Louis Corhay, Renaud E. Louis, and Ingrid Struman. "Sputum exosomes: promising biomarkers for idiopathic pulmonary fibrosis." *Thorax* 74, no. 3 (2019): 309-312.

Organ, L. A., Anne-Marie R. Duggan, Eunice Oballa, Sarah C. Taggart, Juliet K. Simpson, Arthur R. Kang'ombe, Rebecca Braybrooke et al., "Biomarkers of collagen synthesis predict progression in the PROFILE idiopathic pulmonary fibrosis cohort." *Respiratory research* 20, no. 1 (2019): 1-10.

Raghu, G., Martine Remy-Jardin, Jeffrey L. Myers, Luca Richeldi, Christopher J. Ryerson, David J. Lederer, Juergen Behr et al., "Diagnosis of idiopathic pulmonary fibrosis. An official ATS/ERS/JRS/ALAT clinical practice guideline." *American journal of respiratory and critical care medicine* 198, no. 5 (2018): e44-e68.

Rindlisbacher, B., Cornelia Schmid, Thomas Geiser, Cédric Bovet, and Manuela Funke-Chambour. "Serum metabolic profiling identified a distinct metabolic signature in patients with idiopathic pulmonary fibrosis–a potential biomarker role for LysoPC." *Respiratory research* 19, no. 1 (2018): 7.

Wang, Y., Jaswanth Yella, Jing Chen, Francis X. McCormack, Satish K. Madala, and Anil G. Jegga. "Unsupervised gene expression analyses identify IPF-severity correlated signatures, associated genes and biomarkers." *BMC pulmonary medicine* 17, no. 1 (2017): 133.

In: Respiratory Ventilatory Strategies … ISBN: 978-1-53617-847-0
Editor: Antonio M. Esquinas © 2020 Nova Science Publishers, Inc.

Chapter 9

GASTROESOPHAGEAL REFLUX AND CHRONIC LUNG DISEASE

Mo'ath Nassar, MD, Tricia L. Griffiths, MD and Ayman O. Soubani*, MD
Division of Pulmonary, Critical Care and Sleep Medicine, Wayne State University School of Medicine, Detroit, MI, US

ABSTRACT

Gastroesophageal Reflux Disease (GERD) is an important consideration as the direct cause or a contributing factor in patients presenting with pulmonary symptoms. This chapter aims to look at several different pulmonary diseases affected by GERD ranging from upper airway including chronic cough, vocal cord dysfunction, lower airway diseases including COPD, asthma, and bronchiolitis obliterans syndrome, down to parenchymal diseases such as interstitial lung diseases. The chapter will also discuss the potential mechanisms leading to pulmonary disease associated with GERD, the diagnostic approach and different treatment options.

INTRODUCTION

Gastroesophageal Reflux Disease (GERD) is a condition in which reflux of stomach contents causes symptoms and/or complications [1] that could be esophageal like retrosternal "heartburn" or extraesophageal like chronic cough and other pulmonary diseases. It is quite common in western countries with a prevalence of 15-20% [2]. It is

* Corresponding Author's E-mail: asoubani@med.wayne.edu.

known that GERD can cause a spectrum of respiratory diseases, which can be sometimes challenging to diagnose. In this review, we discuss GERD related pulmonary diseases pathophysiology and spectrum as well as their management.

PATHOPHYSIOLOGY

The esophagus and trachea share the same embryological derivation and innervation by vagus nerve. The Esophagus runs by the posterior aspect of trachea and the upper esophageal sphincter lies behind the larynx. In normal individuals, gastro esophageal reflux happens physiologically from the relaxation of lower esophageal sphincter and doesn't cause mucosal injury [3]. However, disease state happens when there is lower esophageal sphincter incompetence causing more frequent reflux and longer duration of exposure [4].

There are three main clinical settings for GERD causing lung disease: first is increased thoracic cavity negative pressure in relation to abdominal cavity during inspiration, which may aggravate pre-existing lower esophageal sphincter incompetence [3]. A study on asthmatic revealed that lower esophageal sphincter relaxation is increased in response to methacholine challenge test which indicates a relationship between obstructive lung disease and lower esophageal sphincter relaxation [5]. Second, is increased intra-abdominal pressure like in obesity and pregnancy. Third, is intrinsic esophageal muscular diseases such as in myopathic diseases and scleroderma [3].

Lung disease happens by two main mechanisms in the setting of GERD. Reflex neural mechanisms caused by reflex events limited to lower esophageal sphincter. A study showed that acid infusion in distal esophagus has resulted in vagally mediated reflexes leading to bronchoconstriction [6]. This also mediates pro-inflammatory mediators release aggravating airway hyperresponsiveness. The second, is direct effect from the gastric content causing upper airway irritation and lung disease if aspirated [3]. This can be in the form of gross aspiration causing acute conditions like recurrent pneumonia, or microaspiration causing more subtle symptoms like chronic cough.

SPECTRUM OF LUNG DISEASE FROM GERD

There are a variety of lung diseases mentioned below that are associated with GERD ranging from upper airway to parenchymal involvement (Figure 1). Some have been shown to affect quality of life while others are linked with mortality if GERD is not well controlled.

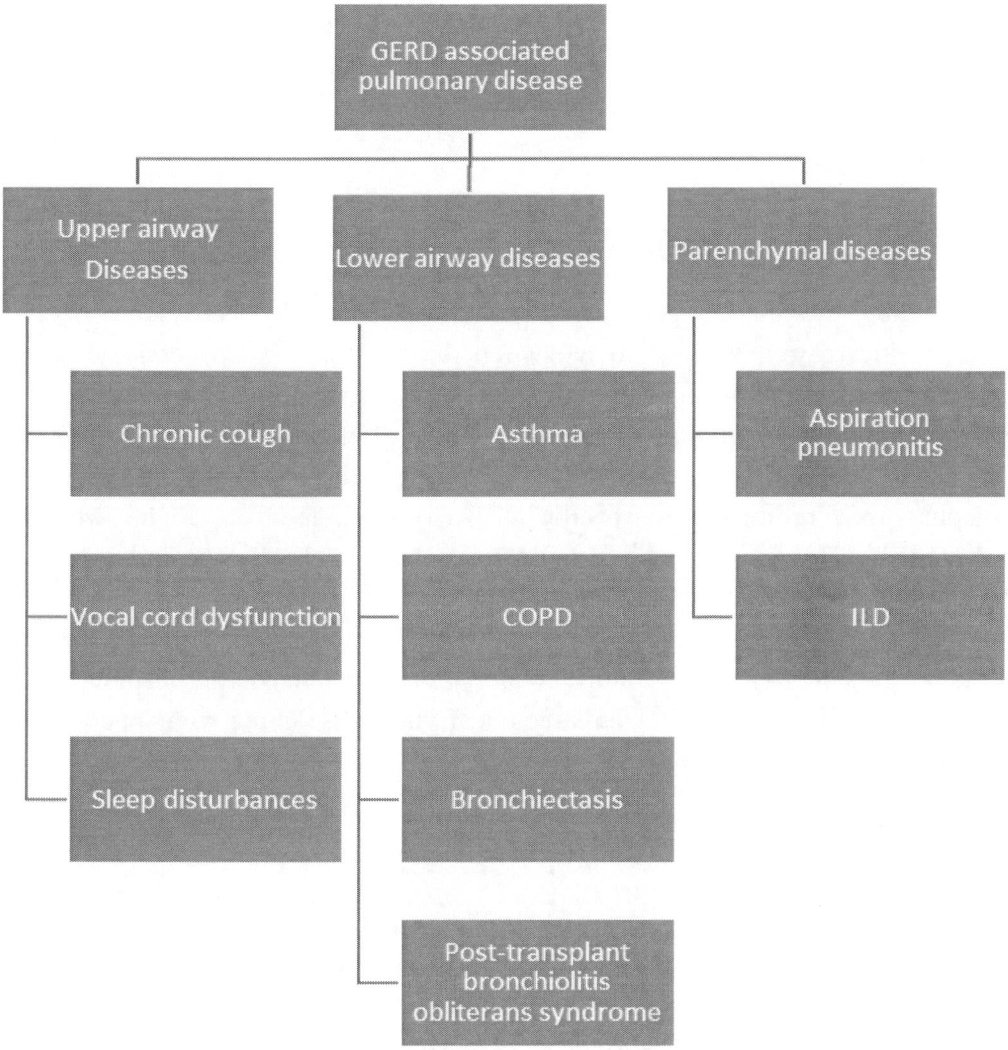

Figure 1. Spectrum of pulmonary manifestations of GERD.

Chronic Cough

Chronic cough, is defined as persistent cough for longer than 8 weeks, often attributed to asthma, upper airway cough syndrome or GERD [7]. GERD causes chronic cough through two different mechanisms: direct stimulation of the afferent limb of cough reflex by irritating the upper airway tract without aspiration or the lower airway tract by mirco or macro aspiration [8]. The second mechanism is by stimulating an esophageal-bronchial cough reflex in which refluxate into the distal esophagus alone is thought to be a sufficient stimulus to cause cough [9]. Clinically, the patient may present with dry or productive cough [8]. The condition can present without GERD symptoms in 75% of the time [10]. The diagnosis is predicted mainly by ruling out other etiologies like symptomatic Asthma, Upper airway cough syndrome and angiotensin-converting enzyme inhibitor induced cough [8]. Dietary and life style modifications as well as acid suppression therapy are the main treatment [8].

Vocal Cord Dysfunction

Vocal cord dysfunction is a syndrome characterized by paroxysms of glottic obstruction due to true vocal cord adduction during inspiration, occasionally during expiration, or both, resulting in symptoms such as dyspnea and noisy breathing [11]. This condition is often misdiagnosed as asthma [12]. True relationship between GERD and Vocal cord dysfunction remains unclear as the laryngoscopic findings used to diagnose laryngopharyngeal reflux are nonspecific [12]. However, 18% of patients with Vocal cord dysfunction are reported to have underlying GERD [11]. The diagnostic criteria for Vocal cord dysfunction include clinical symptoms of noisy breathing and dyspnea, laryngoscopic evidence of vocal cord adduction, and confirmatory pulmonary function test findings of abnormal flow-volume loop (Often flattening of the inspiratory limb) [11]. The treatment is directed towards the underlying cause along with supportive care that may include speech therapy [12].

Sleep Disturbances

Several studies have shown that nighttime reflux is associated with sleep disturbances including insomnia and obstructive sleep apnea [13]. Physiologically, acid reflux postprandially is normal and leads to increase saliva secretion as well as peristalsis of the esophagus. However, those two responses are almost not existent during sleep, which prolongs acid contact time during sleep and attributes to frequent arousals [14]. In patients with symptomatic obstructive sleep apnea, the transient increase in trans-diaphragmatic pressure and decrease in trans-thoracic pressure lead to acid reflux [15]. As the relationship between GERD and sleep disturbance is bidirectional, the vicious cycle can be interrupted by aggressive acid reducing therapy, which is the mainstay of management [13].

Asthma

GERD is known to be associated with asthma symptoms in 30-80% of patients depending on the patient population, diagnostic test, and number of ascertained etiologies [16]. It is known that respiratory symptoms associated with GERD include difficult to treat asthma [16]. One pathogenic mechanism known is microaspiration of gastric contents from the proximal esophagus producing an exudative mucosal reaction in the larynx and in the tracheobronchial tree [16]. In general, there are three main mechanisms for GERD relating to asthma: frank aspiration of gastric contents into the lower respiratory tract, aspiration of contents as far as the pharynx causing the symptoms by stimulation of irritant receptors, and reflux of gastric contents limited to the lower esophagus causing symptoms either by increasing bronchial reactivity, or by bronchoconstriction secondary to a vagal reflex [17]. There is good evidence that receptors in the lower esophagus, when stimulated can cause bronchoconstriction in patients with asthma via a vagal reflex [17]. The majority of nerves innervating the airways are afferent or sensory in nature, and a subset are analogous to nociceptive sensory nerves and when activated, this subset initiates cough, bronchospasm, vascular engorgement, and mucus secretion. Similar reflexes can be initiated by noxious stimuli (acidic solutions, capsaicin) delivered to the esophageal mucosa [18]. Studies have shown episodes of reflux followed by a fall of intra-tracheal pH and episodes with a fall of intratracheal pH result in a marked fall in peak expiratory flow that was several times greater than that observed when reflux was not followed by a change in intratracheal pH [17]. In addition to these mechanisms, asthmatic patients often have hyperinflation, and with the hyperinflation, there is increased intrathoracic pressure by way of increased total lung capacity, and so there may be descent of the diaphragm in this setting which can increase the pressure gradient between the abdomen and chest and can cause herniation of the lower esophageal sphincter into the chest, and so it's barrier function impaired [19]. Asthma and GERD are also associated with obstructive sleep apnea and upper airway obstruction during sleep is associated with an increased trans-diaphragmatic pressure gradient and may lead to gastric content reflux into esophagus [20]. There has been a proposed connection between asthma treatment and GERD where beta agonists relax smooth muscle and thus have potential to reduce lower esophageal sphinctertone and to promote GERD and some studies have shown oral theophylline preparations on GERD have shown some effects on lower esophageal sphincter pressure. In a study on normal subjects, theophylline administrations producing blood levels in a therapeutic range, caused a mean reduction in LES pressure of 25% [16].

Treatment recommendations for GERD related asthma include both treatment of GERD and asthma. Proton pump inhibitors (PPI) and H2 blockers stop or markedly reduce acid production, but studies have been inconclusive about whether they improve asthma symptoms [17]. PPIs should be maintained at the lowest most effective dose [16]. There were 3 large trials done with proton pump inhibitor versus placebo, but none were done with PPI therapy vs H2 blockers. In Japan, a small study with 30 patients looked at peak expiratory flows and asthma control questionnaires on lansoprazole (PPI) vs roxatidine (H2 blocker) and showed there was significant improvement on PPI vs H2 blocker on both peak expiratory flow asthma control questionnaire, but no large trials have been repeated [21]. No large trials have been done solely on H2 blockers either, however GERD treatment medical management includes H2 blockers for mild intermittent symptoms according to the American Gastroenterological Association, but with failure, or more severe symptoms, requires PPI therapy.

The first PPI vs placebo trial was a multicenter randomized control study that evaluated difficult to control asthma associated with GERD. Patients were randomized to Lansoprazole 30mg BID or placebo BID for 24 weeks, and the study concluded that albuterol use, pulmonary function tests, or asthma symptoms were not improved, however the PPI dose did improve asthma exacerbations (8.1% vs 20.4%), and quality of life [22]. The next study done around the same time looked at effect of gastric acid suppression with PPIs on asthma outcomes. 770 subjects were randomized to 40mg esomeprazole BID or placebo BID for 16 weeks and found esomeprazole improved peak expiratory flow in the subjects with asthma, GERD and nocturnal symptoms, but no improvement was seen without GERD symptoms or nocturnal symptoms [23]. Finally, a third study was done with esomeprazole 40mg BID and placebo BID for asthmatics and GERD symptoms, and showed that esomeprazole may improve pulmonary function and asthma related quality of life, but the improvements were of small clinical significance [24].

If when empiric therapy with PPI fails without improvement of GERD or asthma, based on American College of Gastroenterology guidelines, pH testing may be warranted with esophageal pH testing, and referral to a gastroenterologist. Patients may be surgical candidates if they have primarily respiratory symptoms, have demonstrated abnormal gastroesophageal reflux refractory to treatment, and reflux episodes with 24-hour pH monitoring, the patient should also have a positive response to medical therapy [18].

Chronic Obstructive Pulmonary Disease (COPD)

The prevalence of GERD in patients with COPD ranges from 19% to 78% based on multiple studies. This wide range is attributed to the different screening questionnaires and diagnostic modalities used [25]. Patients with COPD are at slightly increased risk for developing GERD [2]. Suggested mechanisms include nicotine induced lower esophageal sphincter relaxation leading to acid reflux, and decreased salivation; prolonging the acid reflux time [26]. Severe hyperinflation may also contribute as the increased inspiratory muscles effort at high lung volumes amplifies the pressure gradient between thorax and abdomen, which impacts lower esophageal sphincter and predisposes to acid reflux [27]. The condition is managed by anti-reflux measures and pharmacologic anti-reflux therapy, which can possibly decrease the risk of COPD exacerbation in this patient population [25].

Bronchiectasis

Bronchiectasis is defined by irreversibly widened bronchi due to damage to the bronchial wall, usually arises from bronchial obstruction and infection [28]. GERD contributes to about 4% of the cases of non-cystic fibrosis bronchiectasis [29]. However, it is not clear how the causal relationship between aspiration and bronchiectasis was established. Upper GI contrast studies and correlation with the location on bronchiectasis has been used in implicating the aspiration [12]. Treatment is with Intensive acid-suppression and prokinetic agents [30].

Post-Transplant Bronchiolitis Obliterans

GERD has been implicated in the pathogenesis of bronchiolitis obliterans and bronchiolitis obliterans syndrome post lung transplantation. The failure of lung transplantation is largely determined by bronchiolitis obliterans syndrome which is a disease process whose pathophysiology is largely unknown and finding modifiable risk factors to avoid or slow progression has become extremely important [31]. Chronic rejection of the lung transplantation typically falls under the umbrella of bronchiolitis obliterans (BO), and bronchiolitis obliterans syndrome (BOS). BO is a histological diagnosis that occurs as a result of macrophage and myofibroblast infiltration of the bronchioles which induces fibrous obliteration and scar formation, seen on biopsy [32]. BOS following lung transplantation is a clinical diagnosis defined as a FEV1 drop by 20% from baseline value and includes early BOS stage with FEV1 81-90% with drop in mid expiratory flow rate without another identifiable cause [33]. GERD has been associated with increased morbidity in lung transplant patients through a proposed pathway of reflux, aspiration, immunomodulation, and allograft injury, culminating in functional decline and rejection [32]. Many studies have proposed that GERD is a risk factor in the development of BOS through silent aspiration of stomach contents leading to direct airway injury and upregulation of the inflammatory response of the lung [32]. Studies have shown almost a 63% prevalence of GERD in end stage lung disease, and numerous other studies showing increased prevalence of GERD post transplantation suggesting that transplant itself worsens GERD [32]. This can also depend on the type of transplant done as bilateral transplants tend to have increased proximal reflux compared to single, and re-transplantation greater than primary transplantation [31]. One hypothesis as to why this happens is extensive dissection during the surgery disrupting the vagal nerve [31]. Other factors include loss of cough reflex, impaired mucociliary clearance, and development of gastroparesis as a side effect of calcineurin inhibitors, steroids, mycophenolate mofetil, and other post-transplant immunosuppression treatments [32].

The central belief is that BOS is a chronic inflammatory and fibrotic process of the small airways, marked by recurrent injury, remodeling, and repair, ultimately resulting in allograft failure typified by obliterative fibrosis. There have been numerous studies supporting these changes which have shown that chronic aspiration of gastroduodenal contents is linked to immunomodulation, including increased local levels of IL-1a, IL-1B, IL-6, IL-10, TNF-a, TNF-B, increased alveolar neutrophils, increased IL-8, increased IL-15, IL-17, basic FGF, TNF-a, and MPO and reduced alpha-1-antitrypsin, augmented allorecognition, and reduced levels of surfactant proteins [32]. This inflammatory environment via the cytokine cascade leads to allograft rejection and dysfunction [33]. There have also been studies looking into the role of pepsin and bile acids in relation with GERD and BOS. Bile acids have been shown to be cytotoxic especially to type II pneumocytes and that highest concentrations of bile acids were found in 70% of patients with early onset and most severe manifestation of BOS suggesting a temporal and dose-related relationship [32].

A similar BOS has been described in allogeneic hematopoietic stem cell transplantation recipients. This is considered the primary manifestation of chronic graft versus host disease and is usually diagnosed after the first 100 days following transplantation. GERD has also been suggested as a potential contributing factor to BOS in this patient population, especially in patients with Graft Versus Host Disease involving the esophagus [34].

It has also been shown that typical symptoms of GERD are not necessarily predictive of the effect or severity of respiratory disease [32]. Diagnostic approach includes 24-hour ambulatory pH testing, pH impedance testing, and even bronchoscopy with bronchoalveolar lavage [31, 32]. The impedance testing was better able to asses for non-acid reflux in presence, direction, and independent of pH, which too is known to cause chronic changes leading to rejection [32]. In terms of bronchoscopy with bronchoalveolar lavage, one study showed that higher amounts of pepsin within the bronchoalveolar lavage was associated with a higher rate of rejection [32]. Treatment of GERD includes medical therapy that decreases the acidity of gastric contents with H2 blockers or proton pump inhibitors. These reduce symptoms, however nonacid reflux can also lead to significant damage and augment GERD associated pulmonary injury [33]. The role of azithromycin has also been brought to attention for GERD and BOS for its for anti-inflammatory and prokinetic properties, although the mechanism remains unclear [31, 33]. At this time, laparoscopic anti reflux surgery is the most successful management of GERD in those with end stage lung disease and after lung transplant [15]. Many transplant surgeons are recommending anti reflux surgery especially fundoplication for those diagnosed with GERD, as it has a low association with morbidity and mortality, and furthermore leads to a reduction in immune modulators associated with development of BOS and preservation in overall lung function [33]. This was seen in a study from Robertson, et al. that looked at 16 lung transplant patients undergoing fundoplication and assessing quality of life, BMI, and pulmonary function. Fifteen of the sixteen patients were satisfied with the results post operatively, there was significant improvement in symptoms, BMI had decreased, and those operated on for deteriorating lung function had a statistically significant decrease in the rate of decline of their lung function post operatively [35]. Another study was from Abassi-Ghadi et al. looking to determine the safety of antireflux surgery for those with lung transplant recipients who looked at histologic evidence of GERD, positive impedance study with symptoms, and declining FEV1.Forty patients underwent Nissen fundoplication. These patients overall did have a slight decline of 2119 to 1967mL and a mean rate of change in FEV1 did improve from -2.42 to -.041 mL/day. The study did show that fundoplication was safe and overall improves rate of change in FEV1 post operatively [36]. Hartwig et al. looked at how fundoplication could prevent GERD related allograft dysfunction. They concluded that transplant patients with abnormal esophageal pH studies attain a lower peak allograft function as well as diminished 1-year FEV1 after transplantation, but with a strategy of early fundoplication (within 90 days), these recipients appear to preserve lung allograft function measured by esophageal pH monitoring as a surrogate for recipient's risk of aspiration and subsequent allograft dysfunction [37]. Only one study by Cantu et al. thus far has shown a survival benefit with early fundoplication (within 90 days of transplant) vs late [33]. The conclusions of this study showed that in 14 patients with early fundoplication, actuarial survival was 100% at 1 and 3 years compared to those with reflux and no intervention (92% and 76%), and further those who underwent early fundoplication had improved freedom from BOS at 1 and 3 years (100% and 100%) when compared with no fundoplication in patients with reflux (96% and 60%) [38].

Aspiration Pneumonitis and Pneumonia

Aspiration pneumonitis occurs upon inhalation of large volume gastric content causing chemical injury in lungs parenchyma. This often happens in the setting of altered consciousness. A comprehensive review of Aspiration Pneumonia was done recently showing that while GERD does not directly cause aspiration pneumonia, it is one of the risk factors by increasing the chance of gastric contents to reach the lung especially in the context of impaired cough reflex or dysphagia as shown by studies looking at elderly populations with dysphagia and GERD or with feeding tubes as well [39]. Superimposed bacterial infection may complicate the condition especially in the presence of acid suppressive therapy [12]. Clinically, this condition manifests with immediate coughing spills, wheezes and may be associated with hypoxemia. Inflammation in lungs parenchyma happens 4-6 hours later [40]. Chest radiography usually shows progressing diffuse air-space opacities in the following 24-47 hours [41]. Diagnosis is suspected when the event of aspiration is witnessed. However, for unwitnessed event, the diagnosis is supported by the presence of particulate matter in the airway during bronchoscopy. For the latter, caution should be exercised so other etiologies for air-space opacities are not missed [41].

The management of aspiration pneumonitis is mainly supportive. Endotracheal intubation is considered if clinically indicated. Bronchodilators can be given for management of bronchospasm [41]. Steroids use may improve radiographic changes, however its use remains controversial [42]. Empiric antimicrobial therapy with broad-spectrum agents should be considered if aspiration happens in the setting of small bowel obstruction or in patients with aspiration pneumonitis that fails to improve within 48 hours [42].

Interstitial Lung Disease (ILD)

GERD and ILD has been a recent topic of controversy, and the two most studied types of ILD with GERD are Idiopathic pulmonary fibrosis and systemic sclerosis related ILD. ILD encompasses a large number of pulmonary disorders characterized by cellular and extracellular infiltrates distal to the terminal bronchiole or acinus: sarcoidosis, pneumoconiosis, hypersensitivity pneumonitis, cryptogenic organizing pneumonitis etc. Idiopathic pulmonary fibrosis, or IPF, in which no evidence of a specific etiology or multisystem disorder exists, a number of proposed initiating mechanisms have been investigated; GERD has been included in this list [43]. IPF is strikingly similar to the lung involvement occurring in scleroderma. Patients with both disorders present with dyspnea, rales, finger clubbing, exercise induced hypoxemia, interstitial and fibrotic radiographic changes, and nonuniform collagen deposition, fibroblastic foci and honeycomb changes on pathology [3]. Recurrent microaspiration has been identified as a potential risk factor for IPF as a recurrent inflammatory stimulus and is postulated as important in the pathogenesis of scleroderma pulmonary fibrosis and IPF based on the observation of frequent esophageal dysfunction in both diseases [44, 3]. One mechanism proposed as to why this happens is that respiratory disorders associated with an increased ventilatory effort can cause an even more negative intrathoracic pressure and a more positive intra-abdominal pressure by flattening of the diaphragm, thereby increasing the thoraco-abdominal gradient making reflux of acidic or non-acidic contents more likely to happen [45]. Gastro esophageal reflux and esophageal diseases alike are reported in other ILDs but are less studied [45] and studies done have shown a higher incidence of gastro esophageal reflux in IPF patients compared to those with ILD of other etiology [43]. The mechanism of fibrosis has been suggested by previous studies done proposing recurrent occult microaspiration may drive the ongoing inflammation [3], and repeated small tracheobronchial aspiration of gastric secretions, and non-acid reflux over a long period of time could lead to IPF [43]. Microaspiration over time can lead to pneumonitis, increased epithelial permeability, stimulation of fibrotic proliferation, and eventual lung fibrosis [46]. Despite these studies, A causal relationship between GERD and IPF has yet to be established [43]. Idiopathic pulmonary fibrosis has been studied with esophageal pH monitoring to assess the prevalence of gastroesophageal reflux, and the results revealed a very high prevalence of gastro esophageal reflux compared with both normal individuals and with other patients with ILD of known cause [43]. This was seen by Tobin et al. who looked at 17 patients with biopsy proven IPF and compared them with controls with ILD other than IPF. Sixteen of seventeen patients with IPF had abnormal acid exposure as seen by ambulatory pH monitoring compared to 4/8 ILD patients without IPF. Most of the IPF patients (75%) did not have GERD symptoms [43]. In terms of systemic sclerosis, because esophageal involvement in systemic sclerosis is so common, it is difficult to determine whether gastro esophageal reflux and ILD when present together are causally related, or if they are merely two of the common manifestations of a systemic illness. One study by Denis, did in fact show decreased lung compliance in those patients with systemic sclerosis that had impaired peristalsis and impaired lower esophageal sphincter function suggesting that GER could enhance pulmonary fibrosis in systemic sclerosis [43].

In terms of treatment, although GERD and microaspiration have been proposed as risk factors for the development and progression of IPF, robust definitive data are few. A recent international guideline conditionally recommended the use of antacid therapy for patients with IPF in the absence of esophageal reflux or symptoms [46]. There are data to suggest that treatment with antacid therapy might be of clinical benefit in terms of slowing chronic disease progression and possibly even survival. Lee et al. looked at three randomized control trials treating IPF patients with PPI and H2 blockers vs placebo where the primary outcome was change in forced vital capacity at 30 weeks and found that 124 patients of 242 were taking either H2 blocker or PPI, and after adjustment for sex, baseline FVC and DLCO, the patients taking ant-acid treatment had a smaller decrease in FVC at 30 weeks [47]. Lee, Ryu, et al. did a regression analysis to investigate the relationship between GER related variables and survival time in IPF patients and found that reported use of GERD medications is associated with decreased radiologic fibrosis and an independent predictor of longer survival time in patients with IPF [48]. More recently, Ghebre and Raghu reviewed trials and articles and stated that PPIs play a beneficial role in IPF despite the ability to control gastric reflux completely, and possibly have another mechanism of down-regulation of fibroinflammatory molecules [49]. Conversely, other reports question the efficacy of antacid therapy, and have suggested that harm cannot be excluded [46]. This was looked at in Kreuter, et al's article which investigated three large phase 3 trials of patients on pirfenidone for IPF.

The patients from the CAPACITY 004, CAPACITY 006, and ASCEND trials were included, and the authors analyzed effects of antacid therapy with pulmonary function, exercise tolerance, survival, and other adverse events for 52 weeks. Primary endpoint was disease progression by 1 year. The findings showed no difference between the groups on antacid therapy and those who were not, higher admission rates in antacid therapy group, and no difference in pulmonary function or exercise [50]. PPIs are not benign medications with side effects such as C. difficile, pneumonia, hip fractures, dementia, cardiovascular events [46]. One other issue with proton pump inhibitors, is that they do not address non-acid reflux which may be important in extraesophageal symptom production and lung disease pathogenesis [44].

Along with lifestyle modifications, anti-acid therapy, if the symptoms persist, refractory reflux disease, laparoscopic fundoplication is the preferred surgical approach for most patients as it reliably decreases esophageal acid contact time, increases lower esophageal sphincter pressure, improves esophageal symptoms, and decreases proximal reflux [3]. There was a study (WRAP-IPF) that looked at laparoscopic anti-reflux surgery for IPF by Raghu et al. that looked to determine whether treatment of GERD with laparoscopic anti-reflux surgery would reduce the rate of disease progression. It was a randomized control trial that enrolled patients with IPF, GERD measured by 24-hour pH monitoring, and preserved FVC with a primary endpoint of change in FVC from randomization to week 48. 29 patients received surgery, and 29 did not. They found that the surgery group had a rate of change in FVC of -0.05L compared to -0.13L in the non-surgery group. Acute exacerbations, hospitalizations, and death was less common in the surgery group. Dysphagia and abdominal distention were the most common adverse events [51].

CONCLUSION

GERD as demonstrated in this review has a wide spectrum of pulmonary manifestations ranging from upper airway, to lower airway, to lung parenchyma, and while in some disease states acts as a risk factor, in others is a direct cause. In most cases, as soon as symptoms arise in the form of pulmonary symptoms, or even GERD like symptoms, treatment of the GERD with either H2 blocker, PPI, or even surgery is generally indicated. Knowledge of these pulmonary complications and maintaining high clinical suspicion are important to prevent long term complications and improving patient quality of life.

REFERENCES

[1] Vakil N, van Zanten SV, Kahrilas P, Dent J, Jones R; Global Consensus Group. The Montreal definition and classification of gastroesophageal reflux disease: a global evidence-based consensus. *Am J Gastroenterol.* 2006 Aug;101(8):1900-20.

[2] Dent J, El-Serag HB, Wallander MA, Johansson S. Epidemiology of gastro-oesophageal reflux disease: a systematic review. *Gut.* 2005 May;54(5):710-7.

[3] Morehead RS. Gastro-oesophageal reflux disease and non-asthma lung disease. *Eur Respir Rev.* 2009 Dec;18(114):233-43.

[4] Dent J, Holloway RH, Toouli J, Dodds WJ. Mechanisms of lower oesophageal sphincter incompetence in patients with symptomatic gastrooesophageal reflux. *Gut.* 1988 Aug;29(8):1020-8.

[5] Zerbib F, Guisset O, Lamouliatte H, Quinton A, Galmiche JP, Tunon-De-Lara JM. Effects of bronchial obstruction on lower esophageal sphincter motility and gastroesophageal reflux in patients with asthma. *Am J Respir Crit Care Med.* 2002 Nov 1;166(9):1206-11.

[6] Stein MR. Possible mechanisms of influence of esophageal acid on airway hyperresponsiveness. *Am J Med.* 2003 Aug 18;115 Suppl 3A:55S-59S.

[7] Irwin RS, Baumann MH, Bolser DC, Boulet LP, Braman SS, Brightling CE, et al. Diagnosis and management of cough executive summary: ACCP evidence-based clinical practice guidelines. *Chest.* 2006 Jan;129(1 Suppl):1S-23S.

[8] Irwin RS. Chronic cough due to gastroesophageal reflux disease: ACCP evidence-based clinical practice guidelines. *Chest.* 2006 Jan;129(1 Suppl):80S-94S.

[9] Irwin RS, Madison JM, Fraire AE. The cough reflex and its relation to gastroesophageal reflux. *Am J Med.* 2000 Mar 6;108 Suppl 4a:73S-78S.

[10] Irwin RS, French CL, Curley FJ, Zawacki JK, Bennett FM. Chronic cough due to gastroesophageal reflux. Clinical, diagnostic, and pathogenetic aspects. *Chest.* 1993 Nov;104(5):1511-7.

[11] Morris MJ, Christopher KL. Diagnostic criteria for the classification of vocal cord dysfunction. *Chest.* 2010 Nov;138(5):1213-23.

[12] Hu X, Lee JS, Pianosi PT, Ryu JH. Aspiration-related pulmonary syndromes. *Chest.* 2015 Mar;147(3):815-823.

[13] Jung HK, Choung RS, Talley NJ. Gastroesophageal reflux disease and sleep disorders: evidence for a causal link and therapeutic implications. *J Neurogastroenterol Motil.* 2010 Jan;16(1):22-9.

[14] Orr WC, Chen CL. Sleep and the gastrointestinal tract. *Neurol Clin.* 2005 Nov;23(4):1007-24.

[15] Ing AJ, Ngu MC, Breslin AB. Obstructive sleep apnea and gastroesophageal reflux. *Am J Med.* 2000 Mar 6;108; Suppl 4a:120S-125S.

[16] Ayres JG, Miles JF. Oesophageal reflux and asthma. *Eur Respir J.* 1996 May;9(5):1073-8.

[17] Kasasbeh A, Kasasbeh E, Krishnaswamy G. Potential mechanisms connecting asthma, esophageal reflux, and obesity/sleep apnea complex--a hypothetical review. *Sleep Med Rev.* 2007 Feb;11(1):47-58.

[18] Oelschlager BK, Pellegrini CA. Surgical treatment of respiratory complications associated with gastroesophageal reflux disease. *Am J Med.* 2003 Aug 18;115 Suppl 3A:72S-77S.

[19] Parsons JP, Mastronarde JG. Gastroesophageal reflux disease and asthma. *Curr Opin Pulm Med.* 2010 Jan;16(1):60-3.

[20] Canning BJ. Role of nerves in asthmatic inflammation and potential influence of gastroesophageal reflux disease. *Am J Med.* 2001 Dec 3;111 Suppl 8A:13S-17S.

[21] Yasuo Shimizu Y, Dobashi K, Kobayashi S, Ohki I, Tokushima M, Kusano M, et al.. A Proton Pump Inhibitor, Lansoprazole, Ameliorates Asthma Symptoms in Asthmatic Patients with Gastroesophageal Reflux Disease. *The Tohoku Journal of Experimental Medicine*. 2006. 209:3: 181-189.

[22] Littner MR, Leung FW, Ballard ED 2nd, Huang B, Samra NK; Lansoprazole Asthma Study Group. Effects of 24 weeks of lansoprazole therapy on asthma symptoms, exacerbations, quality of life, and pulmonary function in adult asthmatic patients with acid reflux symptoms. *Chest.* 2005 Sep;128(3):1128-35.

[23] Kiljander TO, Harding SM, Field SK, Stein MR, Nelson HS, Ekelund J, et al. Effects of esomeprazole 40 mg twice daily on asthma: a randomized placebo-controlled trial. *Am J Respir Crit Care Med.* 2006 May 15;173(10):1091-7.

[24] Kiljander TO, Junghard O, Beckman O, Lind T. Effect of esomeprazole 40 mg once or twice daily on asthma: a randomized, placebo-controlled study. *Am J Respir Crit Care Med.* 2010 May 15;181(10):1042-8.

[25] Lee AL, Goldstein RS. Gastroesophageal reflux disease in COPD: links and risks. *Int J Chron Obstruct Pulmon Dis.* 2015 Sep 14;10:1935-49.

[26] Pandolfino JE, Kahrilas PJ. Smoking and gastro-oesophageal reflux disease. *Eur J Gastroenterol Hepatol.* 2000 Aug;12(8):837-42.

[27] Pauwels A, Blondeau K, Dupont LJ, Sifrim D. Mechanisms of increased gastroesophageal reflux in patients with cystic fibrosis. *Am J Gastroenterol.* 2012 Sep;107(9):1346-53.

[28] McShane PJ, Naureckas ET, Tino G, Strek ME. Non-cystic fibrosis bronchiectasis. *Am J Respir Crit Care Med.* 2013 Sep 15;188(6):647-56.

[29] Pasteur MC, Helliwell SM, Houghton SJ, Webb SC, Foweraker JE, Coulden RA, et al. An investigation into causative factors in patients with bronchiectasis. *Am J Respir Crit Care Med.* 2000 Oct;162(4 Pt1):1277-84.

[30] Li AM, Sonnappa S, Lex C, Wong E, Zacharasiewicz A, Bush A, Jaffe A. Non-CF bronchiectasis: does knowing the aetiology lead to changes in management? *Eur Respir J.* 2005 Jul;26(1):8-14.

[31] Fisichella PM, Jalilvand A. The role of impaired esophageal and gastric motility in end-stage lung diseases and after lung transplantation. *J Surg Res.* 2014 Jan;186(1):201-6.

[32] Hathorn KE, Chan WW, Lo WK. Role of gastroesophageal reflux disease in lung transplantation. *World J Transplant.* 2017 Apr 24;7(2):103-116.

[33] Gulack BC, Meza JM, Lin SS, Hartwig MG, Davis RD. Reflux and allograft dysfunction: is there a connection? *Thorac Surg Clin.* 2015;25(1):97-105.

[34] Soubani AO, Uberti JP. Bronchiolitis obliterans following haematopoietic stem cell transplantation. *Eur Respir J.* 2007 May;29(5):1007-19.

[35] Robertson AG, Krishnan A, Ward C, Pearson JP, Small T, Corris PA, Dark JH, Karat D, Shenfine J, Griffin SM. Anti-reflux surgery in lung transplant recipients: outcomes and effects on quality of life. *Eur Respir J.* 2012 Mar;39(3):691-7.

[36] Abbassi-Ghadi N, Kumar S, Cheung B, McDermott A, Knaggs A, Zacharakis E, et al. Anti-reflux surgery for lung transplant recipients in the presence of impedance-detected duodenogastroesophageal reflux and bronchiolitis obliterans syndrome: a study of efficacy and safety. *J Heart Lung Transplant.* 2013 Jun;32(6):588-95.

[37] Hartwig MG, Anderson DJ, Onaitis MW, Reddy S, Snyder LD, Lin SS, Davis RD. Fundoplication after lung transplantation prevents the allograft dysfunction associated with reflux. *Ann Thorac Surg.* 2011 Aug;92(2):462-8; discussion; 468-9.

[38] Cantu E 3rd, Appel JZ 3rd, Hartwig MG, Woreta H, Green C, Messier R, et al. Maxwell Chamberlain Memorial Paper. Early fundoplication prevents chronic allograft dysfunction in patients with gastroesophageal reflux disease. *Ann Thorac Surg.* 2004 Oct;78(4):1142-51; discussion 1142-51.

[39] Mandell LA, Niederman MS. Aspiration Pneumonia. *New England Journal of Medicine* 2019; 380:651-663.

[40] Kennedy TP, Johnson KJ, Kunkel RG, Ward PA, Knight PR, Finch JS. Acute acid aspiration lung injury in the rat: biphasic pathogenesis. *Anesth Analg.* 1989 Jul;69(1):87-92.

[41] Raghavendran K, Nemzek J, Napolitano LM, Knight PR. Aspiration-induced lung injury. *Crit Care Med.* 2011 Apr;39(4):818-26.

[42] Marik PE. Pulmonary aspiration syndromes. *Curr Opin Pulm Med.* 2011 May;17(3):148-54.

[43] Ing AJ. Interstitial lung disease and gastroesophageal reflux. *Am J Med.* 2001 Dec 3;111 Suppl 8A:41S-44S. Review.

[44] Sweet MP, Patti MG, Hoopes C, Hays SR, Golden JA. Gastro-oesophageal reflux and aspiration in patients with advanced lung disease. *Thorax.* 2009 Feb;64(2):167-73.

[45] Allaix ME, Fisichella PM, Noth I, Mendez BM, Patti MG. The pulmonary side of reflux disease: from heartburn to lung fibrosis. *J Gastrointest Surg.* 2013 Aug;17(8):1526-35.

[46] Johannson KA, Strâmbu I, Ravaglia C, Grutters JC, Valenzuela C, Mogulkoc N, et al. Erice ILD Working Group. Antacid therapy in idiopathic pulmonary fibrosis: more questions than answers? *Lancet Respir Med.* 2017 Jul;5(7):591-598.

[47] Lee JS, Collard HR, Anstrom KJ, Martinez FJ, Noth I, Roberts RS, et al. IPFnet Investigators. Anti-acid treatment and disease progression in idiopathic pulmonary fibrosis: an analysis of data from three randomized controlled trials. *Lancet Respir Med.* 2013 Jul;1(5):369-76.

[48] Lee JS, Ryu JH, Elicker BM, Lydell CP, Jones KD, Wolters PJ, et al. Gastroesophageal reflux therapy is associated with longer survival in patients with idiopathic pulmonary fibrosis. *Am J Respir Crit Care Med.* 2011 Dec 15;184(12):1390-4.

[49] Ghebre YT, Raghu G. Idiopathic Pulmonary Fibrosis: Novel Concepts of Proton Pump Inhibitors as Antifibrotic Drugs. *Am J Respir Crit Care Med.* 2016 Jun 15;193(12):1345-52.

[50] Kreuter M, Wuyts W, Renzoni E, Koschel D, Maher TM, Kolb M, et al. Antacid therapy and disease outcomes in idiopathic pulmonary fibrosis: a pooled analysis. *Lancet Respir Med.* 2016 May;4(5):381-9.

[51] Raghu G, Pellegrini CA, Yow E, Flaherty KR, Meyer K, Noth I, et al. Laparoscopic anti-reflux surgery for the treatment of idiopathic pulmonary fibrosis (WRAP-IPF): a multicentre, randomised, controlled phase 2 trial. *Lancet Respir Med.* 2018 Sep;6(9):707-714.

In: Respiratory Ventilatory Strategies …
Editor: Antonio M. Esquinas ISBN: 978-1-53617-847-0
© 2020 Nova Science Publishers, Inc.

Chapter 10

IDIOPATHIC PULMONARY FIBROSIS COMPLICATIONS

Ken M. Stern**, *MD and Huawei Dong, MD
Division of Pulmonary and Critical Care
University of California, Irvine, Orange, CA, US

ABSTRACT

Idiopathic pulmonary fibrosis (IPF) is usually characterized by a progressive disease course, during which multiple complications may arise that cause significant morbidity and mortality. The most severe complication is idiopathic acute exacerbation of IPF (AEx) which accounts for nearly 40% of mortality in IPF. AEx is characterized by acute worsening of dyspnea with associated radiographic findings and lacks effective treatment. Patients with IPF are also at significantly increased risk of lung cancer, likely due to multiple shared pathogenetic pathways between fibrosis and tumor formation and proliferation. Additional common complications include pneumothorax, pneumomediastinum, bacterial and viral respiratory infections, and thromboembolic disease such as acute coronary syndrome and deep vein thrombosis. In IPF patients presenting with a decline in respiratory status, it is important to consider these entities as they carry important implications for both medical management and clinical outcomes.

Keywords: acute exacerbation of idiopathic pulmonary fibrosis, lung cancer, pneumothorax, pneumomediastinum, infection, thromboembolism

* Corresponding Author's E-mail: kenmstern@gmail.com.

INTRODUCTION

Idiopathic pulmonary fibrosis (IPF) is a progressive and chronic disease with a variable and unpredictable clinical course. It is the most common cause of fibrotic lung disease with an increased prevalence in elderly patients. As such, this population is at risk for various complications. The management of these complications is often equally as important as treating IPF itself. This chapter will focus on the major complications of IPF, such as acute exacerbations of IPF, lung cancer, infections, pneumothorax, and thromboembolic disease. Pulmonary hypertension is another important complication, which is reviewed in chapter 6.

ACUTE EXACERBATIONS OF IDIOPATHIC PULMONARY FIBROSIS

Majority of patients with IPF have a steady decline in pulmonary function and clinical severity over time. However, a minority of patients experience acute episodes of respiratory decline of unidentifiable etiology, termed acute exacerbations of IPF (AEx). These exacerbations not only lead to significant morbidity but also account for as much as 40% of deaths in IPF patients [1].

While the general concept of IPF exacerbation as an acute clinical worsening has been known and utilized for many years, the official definition for AEx of IPF was proposed in 2007 by the National Institutes of Health-Sponsored IPF Clinical Trials Network [2]. The diagnosis of AEx requires all of the following: 1) previous or concurrent diagnosis of IPF, 2) acute worsening or development of dyspnea within 30 days, 3) high-resolution computed tomography (CT) imaging with new bilateral ground-glass opacity and/or consolidation superimposed on a background consistent with usual interstitial pneumonia pattern, 4) no evidence of pulmonary infection by endotracheal aspirate or bronchoalveolar lavage, and 5) exclusion of alternative causes such as cardiac failure or pulmonary embolism. Hence while clinical deteriorations can be often triggered by infection, left heart failure, or pulmonary embolism, an acute exacerbation of IPF is considered idiopathic.

The exact epidemiology of AEx has been difficult to establish due to large differences in previously used diagnostic criteria, variability in study population disease severity and sample size, and overall study design. The proposed incidence of AEx range from 4.0 per 100 patient-years to 20.0 per 100 patient years based on either the strict adherence to the 2007 definition or a more lenient inclusion of both definite and suspected AEx [3]. The difficulty with determining epidemiology was highlighted in a large prospective clinical trial, where only half of acute exacerbations reported by site investigators were eventually classified as definite or suspected AEx by a review committee.

The etiology of AEx remains unclear. Hypotheses have included a natural acceleration of the patient's underlying IPF, a distinct biologic process in response to an environmental insult that remains undiagnosed and leads to acute lung injury (ALI), or the result of direct lung injury that accelerates the ongoing fibroproliferative process [2]. Both ALI, also known as acute respiratory distress syndrome (ARDS), and AEx share multiple clinical characteristics including increased oxygen requirements, bilateral ground glass opacities or consolidations on imaging. In vivo surgical biopsies and autopsies of IPF patients with AEx have demonstrated diffuse alveolar damage on histopathology, which is indistinguishable from those changes seen in ALI. Such comparisons have raised the question of a common pathophysiology between these two conditions.

The usual causes of ALI include drugs, aspiration, infection, trauma, and massive transfusion. Multiple studies have suggested these similar causes can be seen in AEx as well. It has been shown that AEx occurs more frequently in the winter and spring seasons, and that occult respiratory infections can be demonstrated on post-mortem analyses. A post hoc analysis of clinical trials revealed that AEx only occurred in subjects not on anti-acid therapy, supporting the hypothesis that aspiration of gastric contents may trigger an AEx [4]. Procedures such as surgical lung biopsy and bronchoalveolar lavage have also been seen to trigger AEx. Rather than being a mainly idiopathic condition as the current 2007 definitions suggest, perhaps a much larger proportion of AEx results from one of these similar triggers that was either not clinically apparent or not able to be identified.

The pathobiology of AEx is remains a continued area of active research. Current evidence suggests an interplay of chronic epithelial cell dysfunction and fibroblast activation and acute lung injury, as responsible for its pathogenesis. Several risk factors have been identified in the development of AEx. Though AEx can be seen at any time in the disease course, most consistent risk factor identified is low forced vital capacity (FVC). Other major risk factors include low diffusing capacity for carbon monoxide (DLCO), low 6-minute-walk distance, poor baseline oxygenation, pulmonary hypertension, higher Modified Medical Research Council scale, and a decline of FVC by at least 10% at 6 months. Age and smoking status, on the other hand, have not consistently been shown to be a risk factor for development of AEx.

Clinically, patients present with an acute to subacute worsening of dyspnea, usually within 30 days. Additional signs can include cough, fever, and flulike symptoms. Majority of patients will have an increased requirement for oxygen supplementation, and many may require further respiratory support such as non-invasive and invasive mechanical ventilation. Rarely, an AEx can be the first presentation of IPF for a patient. On radiographic imaging, diffuse ground glass opacities can be seen on plain chest films, while high-resolution CT of the chest will demonstrate new bilateral ground-glass opacity and/or consolidation superimposed on a background of Usual interstitial pneumonia (UIP) pattern, consisting of bibasilar subpleural reticular changes, traction bronchiectasis and honeycombing.

The diagnosis of AEx remains a clinical one using the 2007 definition and practitioner evaluation. Laboratory tests specific to the diagnosis of AEx have yet to be developed. Several serum biomarkers to assist with prognostication have been proposed, such as Krebs von Lungen-6 (KL-6), thrombomodulin, and creactive protein, though these have yet to be made part of routine clinical practice. Almost universally, significant gas exchange abnormalities are seen with low PaO2/FIO2 ratio. A central component in the evaluation of AEx is the evaluation for reversible conditions including: pulmonary embolism, heart failure, fluid overload, infection, pneumothorax, and pleural effusion. Bronchoscopy may not be feasible during AEx, but when obtained, an increase in bronchoalveolar lavage neutrophils has been reported. However, this finding is not specific for AEx and the main utility of bronchoscopy remains in the assessment of possible infectious triggers. Transbronchial biopsies during AEx are of limited benefit given the small amount of tissue sampled. Surgical lung biopsies to demonstrate histopathological diffuse alveolar damage are infrequently performed due to the high morbidity in this setting.

Outside of managing potentially reversible triggers, the treatment of AEx remains supportive. Though no randomize controlled trials for use of invasive and noninvasive positive-pressure ventilation have been performed, oxygen supplementation is generally titrated to an oxygen saturation (SpO2) above 88% is advised and a trial of noninvasive positive-pressure ventilation to achieve this is reasonable [5]. Unfortunately, patients with IPF and respiratory failure, including AEx, who undergo mechanical ventilation have an extremely high hospital mortality, often greater than 80%. Therefore, given the high morbidity and mortality, it is crucial for practitioners to carefully discuss the risk and benefits of any invasive intervention with the patient and family. In clinical settings where lung transplant is feasible, discussions with the lung transplant team can be initiated on a case to case basis. Palliative, psychological and spiritual support, as well as end of life support when appropriate, should be offered to all patients and families.

No medical treatments have been definitively proven to improve outcomes in AEx. Current American Thoracic Society (ATS)/European Respiratory Society (ERS) guidelines make a weak recommendation for high-dose corticosteroids [6], yet no specific dose, route, or duration has been established. Broad spectrum respiratory antibiotics are also generally initiated. Many experts consider the combination of corticosteroids and antibiotics as low risk but potentially beneficial in the setting of a highly lethal condition. While anti-fibrotic therapies have been demonstrated to reduce the rate of functional decline in IPF, they have not been shown to affect the incidence or outcomes of AEx. If the patient is already receiving anti-fibrotic therapy, this can be continued, but it is not advised to initiate anti-fibrotic therapy during an AEx. Studies have looked at other therapies such as polymyxin-B-immobilized fiber column, azithromycin, rituximab, plasma exchange, intravenous immunoglobulin, tacrolimus, and recombinant human thrombomodulin, but all were limited by small cohorts and by study design and not currently recommended for use.

The prognosis of respiratory failure from AEx is poor. The median survival after an AEx is only 3 to 4 months, while in-hospital mortality is upward of 50% and even worse if mechanical ventilation is required. A recently proposed staging system groups AEx patients into limited versus extensive disease-stage groups based on four composite parameters: serum lactate dehydrogenase, KL-6, ratio of partial pressure of oxygen and fraction of inspiratory oxygen, and total extent of abnormal findings on high-resolution computed tomography of the chest. The extensive stage group not only more frequently required mechanical ventilation but also had a significantly worse 3-month mortality of 80.6% versus 54.5% in the limited stage group [7]. Given this grim prognosis, discussions regarding end of life care should preferably be held with the patient, family, and provider prior to hospitalizations for AEx and perhaps even at the time of diagnosis.

Lung Cancer

Growing evidence suggest that the progressive fibrosis in IPF is not only a risk factor but also a potential pathogenic cause for the development of lung cancer. Compared to the general population, IPF confers a roughly fivefold increase in risk for lung cancer. In addition, IPF and lung cancer share multiple common pathogenetic mechanisms including alterations in genetics, epigenetics and signal transduction pathways.

Epidemiologic studies suggest that patients with IPF exhibit a greater risk for lung cancer development. The prevalence of lung cancer in IPF has been reported to be from 2.7% to 48%. Cumulative incidence has also varied, with some studies showing 3.3%, 15.4%, and 54.7% after 1,5, and 10 years of follow-up of IPF, while others showing a cumulative incidence of 41% and 82% at 1 and 3 years, respectively [8]. Age and smoking status may confound these data, as IPF and lung cancer share common environmental risk factors.

Though adenocarcinoma is the most common histotype of lung cancer in the general population, most studies have shown squamous cell carcinoma as most common in patients with IPF. Tumors tend to be localized to the periphery of the lung, with some reports supporting a lower lobe predilection. Given the overlap of the epidemiology, risk factors and co-location of fibrosis and lung cancer in these patients, the concept of "scarcinoma" has been developed [9]. "Sarcinoma" describes this distinct subtype of lung cancer where 1) squamous metaplasia atypically develops in the lung periphery, 2) close proximity to areas of fibrosis, and 3) tumors deriving from hyperproliferative regions of the bronchiolar epithelium within honeycomb cysts.

Recent studies have implicated several genetic variations with increased risk of IPF development, such as Muc5b and genes involved in both surfactant production and telomere maintenance [10]. Mutations in telomere maintenance genes such as TERC (telomerase RNA component) and TERT (telomerase reverse transcriptase) results in genomic instability and cellular senescence, and is commonly found in familial pulmonary fibrosis. In contrast, patients with longer than usual telomeres are at increased risk for lung cancer, irrespective of other risk factors. Abnormalities in surfactant protein genes such as SFTPA1 and SFTPA2 leads to altered protein secretions in the alveoli, endoplasmic reticular stress and apoptosis, and have also been reported in bronchoalveolar cell carcinoma and adenocarcinoma [9].

While most genetic changes in IPF tend to be germline mutations, lung cancer usually develops through a different mechanism of mutation accumulation within tumor suppressor genes or oncogenes in the tissue over time. However, these typical tumor suppressor genes and oncogenes such as p53, EGFR (epidermal growth factor receptor), and KRAS, as well as micro-satellite instability, and loss of heterozygosity have been identified in IPF.

Altered signal transduction pathways are crucial in the pathogenesis of both diseases. The Wnt/β-catenin signaling pathway increases nuclear accumulation of β-catenin at different sites of lung tissues and is involved in cancer progression and IPF. The phosphoinositide 3-kinase (PI3K)/protein kinase B (AKT) oncogenic signaling pathway has been shown to activate several pro-fibrotic mediators and involved in cancer invasion. Additionally, tyrosine kinase signaling, a key regulatory pathway in cell growth, differentiation, adhesion, cell death, and angiogenesis, is involved in both the development and progression of fibrosis and cancer. Nintedanib, one of the only two currently approved anti-fibrotic therapies, is a tyrosine-kinase inhibitor and an anti-neoplastic agent. Lastly, immune checkpoint inhibition of programmed cell death 1 (PD-1)/programmed death ligand-1 (PD-L1) has been established as first-line treatment in advanced non-small cell lung cancer (NSCLC). As PD-1/PD-L1 is also overexpressed in IPF compared to non-IPF lung tissue samples in recent studies, this pathway may serve as a therapeutic target in the future [11].

There are additional commonalities between IPF and lung cancer in various biological areas. In epigenetics, genome-wide methylation analysis have shown similar methylation profiles in both IPF and lung cancer samples [12]. Elevated expression of certain noncoding microRNAs have also identified in both IPF patients, as found to be associated with poorer survival and increased recurrence in NSCLC patients. In epithelial mesenchymal crosstalk, abnormal myofibrolasts in IPF have many cancer-like properties such as increased cellular proliferation, resistance to apoptosis and glycolytic reprogramming. This may contribute to the initiation and progression of cancer in IPF.

The data regarding the optimal therapy for patients diagnosed with both IPF and lung cancer remains limited. The majority of existing studies show the coexistence of both conditions can lead to shorter survival than patients with lung cancer alone, even in those with stage I disease amenable to resection [8]. This may be due to a variety of factors including a higher risk of a new primary lung cancer after resection and higher postoperative morbidity in patients with IPF. The utilization of usual treatment modalities for lung cancer also proves challenging in IPF patients as both surgical resection and radiation therapy can lead to acute exacerbations, and multiple chemotherapeutic agents are known to cause drug-induced pneumonitis, both of which can be harmful in patients with existing respiratory compromise. While surgical resection for early stage lung cancer should be considered in a carefully selected subgroup of IPF patients, there is no consensus on the recommended approach to cancer therapy in patients with advanced or inoperable lung cancer.

Spontaneous Pneumothorax and Pneumomediastinum

Secondary spontaneous pneumothorax (SSP) is a rare but well-known complication in IPF. While the pathogenesis is unclear, it has been hypothesized to be due to increased intrapulmonary pressure during cough, leading to a rupture of alveoli within the honeycombed subpleural areas [13]. Subsequent air tracking along the vascular sheath leads to accumulation in the mediastinum and pneumomediastinum. Due to chronic inflammation, the lung may partially adhere to the chest wall, resulting in unusual configuration and/or loculations of the pleural air collections. Drainage with tube thoracostomy is indicated if the air collection exceeds 25% of the volume of one hemithorax, if there is severe chest pain or dyspnea, or a persistent air leak. However, management of SSP in IPF is challenging as high negative pressures are required to re-expand the rigid and fibrotic lung. The resultant response to drainage may be suboptimal and there is a high rate of recurrence and intractable cases.

Risk factors for development of SSP in IPF include lower body mass index and extensive reticular abnormalities. Most importantly, the development of SSP has prognostic implications. A retrospective review found a median survival of 40.3 months in IPF patients with SSP compared to 53.0 months in those who did not develop SSP [14]. In this study, the cumulative incidence of SSP has been reported to exceed 17% over three years. In addition, 70.6% of the patients who developed SSP experienced recurrences and 41.2% had intractable pneumothorax requiring chest drainage to the time of death. The observed worsened survival associated with the development of SSP in IPF is not surprising, as this complication not only dramatically worsens the pulmonary function in patients with already compromised respiratory reserve, but also exposes them to invasive intra-thoracic procedures.

INFECTIONS

IPF is associated with an increased incidence of pneumonia and infectious complication is the second leading cause of AEx and the cause of death in 2-4% of patients. Infections, both bacterial and viral, have been implicated in the pathogenesis, progression and acute exacerbation in IPF. Epidemiologic and microbiologic studies suggest a potential correlation between IPF and viruses such as hepatitis C, cytomegalovirus, Epstein-Barr virus, human herpes virus and herpes simplex virus [15]. Influenza virus is also a known trigger of acute lung injury and AEx. Bacteria remains the most common causative organisms in AEx, and frequently identified species include *Haemophilus influenzae*, *Pseudomonas aeruginosa*, *Staphylococcus aureus*, and *Klebsiella pneumoniae* [16]. There is also an increased incidence of both tuberculosis and non-tuberculous mycobacteria in IPF patients, however opportunistic infections have rarely been identified [17]. Advancements in microbiome have also demonstrated that IPF patients have a higher respiratory bacterial burden and this was associated with a reduced progression-free survival. However, it remains unclear if the causation is alterations in microbial diversity or the prevalence of a particular species. Given the high incidence of infections in AEx, all IPF patients with an acute respiratory decline should undergo microbiologic investigation through either sputum or bronchoalveolar lavage sampling.

CARDIOVASCULAR AND THROMBOEMBOLIC DISEASE

Large epidemiologic studies have shown an increased risk of both acute coronary syndrome and deep-vein thrombosis in the IPF population [18]. In addition, pulmonary embolism causes 3-7% of deaths in IPF. There are multiple hypotheses regarding this relationship. Chronic hypoxia may be a trigger for acute coronary syndrome, while deconditioning and poor mobility in may cause thromboembolic disease. More likely, there are shared etiological factors such as smoking and environmental exposures. There is also evidence that lung fibrosis activates clotting cascade. This potential pathogenesis led to the ACE-IPF trial which examined the effectiveness of warfarin as a treatment for IPF [19]. This study was terminated early due to higher mortality seen in the warfarin group. While anticoagulation should not be prescribed for IPF patients without a thromboembolic indication, pulmonary embolism causes 3-7% of deaths in IPF and remains an important trigger for AEx that should be investigated.

Summary

Patients with IPF are at risk for multiple complications including acute exacerbations, lung cancer, pneumothorax, infection, and thromboembolic disease. In a patient with IPF presenting with a decline in respiratory status, it is important to consider these entities as each complication carries significant implications for morbidity and mortality.

Key Points

- Various complications are common in IPF and are associated with significant morbidity and mortality.
- Acute exacerbations are a common cause of death in IPF with no known effective medical therapy. A thorough evaluation for reversible causes such as infection, pulmonary embolism and pulmonary edema should be undertaken.
- Patients with IPF have an increased risk for lung cancer, of which squamous cell carcinoma is the most common histotype. They carry a worse prognosis compared to non-IPF patients and usual treatment modalities can pose further risks in this population.
- Patients with IPF also have an increased risk pneumothorax, pulmonary infections, and thromboembolic disease.

References

[1] Ley, B, Collard, HR and King, TE. 2011. "Clinical Course and Prediction of Survival in Idiopathic Pulmonary Fibrosis." *American Journal of Respiratory and Critical Care Medicine* 183(4):431–440. doi: 10.1164/rccm.201006-0894CI.

[2] Collard, HR et al., 2007. "Acute exacerbations of idiopathic pulmonary fibrosis." *American Journal of Respiratory and Critical Care Medicine* 176(7):636–43. doi: 10.1164/rccm.200703-463PP.

[3] Collard, HR et al., 2016. "Acute exacerbation of idiopathic pulmonary fibrosis an international working group report." *American Journal of Respiratory and Critical Care Medicine* 194(3):265–275. doi: 10.1164/rccm.201604-0801CI.

[4] Lee, JS, Collard, HR, Anstrom, KJ, Martinez, FJ, Noth, I, Roberts, RS, Yow, E and Raghu, G. 2013. "Anti-acid treatment and disease progression in idiopathic pulmonary fibrosis: An analysis of data from three randomised controlled trials." *The Lancet Respiratory Medicine* 1(5):369–376. doi: 10.1016/S2213-2600(13) 70105-X.

[5] Maher, TM, Whyte, MKB, Hoyles, RK, Parfrey, H, Ochiai, Y, Mathieson, N, Turnbull, A, Williamson, N and Bennett, BM. 2015. "Development of a Consensus Statement for the Definition, Diagnosis, and Treatment of Acute Exacerbations of Idiopathic Pulmonary Fibrosis Using the Delphi Technique." *Advances in therapy* 32(10):929–43. doi: 10.1007/s12325-015-0249-6.

[6] Raghu, G et al., 2011. "An official ATS/ERS/JRS/ALAT statement: idiopathic pulmonary fibrosis: evidence-based guidelines for diagnosis and management." *American journal of respiratory and critical care medicine* 183(6):788–824. doi: 10.1164/rccm.2009-040GL.

[7] Kishaba, T, Tamaki, H, Shimaoka, Y, Fukuyama, H and Yamashiro, S. 2014. "Staging of Acute Exacerbation in Patients with Idiopathic Pulmonary Fibrosis." *Lung* 192(1):141–149. doi: 10.1007/s00408-013-9530-0.

[8] Karampitsakos, T, Tzilas, V, Tringidou, R, Steiropoulos, P, Aidinis, V, Papiris, SA, Bouros, D and Tzouvelekis, A. 2017. "Lung cancer in patients with idiopathic pulmonary fibrosis." *Pulmonary Pharmacology and Therapeutics* 451–10. doi: 10.1016/j.pupt.2017.03.016.

[9] Tzouvelekis, A, Gomatou, G, Bouros, E, Trigidou, R, Tzilas, V and Bouros, D. 2019. "Common Pathogenetic Mechanisms Between IPF and Lung Cancer." *Chest* doi: 10.1016/j.chest.2019.04.114.

[10] Wolters, PJ. 2017. "A recurring theme in pulmonary fibrosis genetics." *European Respiratory Journal* 49(5):1700545. doi: 10.1183/13993003.00545-2017.

[11] Montgomery, CG et al., 2018. "PD-1 up-regulation on CD4 + T cells promotes pulmonary fibrosis through STAT3-mediated IL-17A and TGF-β1 production." *Science Translational Medicine* 10(460):eaar8356. doi: 10.1126/scitranslmed.aar8356.

[12] Rabinovich, EI, Kapetanaki, MG, Steinfeld, I, Gibson, KF, Pandit, K V., Yu, G, Yakhini, Z and Kaminski, N. 2012. "Global methylation patterns in idiopathic pulmonary fibrosis." *PloS one* 7(4):e33770. doi: 10.1371/journal.pone.0033770.

[13] Porcel, JM. 2018. "Secondary spontaneous pneumothorax in idiopathic pulmonary fibrosis: Grim news." *Respirology (Carlton, Vic.)* 23(5):448–449. doi: 10.1111/resp.13253.

[14] Nishimoto, K, Fujisawa, T, Yoshimura, K, Enomoto, Y, Enomoto, N, Nakamura, Y, Inui, N, Sumikawa, H, Johkoh, T, Colby, T V. and Suda, T. 2018. "The prognostic significance of pneumothorax in patients with idiopathic pulmonary fibrosis." *Respirology* 23(5):519–525. doi: 10.1111/resp.13219.

[15] Jenkins, G. 2017. "IPF: Moving from Idiopathic to Infectious Pulmonary Fibrosis?" *American Journal of Respiratory and Critical Care Medicine* 196(2):125–127. doi: 10.1164/rccm.201702-0387ED.

[16] Yamazaki, R, Nishiyama, O, Sano, H, Iwanaga, T, Higashimoto, Y, Kume, H and Tohda, Y. 2016. "Clinical Features and Outcomes of IPF Patients Hospitalized for Pulmonary Infection: A Japanese Cohort Study." *PLOS ONE* 11(12):e0168164.

[17] Park, S-W, Song, JW, Shim, TS, Park, M-S, Lee, H-L, Uh, S-T, Park, C-S and Kim, DS. 2012. "Mycobacterial pulmonary infections in patients with idiopathic pulmonary fibrosis." *Journal of Korean medical science* 27(8):896–900. doi: 10.3346/jkms.2012.27.8.896.

[18] Hubbard, RB, Smith, C, Le Jeune, I, Gribbin, J and Fogarty, AW. 2008. "The association between idiopathic pulmonary fibrosis and vascular disease: A population-based study." *American Journal of Respiratory and Critical Care Medicine* 178(12):1257–1261. doi: 10.1164/rccm.200805-725OC.

[19] Noth, I, Anstrom, KJ, Calvert, SB, De Andrade, J, Flaherty, KR, Glazer, C, Kaner, RJ and Olman, MA. 2012. "A placebo-controlled randomized trial of warfarin in idiopathic pulmonary fibrosis." *American Journal of Respiratory and Critical Care Medicine* 186(1):88–95. doi: 10.1164/rccm.201202-0314OC.

In: Respiratory Ventilatory Strategies …
Editor: Antonio M. Esquinas

ISBN: 978-1-53617-847-0
© 2020 Nova Science Publishers, Inc.

Chapter 11

FUNCTIONAL CAPACITY ASSESSMENT IN IDIOPATIC PULMONARY FIBROSIS

Angelo Petroianni*[1,*]*, MD, PhD,
Arianna Sanna*[2,†]*, MD
and Gregorino Paone*[3,‡]*, MD
[1]Department of Cardiovascular and Respiratory Diseases,
Respiratory Diseases Unit, Umberto I Policlinic, Rome, Italy
[2]Respiratory Diseases Unit, Sapienza University of Rome, Rome, Italy
[3]Department of Internal Medicine and Infectious Diseases,
Respiratory Diseases Unit, Sapienza University of Rome,
Rome, Italy

ABSTRACT

Lung function tests in patients with Idiopathic Pulmonary Fibrosis (IPF) show a characteristic restrictive pattern with a decrease of Diffusing Capacity for Carbon Monoxide (DLCO) and moderate hypoxemia and hypocapnia at rest, which, in the more advanced stages, develops into persistent respiratory failure. International recommendations on IPF remark the importance of lung function testing in the control of this disease. Clinical trials testing new drugs for the treatment of IPF have adopted Forced Vital Capacity (FVC) and DLCO as primary variables for confirming clinical efficacy. FVC was a standard spirometric measure of pulmonary function in IPF for many decades. Change over time in serial measures of FVC is a widely accepted reflection of disease progression and several studies have identified change in predicted FVC as an independent predictor of mortality in patients with IPF. A reduction in static

* Corresponding Author's E-mail: angelo.petroianni@uniroma1.it.
† Corresponding Author's E-mail: ariannasanna1990@gmail.com.
‡ Corresponding Author's E-mail: gregorino.paone@uniroma1.it.

(Total Lung Capacity) and dynamic lung volumes is typical in patients with IPF as in other Interstitial Lung Diseases. In patients with IPF, the DLCO and the value of gas exchange per unit of lung volume (KCO) are both reduced, because of the coexisting alterations on alveolar membrane and on capillary vessels. In addition, the 6-minute walking test and the distance assessed during exercise represent mortality predictors.

Keywords: spirometry, FVC, DL_{CO}, 6MWT, CPET

ABBREVIATIONS

6MWT	6-minute walking test
CPET	Cardio-Pulmonary Exercise Testing
CPI	Composite Physiologic Index
DL_{CO}	Diffusing Capacity for Carbon Monoxide
DL_{NO}	Diffusing Capacity for Nitric Oxide
FEV1	Forced Expiratory Volume in 1 second
FRC	Functional Residual Capacity
FVC	Forced Vital Capacity
GAP	Gender-Age-Physiology
HRCT	High-resolution computed tomography
ILD	Interstitial Lung Disease
IPF	Idiopathic Pulmonary Fibrosis
PFTs	Pulmonary Function Tests
PH	Pulmonary Hypertension
RR	Respiratory Rate
RV	Residual Volume
TLC	Total Lung Capacity
VC	Vital Capacity
VD/VT	Dead space to tidal volume ratio
V′E	Minute ventilation

INTRODUCTION

Idiopathic Pulmonary Fibrosis (IPF) is a progressive pulmonary disease characterized by a gradual worsening of symptoms and physical functional capacity that mainly affects older adults, especially those in their sixth and seventh decades. Even though novel antifibrotic agents may attenuate the progressive decline in lung function and the risk of death, IPF remains in any way a severe disease, and the clinical decline is a common event [1, 2]. Variations in symptoms, from exertional dyspnea in early stage to respiratory failure in late phase, are directly related to worsening of respiratory function that occur throughout the progression of the disease [3].

With this as background, as for all other Interstitial Lung Disease (ILD) conditions, Pulmonary Function Tests (PFTs) represent a fundamental element in the initial evaluation of the disease, estimating the grade of functional impairment. They also demonstrated a central role in predicting disease severity and mortality at baseline and in evaluating disease progression and treatment response during follow-ups [4]. There is a wide range of PFT variables that can be measured in daily routine, such as spirometric volumes, plethysmographic volumes, values of gas transfer and gas exchange, the 6-minute walking test (6MWT) and maximal exercise variables.

Lung compliance describes the ability of the lung to expand and is defined as the change in lung volumes divided by the change in transpulmonary pressure. Reduction in lung compliance occurs early in IPF, and may be closely correlated with the degree of lung fibrosis. Lung compliance is the major determinant of the load of the respiratory muscles and consequently of the work of breathing [5]. These mechanical changes relate to clinical features such as dyspnoea. The symptom burden is heavy in IPF patients and shortness of breath and cough are the most common symptoms [6].

Spirometry

Spirometry is the most common PFT and assesses lung function, in terms of volume and/or flow of air that can be inhaled and exhaled. Main advantages that make spirometry particularly important in the follow-up of IPF are represented by its simplicity and good reproducibility. This technique allows monitoring the disease course that induces alterations in lung distension and in gas exchange. In advanced cases of IPFs, alterations can be easily demonstrated at spirometry and High-resolution computed tomography (HRCT). On the other hand, the management of patients with early disease, without significant alterations on chest x-ray and with mild symptoms, is more complicated; in these situations, PTFs represent the indicator that may guide the physician towards further assessments, such as HRCT, and management decision [6]. Plethysmography is the gold standard for measuring pulmonary volumes. Plethysmographic technique is based on Boyle's law applied to the volume of gas present in the lungs: $PV = k$ (P = gas pressure V = volume occupied by the gas). Based on this law, at a constant temperature, the volume of gas in a container varies inversely with changes of pressure and the product of pressure and volume in the system is constant. From the Functional Residual Capacity (FRC) it is easy to obtain Total Lung Capacity (TLC) and Residual Volume (RV) with a simple maneuvre. Also by the plethysmography it is possible to measure airway resistances (Raw) and derived parameters such as specific resistances (sRaw), conductance (Gaw) and specific conductance (sGaw). Carrying on, the diffusing capacity of the lungs for carbon monoxide (DL_{CO}), originally described by Krogh in 1915, estimates the transfer of oxygen from alveolar gas to red cells. The process of carbon monoxide uptake can be simplified into two transfer properties: the membrane conductivity (D_M), which reflects the diffusion properties of the alveolar capillary membrane, and the binding of carbon monoxide with Hb, represented as the product of the carbon monoxide–Hb chemical reaction rate (θ) and the volume of alveolar capillary blood (V_C). In 1957 Roughton and Forster partitioned the total transfer resistance into two approximately equal parts, with half the resistance being in a membrane component ($1/D_{M,CO}$ = alveolar–capillary membrane resistance for CO), and half in pulmonary capillary blood ($1/\theta_{CO}\cdot V_C$ = pulmonary capillary blood resistance for CO), proposing the equation: $1/DL_{CO} = 1/D_{M,CO} + 1/\theta_{CO}\cdot V_C$ [7].

Severity Assessment

Restrictive pattern represents the typical alteration in patients with IPF, because of a wide range of causes, such as loss of volume, reduced alveolar surface and elasticity and increased surface tension. This alteration is characterized by a decrease of static lung volumes such as total lung capacity (TLC), vital capacity (VC), functional residual capacity (FRC), and increased FEV_1/FVC ratio; the residual volume (RV) may be usually normal instead [3, 4]. FVC is a reproducible and reliable indicator of the clinical status and of future IPF progression. It robustly predicts mortality and has been used as the primary endpoint of numerous clinical trials in IPF. DL_{CO} test is based on a single breath that a patient realizes after the inhalation of a gas mix comprising an insoluble gas such as methane (CH_4) combined with carbon monoxide (CO). This test allows the calculation of alveolar volume (VA) and the transfer constant of carbon monoxide (K_{CO}), basing on the reduction of CH_4 and CO in exhaled breath. An average normal value is 20-30 mL/min/mmHg. Specifically, DL_{CO} represents the capacity of the whole lung to make gas exchange, while K_{CO} represents the value of gas exchange per unit of lung volume. These two values are usually both reduced in patients with IPF because of the coexisting alterations on the alveolar membrane and on capillary vessels, and this aspect is also related to the entity of parenchymal damage found at CT imaging [3]. DL_{CO} reduction reflects the pulmonary damage more accurately than K_{CO} variations: normal K_{CO} values cannot exclude an alveolar damage, since the damage on certain areas of pulmonary parenchyma may induce an increased ventilation on other healthy areas, preserving normal K_{CO} values [3]. DL_{NO} measures the ratio of the diffusing capacities of the lung for nitric oxide (NO). DL_{NO}, known as the transfer factor, mostly reflects the D_M or membrane component. In IPF the measure of DL_{NO} can be helpful with the simultaneous measure of DL_{CO} and the DL_{NO}/DL_{CO} ratio [8]. As DL_{NO} is weighted by D_M and DL_{CO} is weighted by V_C, the DL_{NO}/DL_{CO} ratio reflects a relative change in the membrane-to-capillary components of uptake. A low DL_{NO}/DL_{CO} ratio (≤95%) characterizes interstitial lung disease with fibrosis [9].

Gas exchange impairment is a further typical feature of IPF: this is a result of ventilation/perfusion mismatch and diffusion limitation. Previous studies have proposed DL_{CO} as a staging parameter, using a threshold of 39% of predicted to sort out between limited and extensive IPF; 39% was also the threshold below which transplantation should be considered [6]. According to another study, for DL_{CO} level less than 35% of predicted lung biopsy has limited prognostic value. When compared with histologic samples, spirometric functional parameters (DL_{CO} in particular) have shown significant relationship with the severity of morphologic alterations, while no significant relationship was demonstrated with the grade of inflammation [6]. DL_{CO} has also shown the strongest relationship with the extension of disease on HRCT, compared to other spirometric variables at rest, and for that reason it represents the most essential item in order to assess the severity of IPF. In a possible scenario the coexistence of IPF and obstructive disorders, such as pulmonary emphysema, may lead to mixed spirometric pattern: combined restrictive-obstructive alterations.

Disease Progression and Prognostic Value

Even in consideration of the simple execution, a diffuse application of PFTs to all population as a screening method for early IPF is not feasible, because of the low prevalence of the disease [6]. In absence of clinical signs of disease progression, spirometric follow-up is recommended every 3 – 6 months. FVC and/or DL_{CO} variations represent the main parameters most commonly used in clinical practice to monitor the severity and the progression of the disease and the response to treatment. According to several studies, FVC reduction, more than serial DL_{CO} data, better describes an increased disease severity with higher mortality rates; this aspect may be due to the greater inner variability in DL_{CO} assessments [3, 4]. Nevertheless, other studies suggested that baseline DL_{CO} assessment is a superior prognostic factor compared to baseline FVC, especially in patients with specific risk factors that are responsible for a worse prognosis, such as coexisting emphysema or pulmonary hypertension [10, 11]. Concomitant changes of both measurements above the respective thresholds indicate progression of the disease, even if symptoms are stable. On the other hand, in case of worsening of clinical symptoms, non-significant changes of both parameters between two subsequent controls should not be considered as clinically insignificant.

Values indicating significant changes in FVC performance are still uncertain; in particular, it is difficult to determine if longitudinal changes during subsequent follow-ups is due to test variability or represents a true change in lung function. According to recent studies, a decline in absolute-value FVC greater than or equal to 10% at 6 months is associated with a considerable increase of mortality rates during the next year (about five times greater) [10]. Another study proposed the use of relative rather than absolute decrease in 10% of the FVC in order to maximize the chance of detecting disease progression with similar prognostic accuracy [12].

Moreover, marginal changes (between 5 and 10%) are difficult to interpret: while these values were previously just considered as a condition of disease stability, recent evidence demonstrated that they can be associated with higher mortality rates (greater than 2 times during the next year) [13].

Diffusion capacity for carbon monoxide (DL_{CO}) is typically reduced. IPF and other IDLs are characterized by a reduction of both DL_{CO} and DL_{CO}/VA ratio (K_{CO}), due to damage on pulmonary architecture. Because of the greater inner variability, it has been established a DL_{CO} threshold of 15% from baseline values for significant change. A decrease greater than 15% DL_{CO} is a reliable threshold for mortality prediction [10]. In addition, a disproportionate reduction of DL_{CO} such as $\%FVC/\%DL_{CO} > 1.6$ is usually associated with secondary Pulmonary Hypertension (PH) [4]. However, if the vital capacity is below 1500ml the DL_{CO} value can be unreliable with the single breath method (Table 1).

Table 1. Severity of the decrease in Total Lung Capacity (TLC), Diffusing Capacity for Carbon monoxide (DLCO) and Parameters associated with mortality in IPF

Degree of severity	
TLC % pred	
Mild	70 - 80%
Moderate	60 - 70%
Moderately severe	50 - 60%
Severe	< 50%
DL_{CO} % pred	
Mild	> 60% and <LLN
Moderate	40 - 60%
Severe	< 40%
Prognostic Parameters	
FVC reduction > 10% of absolute value (follow-up)	
DL_{CO} reduction > 15% of absolute value (follow-up)	
DL_{CO} <40% pred	
Desaturation < 88% during 6MWT	
Peak V'O2 < 8,3 mL/Kg/min on CPET	
% pred = % predicted; LLN = lower limits of normal.	

Exacerbations

Acute exacerbations of IPF often constitute the primary cause of death in patients with IPF. Acute exacerbations (AE) have been defined as an acute clinically significant deterioration. Diagnostic criteria was published in 2007 and revised in 2016 with the intent to improve the management of IPF [6]. Criteria included a previous or concurrent diagnosis of IPF, unexplained worsening of dyspnoea within the past 30 days, high-resolution computed tomography evidence of new bilateral ground-glass opacities or consolidation, and exclusion of alternative causes, including pulmonary infection by endotracheal aspirate or bronchoalveolar lavage.

Severe IPF is associated with higher risk of acute exacerbations and spirometry, highlighting the delay in the loss of FVC, allows the evaluation of the response to antifibrotic therapy that might lead to a delay in the interval of time between exacerbations. In case of coexistence of emphysema and IPF (in which lung volumes are preserved), disease progression would not be highlighted by serial FVC measurements, except for advanced IPF. For that reason in these patients, serial FEV_1 or DL_{CO} assessments show a more accurate relationship with prognosis [10].

Arterial Blood Gas

Hypoxemia, under exercise in early stage and at rest in later phases, is a typical condition in patients with IPF and is caused by alterations of pulmonary mechanical properties, pulmonary vascular system and altered gas exchange. The effect is an impaired gas diffusion and ventilation/perfusion ratio (V′ /Q′), and an increase in dead space ventilation and in the alveolar–arterial oxygen tension difference (PA–aO2) [3].

In early cases, arterial blood gas values are usually within limits, while arterial hypoxemia is a common finding in advanced disease. Moreover, prior studies demonstrated that arterial hypoxemia represents a strong prognostic predictor in patients with advanced IPF but showed less reliable results in patients with mild or moderate disease. Hypocapnia or normocapnia is a normal evidence in mild and moderate IPF. Hypercapnia is rarely seen in patients with IPF, with the exception of end-stage disease, when this value is an indicator of respiratory muscle failure [3].

Six-Minute Walking Test

Dyspnoea is the most common and disabling symptom in patients with IPF. It becomes even more evident during physical activity and negatively impacts the exercise capacity. Exercise test is an important tool for evaluating the degree of exertional dyspnoea, providing additional information to data collected by PFTs.

The six-minute walking test (6MWT) is a simple test that is widely used to assess functional exercise capacity in patients with IPF. This exam is highly reproducible and denotes the level of exercise in routine daily activities, since it is based on self-paced submaximal effort. Parameters such as six-minute walk distance (6MWD) and desaturation, assessed during exercise, represent mortality predictors as a result of ventilatory and circulatory impairments. However, other factors that are independent from the disease may influence these values, such as age, BMI or other comorbidities [14]. It is important to consider that 6MWT has some limitations when used as a marker of functional status: it provides no indication about the cause of limitation and does not provide information about the overall day-to-day functional status of the patient.

In any case, oxygen desaturation <88% during the 6MWT or a >50-meter decline of walking distance over 6 months both proved to be predictors of mortality in patients with IPF [15]. This test can be also used to identify an underlying condition of pulmonary hypertension (PH), leading to decision to perform echocardiography for PAPS measurement, or to evaluate patient candidacy to lung transplantation. In particular, the 6MWD has a primary role as independent predictor of mortality among patients listed for lung transplantation: patients with IPF who cannot walk more than 207 m in 6 min have a high mortality rate without lung transplantation. Moreover, 6MWD is a better predictor of death at 6months than FVC% predicted [16].

Cardio-Pulmonary Exercise Testing (CPET)

The Cardio-Pulmonary Exercise Testing (CPET) is considered the gold standard for the evaluation of exercise intolerance: this approach considers cardiac, respiratory and musculoskeletal systems, giving a complete assessment of response to exercise. CPET allows us to determine the cause of dyspnea reported by patients affected by IPF, thanks to a wide range of different parameters that can be measured, like V′O2, V′CO2, VT and V′E, as well as other values such as arterial blood pressure and oxygen saturation. However, as for 6MWT, it is still not clear how reduced exercise tolerance reflects day-to-day functional status or how it guides the development of therapeutic management [17].

Even if CPET is a well-known technique, it has only been recently introduced in clinical practice for the evaluation of patients with IPF. CPET can be performed according to two different modalities. First, incremental exercise testing (at least 10 - 12 minutes long) mainly indicates performance levels at maximal exercises; this approach requires a gradual increase of load throughout the exam, until the optimal level is reached, with the exceptions of the onset of complications (angina, ECG alterations, uncontrolled hypertension, <80% desaturation, dizziness or confusion). Second, constant exercise testing is more commonly used to assess disease progression and to evaluate treatment response; after a 1 – 3 minute warm-up, the patient undergoes an abrupt increase of load up to a 75 – 80% of his maximal work rate, until the onset of symptoms.

Typical CPET findings in IPF patients include very high respiratory rate (RR) (often >55 breaths/min), increased minute ventilation (V′E) with scarce or absent breathing reserve, increased dead space to tidal volume (VD/VT) ratio, oxygen desaturation and elevated lung CO_2 concentration. In IPF patients under mild and moderate exercise, the VD/VT usually remains stable or increases instead of decreasing, reducing the ability of the lungs to eliminate CO_2. For that reason the ventilatory response to increasing carbon dioxide output ($V'CO_2$) during exercise is abnormally increased in IPF subjects during exercise [17].

Interstitial fibrosis, caused by thickening of alveolar capillary membrane and destruction of capillary vessels, determines the alteration of gas diffusion: as already seen at rest, ventilation/perfusion (V/Q) alteration determines hypoxemia and an increase of $PA\text{-}aO_2$.

Hypoxemia may also depend on reduced cardiac output and increased oxygen extraction by working skeletal muscles. At the same time, the increase of RR and V′E maintain eucapnia: in fact, hypercapnia is not typical in patients with IPF. Despite this abnormal ventilatory pattern, respiratory mechanics don't seem to be the unique contributors to exercise limitation in ILD patients. Two studies performed in ILD patients with different diagnoses reported that a number of participants had a largely preserved ventilatory reserve at the end of exercise, despite reduced exercise performance. Furthermore, the administration of oxygen during CPET or 6MWT improved both performance and oxygen uptake (V′E), suggesting the occurrence of other factors in limiting maximal exercise performance [18].

Composite Physiologic Indices

IPF is a fibrotic lung disease of unknown origin that is chronic, progressive, and eventually fatal. As for other ILD conditions, IPF currently represents a challenging disease as for diagnosis and clinical management. IPF has still a high mortality with a median survival time of 2.5 – 3.5 years, despite the recent introduction of new drugs such as pirfenidone and nintedanib [1, 2]. Nevertheless, the trend of the disease is different among patients: some subjects have extremely changing trend, with frequent exacerbations that rapidly lead to death; others remain stable over time [1, 6]. It is important to predict the clinical evolution of the disease in order to plan therapy and follow-up for each patient. For that reason, in recent years, the need for a multidisciplinary team, including the figures of radiologist, pathologist, and pulmonologist, has emerged and Composite physiologic index (CPI) and gender-age-physiology (GAP) models have been used to predict IPF progression [19].

Composite Physiologic Indexes (CPIs) were recently introduced because of the complexity of the IPF. Through the integration of different variables, these scores guide the clinician in the management and in predicting the severity of the disease. In 2003, Wells et al. demonstrated that CPI is a stronger prognostic marker for mortality than individual PFT variables considered separately ($p < 0.0005$) [20].

Different parameters can be introduced for CPI, such as:

- Patient-related characteristics (age, gender, smoking habit, dyspnea, finger clubbing, 6MWD, hospitalization, pulmonary hypertension);
- PFTs;
- Imaging findings at HRCT;
- Molecular biomarkers (C-Reactive Protein (CRP) and metalloproteinase-7);
- Pathologic finding.

Thanks to the integration of all these different variables that the clinician would consider separately, CPIs have the advantage of "smoothing" the error of each single variable, providing a more accurate assessment of the disease severity. Some of these indexes are characterized by a relatively great simplicity, containing only spirometric volumes and DL_{CO} values. The following formula is an example of composite index that could be routinely performed:

$$CPI = 92.1 - (0.68 * \%predicted\ DL_{CO}) - (0.53 * \%predicted\ FVC) + (0.35 * \%predicted\ FEV_1)$$

In a recent cohort study, GAP stage and CPI showed significant capabilities to predict mortality. In particular, CPI was more accurate than GAP stage in predicting mortality at 1, 2, and 3 years [19].

During last 10 years, several successes have been achieved in the field of IPF, although it still remains a disease with many unsolved questions. The purpose for the next years would be to improve the therapeutic approach and to facilitate patient management with the purpose of increase survival and quality of life.

KEY MESSAGES

The lung compliance reduction occurs early in IPF and is correlated with the degree of lung fibrosis. It results the major determinant of the load of the respiratory muscles and of the work of breathing. Restrictive pattern is the typical functional alteration in IPF patients because of the loss of volumes, the reduction of alveolar surface and elasticity, and the increase of surface tension.

FVC is a reproducible and reliable indicator of the clinical status and future progression and IPF mortality. The decline greater than10% over 6 months predicts 1year mortality, with a minimal clinically important difference (MCID) of FVC absolute change of 2 – 6%. DLCO is another essential physiological parameter for IPF, and a reduction greater than 15% is a useful threshold to predict mortality. In addition, an excessive reduction of DLco such as %FVC/%DLco > 1.6 can be associated with secondary PH.

Measures of exertional dyspnoea and exercise intolerance, through 6MWT and CPET, represent an important tool for evaluating patients with IPF, providing additional information to data collected by spirometry. In addition, 6MWD is an independent predictor of mortality among IPF patients listed for transplantation, better than FVC % predicted.

Multi-dimension index such as composite physiologic index (CPI) and gender-age-physiology (GAP) models are useful predictors of IPF progression and mortality. CPI was more accurate than GAP stage in predicting accurate prognoses for IPF patients.

REFERENCES

[1] Rogliani, P., Calzetta, L., Cavalli, F. et al. Pirfenidone, nintedanib and N-acetylcysteine for the treatment of idiopathic pulmonary fibrosis: a systematic review and meta-analysis. *Pulm. Pharmacol. Ther.,* 2016; 40: 95 - 103.

[2] Fisher, M., Nathan, S. D., Hill, C. et al. Predicting life expectancy for pirfenidone in idiopathic pulmonary fibrosis. *J. Manag. Care Spec. Pharm.,* 2017; 23: Suppl. 3b, S17 - S24.

[3] Plantier, L., Cazes, A., Dinh-Xuan, A. T. et al. Physiology of the lung in idiopathic pulmonary fibrosis. *Eur. Respir. Rev.,* 2018 Jan. 24; 27(147). pii: 170062.

[4] Kishaba, T. Evaluation and management of Idiopathic Pulmonary Fibrosis. *Respir. Investig.*, 2019 Jul.; 57(4):300 - 311.

[5] Nava, S., Rubini, F. Lung and chest wall mechanics in ventilated patients with end stage idiopathic pulmonary fibrosis. *Thorax,* 1999; 54:390 - 395.

[6] Raghu, G., Rochwerg, B., Zhang, Y. et al. An official ATS/ERS/JRS/ALAT clinical practice guideline: treatment of idiopathic pulmonary fibrosis. An update of the 2011 clinical practice guideline. *Am. J. Respir. Crit. Care Med.,* 2015; 192(2): e3 - 19.

[7] Roughton, F. J. W., Forster, R. E. Relative importance of diffusion and chemical reaction in determining rate of exchange of gases in the human lung. *J. Appl. Physiol.,* 1957; 11:290 - 302.

[8] Zavorsky, G. S., Hsia, C. C., Hughes, J. M. et al. Standardisation and application of the single breath determination of nitric oxide uptake in the lung. *Eur. Respir. J.,* 2017 Feb. 8; 49(2). pii: 1600962.

[9] Hughes, J. M., van der Lee I. The TL,NO/TL,CO ratio in pulmonary function test interpretation. *Eur. Respir. J.,* 2013; 41: 453 - 461.

[10] Robbie, H., Daccord, C., Chua, F., Devaraj, A. Evaluating disease severity in idiopathic pulmonary fibrosis. *Eur. Respir. Rev.,* 2017 Sep. 6; 26(145). pii: 170051.

[11] Taylor Gonzalez, A., Maher, T. Predicting mortality in idiopathic pulmonary fibrosis. Which parameters should be used to determine eligibility for treatment? Analysis of a UK prospective cohort. *Eur. Respir. J.,* 2016; 48: suppl. 60, OA282.

[12] Richeldi, L., Ryerson, C. J., Lee, J. S. et al. Relative versus absolute change in forced vital capacity in idiopathic pulmonary fibrosis. *Thorax,* 2012; 67: 407 - 411.

[13] Du Bois, R. M., Weycker, D., Albera, C. et al. Forced vital capacity in patients with idiopathic pulmonary fibrosis: test properties and minimal clinically important difference. *Am. J. Respir. Crit. Care Med.,* 2011 Dec. 15; 184(12):1382 - 9.

[14] Lancaster, L. H. Utility of the six-minute walk test in patients with idiopathic pulmonary fibrosis. *Multidiscip. Respir. Med.,* 2018 Dec. 13;13:45.

[15] Lederer, D. J., Arcasoy, S. M., Wilt, J. S. et al. Six-minute walk distance predicts waiting list survival in idiopathic pulmonary fibrosis. *Am. J. Respir. Crit. Care Med.,* 2006 Sep. 15; 174(6):659 - 64.

[16] Du Bois, R. M., Albera, C., Bradford, W. Z. et al. 6-Minute walk distance is an independent predictor of mortality in patients with idiopathic pulmonary fibrosis. *Eur. Respir. J.,* 2014 May; 43(5):1421 - 9.

[17] Bonini, M., Fiorenzano, G. Exercional dispnoea in interstitial lung diseases: the clinical utility of cardiopulmonary exercise testing. *Eur. Respir. Rev.,* 2017 Feb. 21; 26(143).

[18] Triantafillidou, C., Manali, E., Lyberopoulos, P. et al. The Role of Cardiopulmonary Exercise Test in IPF Prognosis. *Pulm. Med.,* 2013; 2013:514817.

[19] Lee, S. H., Park, J. S., Kim, S. Y. et al. Comparison of CPI and GAP models in patients with idiopathic pulmonary fibrosis: a nationwide cohort study. *Sci. Rep.,* 2018 Mar. 19; 8(1):4784.

[20] Wells, A. U. et al. Idiopathic pulmonary fbrosis - A composite physiologic index derived from disease extent observed by computed tomography. *Am. J. Resp. Crit. Care,* 2003; 167, 962 - 969.

In: Respiratory Ventilatory Strategies …
Editor: Antonio M. Esquinas
ISBN: 978-1-53617-847-0
© 2020 Nova Science Publishers, Inc.

Chapter 12

ACUTE RESPIRATORY FAILURE IN CHRONIC INTERSTITIAL LUNG DISEASE

Samantha Baah, MD, David J. Nagel, MD, PhD, Aleksandr Kalininskiy, MD and R. Matthew Kottmann*, MD
University of Rochester Medical Center, Department of Pulmonary and Critical Care Medicine, Rochester, NY, US

ABSTRACT

Interstitial lung diseases are a heterogeneous group of chronic lung diseases. Several hundred disorders are known to cause interstitial lung disease. Overall approximately one third of ILDs have known etiologies but the majority are idiopathic. Epidemiologic data, derived primarily from patient registries, suggest that the prevalence of ILD in the U.S.s ranges from 67 per 100,000 in women to 81 per 100,000 in men. However, there are significant variations in prevalence among different geographic populations, likely reflecting a combination of genetic and environmental differences. Certain risk factors, including exposure to cigarette smoke or environmental toxicants (asbestos, silica, coal dust, and air pollution), genetic mutations, and single nucleotide polymorphisms, have all been associated with developing interstitial lung disease. While the cause of the interstitial lung disease may vary, common characteristics include impaired alveolar gas exchange and symptoms of breathlessness and a non-productive cough. Patients with ILD are prone to the development of acute respiratory failure, which is an acute exacerbation of the underlying lung disease. The combination of pre-existing lung impairment combined with a superimposed acute injury can often be fatal. In this chapter, we review the definition of an acute exacerbation, discuss the underlying pathophysiology, and highlight salient features related to the diagnosis and treatment of acute interstitial lung disease exacerbations.

* Corresponding Author's E-mail: Matt_Kottmann@URMC.Rochester.edu.

INTRODUCTION

Interstitial lung diseases (ILD) are a group of over 200 disorders that often arise in association with identifiable causes such as connective tissues diseases, environmental exposures or medications. However, those without an identifiable etiology are categorized as idiopathic interstitial lung diseases, the most notable of which is idiopathic pulmonary fibrosis (IPF)). Regardless of the etiology, ILDs are characterized by abnormal pulmonary parenchymal scarring and/or inflammation which leads to impairment of alveolar gas exchange, dyspnea, cough, and exercise intolerance (Faverio et al. 2018). In certain ILDs, the parenchymal abnormalities are progressive and eventually contribute to respiratory failure.

In general, there are three ways in which respiratory decline can occur in patients with ILD: (1) slow progression (months to years), (2) rapid progression (weeks to months), and (3) acute exacerbations (days to weeks). In these contexts, respiratory failure presents as a continuum of functional limitations to fulminant acute life-threatening respiratory failure necessitating assisted ventilation. While respiratory failure in the general population is associated with significant morbidity and mortality, it is particularly devastating in patients with underlying interstitial lung disease. This is largely secondary to the existing burden of chronic ventilatory impairment and limited respiratory reserve.

One of the main causes of respiratory failure and mortality in patients with any ILD is an acute exacerbation of the underlying interstitial disease. The etiologies of acute exacerbations of ILD are poorly understood and are therefore difficult to predict. In addition, most of the limited clinical data regarding acute exacerbations is derived from observational studies in patients with IPF. An international working group recently revised the definition of an acute IPF exacerbation and recommended distinguishing triggered exacerbations (infection, micro-aspiration, thromboembolic disease, acute heart failure, and post-pulmonary procedure) from idiopathic exacerbations where no precipitating event is readily identifiable (Collard et al. 2016). In addition to the aforementioned triggers, exacerbations may also occur after exposure to environmental antigens that can precipitate an acute or subacute hypersensitivity pneumonitis. Causative antigens may be difficulty to identify, and chronic exposure to environmental agents can also drive the progression of pulmonary fibrosis which can be difficult to differentiate from IPF. In addition to the various extrinsic exacerbating factors, patients with connective tissue associated interstitial lung disease (CT-ILD) can experience exacerbations due to a flare of the underlying rheumatologic disorder. Acute exacerbations are known to occur in patients with Sjogren's syndrome, Rheumatoid Arthritis and Systemic Lupus Erythematosus.

The aim of this chapter is to provide up to date definitions, diagnostic workup, and management recommendations that reflect current expert opinion guidelines. We will discuss what is known about the pathophysiology of acute ILD exacerbations, highlight salient clinical and radiographic features of both acute exacerbations of IPF (AE-IPF) and other ILDs (AE-ILD), review general principles of diagnosing and managing AE-ILDs, and explore exciting future directions in the field.

PATHOPHYSIOLOGY

The classic histologic pattern associated with IPF is usual interstitial pneumonia (UIP). Hallmark findings include spatial and temporal heterogeneity of active fibrosis, the presence of fibroblastic foci, peripheral and basilar predominant fibrosis within secondary lobules, honeycomb changes, and destruction of alveolar architecture (Hashisako and Fukuoka 2016). In contrast to UIP, the pathology of NSIP is comprised of both fibrosis and varying degrees of inflammation. The fibrotic changes in NSIP are more homogenous and diffusely spread throughout pulmonary lobules. The lung architecture is also largely maintained (Hashisako and Fukuoka 2016). Organizing pneumonia (OP) consists of fibroblast proliferation within airspaces and is characterized by fibrosis and varying degrees of inflammation. There is often accompanying edema and infiltration of inflammatory cells. Lung involvement is typically patchy with normal adjacent lung parenchyma (Hashisako and Fukuoka 2016). Hypersensitivity pneumonitis involves bronchocentric inflammation with giant cells and poorly formed non-necrotizing granulomas. Chronic hypersensitivity pneumonitis (CHP) occurs with prolonged exposure to environmental antigens and is characterized by airway-centered interstitial fibrosis. In some circumstances, CHP may be difficult to distinguish from UIP (Morisset et al. 2018). Non-specific interstitial pneumonia (NSIP), organizing pneumonia (OP), and chronic hypersensitivity pneumonitis (CHP) are all forms of ILD that may progress to respiratory failure.

Other types of lung pathologies that may result in acute respiratory failure include eosinophilic pneumonia (EP), acute lung injury (ALI), and acute interstitial pneumonia (AIP). Eosinophilic pneumonia is characterized by invasion of eosinophils into the interstitium and alveolar space with or without associated diffuse alveolar damage (DAD), the absence of granulomas or hemorrhage, and preservation of the alveolar architecture (Sohn 2013). Diffuse alveolar damage is a relatively generalizable finding with several forms of acute lung injury. It is characterized by interstitial edema and hyaline membrane formation. Hyaline membranes are thought to form as the result of epithelial and injury/hyperplasia of type II pneumocytes. As DAD evolves, the pulmonary interstitium may be thickened by myxoid fibroblastic tissue which can further impair gas exchange and create a ventilation-perfusion mismatch (Kaarteenaho and

Kinnula 2011). Diffuse alveolar damage is found on lung biopsy on many types of acute lung injury and AIP, often being the only pathology evident. ALI and AIP are often related to infection, aspiration, sepsis, blood transfusions and/or inhalation of smoke or toxic gases. DAD may also be seen in patients with AE-IPF and AE-ILD. In these instances, DAD is superimposed on the existing interstitial pathology. DAD is more commonly seen in AE-IPF, but similar pathologic findings are found in AEs of CT-ILD, fibrosing NSIP, and CHP (Kaarteenaho and Kinnula 2011).

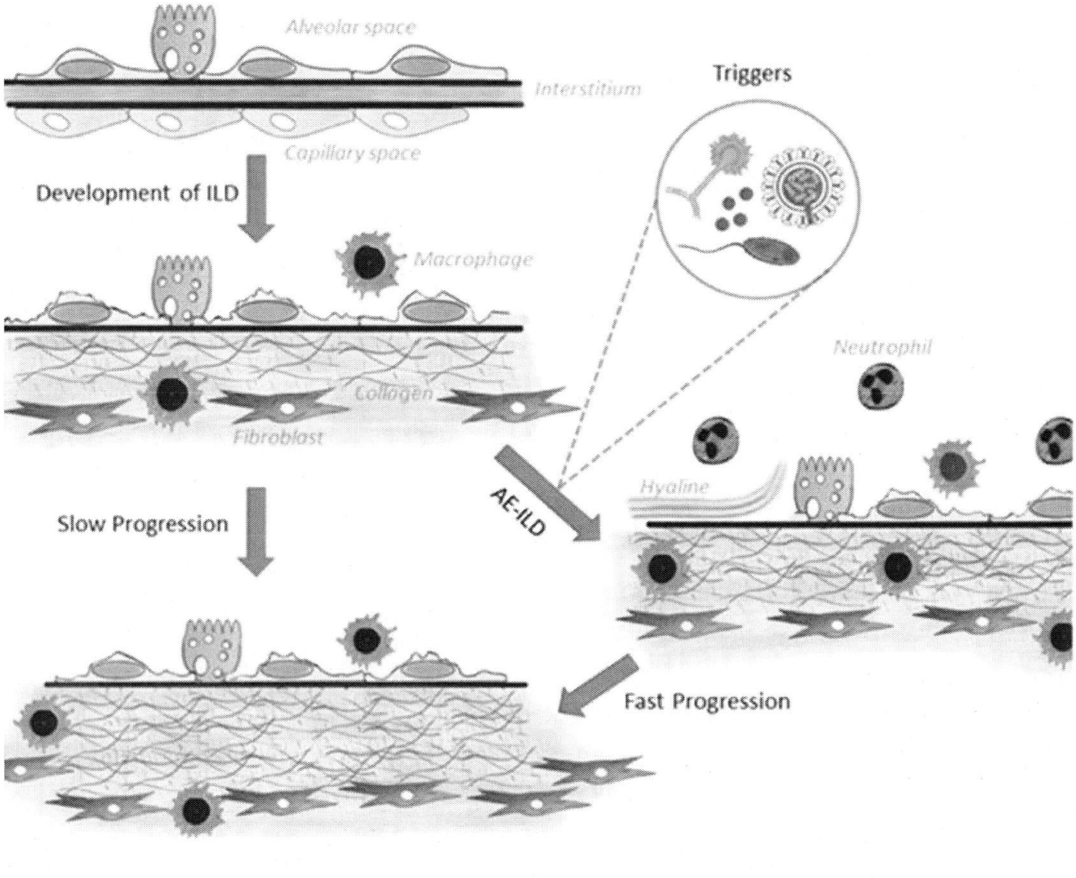

Figure 1. Pictorial representation of an acute ILD exacerbation. Development of ILD often involves a change to a fibrotic phenotype marked by increased extracellular matrix deposition, lung remodeling, and scar formation. Exacerbations speed up this process, cause hyaline membrane formation, inflammatory cell migration, and interstitial edema. Figure adapted from: Collard, H.R., et al. (2016). "Acute Exacerbation of Idiopathic Pulmonary Fibrosis. An international Working Group Report." *American Journal of Respiratory and Critical Care Medicine* 194(3): 265-275.

ACUTE EXACERBATION OF IPF

Idiopathic pulmonary fibrosis is characterized by progressive, irreversible fibrotic parenchymal changes, which cause a decline in forced vital capacity and diffusion of lung for carbon monoxide (DLCO) over time. It is the most common form of idiopathic ILD accounting for about 25% of all idiopathic interstitial pneumonias. The median survival from the time of diagnosis is approximately 3 years with a mortality rate of 6.43 deaths per 100,000 in men and 5.84 deaths 100,000 in women (Olson et al. 2007), though there is some pooled evidence that suggest the anti-fibrotic medications may prolong survival (King, T. E., Jr., et al. (2014); Lancanster, L, et al. (2019)).

The most recent working group guideline defines an AE-IPF as: "an acute, clinically significant respiratory deterioration characterized by evidence of new widespread alveolar abnormality" (Collard et al. 2016). The recommended diagnostic criteria include: (1) previous or concurrent diagnosis of IPF, (2) acute worsening, or the development of, dyspnea (typically of less than one month duration from symptom onset), (3) new bilateral ground glass opacity and/or consolidation superimposed on a background pattern consistent with UIP, and (4) respiratory deterioration that cannot be fully explained by cardiac failure or fluid overload (Collard et al. 2016). Identifiable causes of respiratory failure such as pulmonary embolism, infection (viral, bacterial, or fungal), congestive heart failure, microaspiration, cancer or pneumothorax must be excluded (Leuschner and Behr 2017). Acute exacerbations of IPF are responsible for over half of IPF-related respiratory hospitalizations (Song et al. 2011). They are the second leading cause of mortality in IPF patients (Ley, Collard, and King 2011), and account for up to 40% of IPF-related mortality (Natsuizaka et al. 2014). Once hospitalized, mortality can be as high as 50% in mild exacerbations and may increase up to 90% for patients admitted to the intensive care unit (Faverio et al. 2018). The median survival time after an AE-IPF is only 3 to 4 months (Collard et al. 2016).

AE-IPF tend to occur in the more severe stages of the disease but can manifest at any time during the course of IPF. A reduced forced vital capacity (FVC) is the most well-defined risk factor for AE-IPF. Additional risk factors include a decline in DLCO (>15%), decline in FVC (>10%), low six-minute walk distances (6MWD, < 180 m), greater dyspnea (UCSD SOBQ and SGRQ), and hypoxia ($PaO2 < 62$ on ambient air) (Collard et al. 2013). Other important epidemiological risk factors include male gender, lifelong non-smokers, younger age at time of diagnosis, a history of prior exacerbation, a co-existing diagnosis of at least moderate pulmonary hypertension, coronary artery disease, gastroesophageal reflux disease, and obesity. Interestingly, the incidence of developing acute exacerbations of IPF following lung biopsy can be as high as 23% (Sato et al. 2018) compared to approximately 4% in patients who do not undergo lung biopsy (Collard et al. 2016). The risk of post-operative complications led to the recent ATS/ERS/JRS/ALAT guideline recommendation to avoid surgical lung biopsy in patients with a high-resolution CT pattern defined as typical UIP or probable UIP (Raghu et al. 2018).

Rapidly Progressive IPF

A distinct group of IPF patients develop a more rapid and progressive decline in lung function. This subgroup of patients does not develop DAD as seen in patients with an AE-IPF. Rather they exhibit accelerated production and deposition of extracellular matrix proteins, which functionally leads to respiratory failure. Compared to the majority of patients with IPF, patients exhibiting rapid progression have a significant increase in morbidity and mortality within 6 months of initial onset of symptoms (approximate 65% survival rate at 24 months in rapidly progressive disease versus 99% in slowly progressive disease). This increase in mortality is seen despite similar baseline pulmonary function tests and histologic/radiographic findings at the time of diagnosis when compared to patients diagnosed with slowly progressive IPF (Selman et al. 2007).

The complex interplay of biological mechanisms that underlie the rapid progression of pulmonary fibrosis in this subset of IPF patient population remains unclear. Previous data suggest that this cohort may have distinct genetic polymorphisms compared to patients with slower progression. Transcriptional profiling of patients with rapidly progressive disease has identified a significant over-expression of genes involved in morphogenesis, cancer, oxidative stress, apoptosis, cell migration and proliferation (Selman et al. 2007). One enhanced gene in the rapidly progressing cohort is the adenosine A2B receptor gene. A2B promotes myofibroblast differentiation, thus potentiating the progression of fibrosis. Anti-fibrinolytic genes beta3-endonexin, serine protease inhibitor (kazal type), and plasminogen activator inhibitor-1 are also upregulated in the lung tissue of patients with rapid progression (Leuschner and Behr 2017, Selman et al. 2007). In addition, single nucleotide polymorphisms associated with rapidly progressive disease and increased mortality are found in the Toll-like interacting protein (TOLLIP) rs5743894 (Noth et al. 2013).

Acute Exacerbations of Non-IPF ILD

As with IPF, the most common cause of respiratory failure in non-IPF interstitial lung disease is an exacerbation of the underlying interstitial process (Leuschner and Behr 2017). While an AE-IPF has been formally defined, there is no clear definition of an acute exacerbation in non-IPF ILD. Although there are no formal recommendations regarding evaluation and management of AE-ILDs, exclusion of exacerbating factors similar to those outlined for AE-IPF is recommended. AE-ILDs share strong similarities to AE-IPF and include acute presentation of dyspnea, impaired gas exchange and acute on chronic radiographic findings. Connective tissue disorders are one sub-group of non-IPF ILDs that are associated with acute exacerbations. Similar to AE-IPF, acute respiratory failure in patients with an underlying connective tissue disorder is associated with common bacterial and opportunistic infections, diffuse alveolar hemorrhage, and exacerbation of the primary interstitial process. In addition to acute hypoxic respiratory failure, certain ILDs, such as dermatomyositis, are associated with hypercapnic respiratory failure due to acute on chronic respiratory muscle weakness (Papiris et al. 2016).

While there is much less rigorous epidemiologic data on AE-ILD, the incidence varies depending on the ILD subtype. For example, the overall annual incidence AE-ILD exacerbations is estimated to be approximately 1-4% as compared to up to 19% in patients with IPF. Exacerbations of NSIP (fibrosing) are estimated to have a yearly incidence of 4.2% whereas an AE of CT-ILD ranges from 1.25 to 3.3% (Leuschner and Behr 2017), where the highest exacerbation rates occur in patients with rheumatoid arthritis associated ILD (RA-ILD).

In comparison to IPF, acute exacerbations of non-IPF ILDs generally have a better prognosis and more favorable overall survival. The improved outcomes may be largely associated with the expected improvement in acute lung inflammation after treatment with systemic glucocorticoids. In one study, patients admitted to the hospital for an exacerbation AE-ILD, had a 67% survival rate of one month post discharge, and a survival rate of 40% three months post discharge. The rate of in-hospital CT-ILD mortality is also quite high ranging from 50-100% however the highest overall in-hospital mortality rates are seen in acute exacerbation of hypersensitivity pneumonitis (75-100%) (Kolb et al. 2018). Mortality rates associated with other non-IPF ILDs range from 34 to 83% (Kolb et al. 2018).

Other Lung Diseases Associated with Respiratory Failure

Acute eosinophilic pneumonia (AEP) is a rapidly progressive disease that can be fatal. Patients typically present with the acute onset of fevers, night sweats, dyspnea, cough, and wheezing. Diagnosis can be delayed because symptoms often mimic those of severe bacterial pneumonia. The exact cause of AEP is often unknown, but some presentations are caused by inhalation of smoke, dust, or illicit substances (Sohn 2013). The diagnostic hallmark characteristic is > 25% eosinophil content on bronchoalveolar lavage. Treatment comprises systemic corticosteroids and rapid clinical improvement is often observed. Although AEP most often resolves completely after treatment with systemic steroids, relapses can occur thus leading to chronic eosinophilia pneumonia (CEP). CEP occurs in up to 50% of patients with AEP. CEP is a rare disorder of unknown etiology characterized by persistence of eosinophils in the pulmonary interstitium and alveolar spaces. CEP typically occurs in healthy individuals, although some patients report a history of asthma. The incidence of CEP is higher in women and non-smokers. Radiographically, eosinophilic pneumonia manifests with peripheral alveolar infiltrates ranging from ground glass opacities to areas of consolidation with air bronchograms. These findings can be migratory in nature. The clinical course of CEP is often punctuated by exacerbations which most often occur during or after the taper of systemic corticosteroids (Marchand and Cordier 2006).

Hypersensitivity pneumonitis (HP), also known as allergic alveolitis, is an interstitial process associated with repeated exposure(s) to an environmental antigen. In predisposed individuals, this triggers a hypersensitivity reaction which causes a diffuse infiltration of mononuclear cells into the terminal bronchioles, alveolar wall, alveoli, and interstitium. The inflammation is followed by the formation of granulomas and possible fibrosis (Sharma and Fujimura 1995). To date, over 300 different exposures are associated with the development of HP. Some well-known exposures include organic dusts, enzyme detergents, molds, birds, medications, chemicals, and paint catalysts. The prevalence of HP varies widely, ranging from less than 2% in the United States to up to 15% in Europe and Brazil (Riario Sforza and Marinou 2017). This variability is related to the high likelihood of misdiagnosis, geographical conditions, magnitude of individual exposures, and lack of a widely accepted definition. Although HP can be self-limiting, repeated and prolonged exposure to the offending agent can induce interstitial fibrosis and/or acute exacerbations of the underlying lung disease. The two-year incidence of acute exacerbations of HP is estimated to be 11.5% (Leuschner and Behr 2017). Radiographically, fibrotic HP is characterized by macronodular diffuse parenchymal opacities, typically of upper lobe predominance, reticulation, traction bronchiectasis and volume loss, and may even have evidence of honeycomb changes (Kouranos et al. 2017). As mentioned above, respiratory failure in acute on chronic HP has one of the highest mortality rates among non-IPF interstitial lung diseases.

There are more than 350 medications known to cause drug-induced pulmonary disease (Disayabutr et al. 2015). A diagnosis of a medication induced ILD is supported by the temporal initiation of the medication in relation to the onset of symptoms. Symptoms often improve or resolve following discontinuation of the drug. However, in some cases the medication induces irreparable parenchymal changes. Because drug toxicity may be idiosyncratic, identification of medication-induced pulmonary toxicity can be quite challenging. Ascertainment of a complete medical history is critical and should include evaluation of current and prior medication usage (Faverio et al. 2018). "Pneumotox" (https://www.pneumotox.com/drug/index) is a regularly updated database of medications reported to induce various forms of lung disease. It is readily accessible on the web and may assist in the identification of which medications may be associated with an ILD diagnosis or acute exacerbation.

Diagnostic Approach

Despite the poor prognosis of acute respiratory failure in interstitial lung disease, a personalized diagnostic algorithm may expedite the etiology of an exacerbation and improve a given patient's overall outcome (Faverio et al. 2018). The diagnostic work up for acute respiratory failure in patients with chronic ILD entails a tailored approach to exclude etiologies such as pulmonary emboli, pneumothorax, infection, and heart failure. A detailed medication review should regularly be performed. CT pulmonary angiography is a useful imaging modality as it allows the exclusion of pulmonary embolism and direct evaluation of parenchymal abnormalities. Other potential diagnostic tools include an echocardiogram to evaluate cardiac function and bronchoalveolar lavage (BAL) to assess for infection or inflammation. Although routine BAL is not required in most diagnostic work up algorithms, it can be helpful in excluding rare etiologies of respiratory failure such as diffuse alveolar hemorrhage and pulmonary alveolar proteinosis. BAL analysis may also be helpful in identifying an infectious etiology of the exacerbation (Faverio et al. 2018). Furthermore, cellular profile analysis of alveolar fluid may be helpful. Alveolar fluid cell counts (neutrophils v. lymphocytes) may help differentiate specific ILD subsets and/or predict the relative responsiveness to corticosteroids (Faverio et al. 2018). However, the decision to pursue bronchoscopy must weigh the potential burdens and benefits of the procedure for each patient.

General Management Principles

ILD specific treatments and management of comorbidities may be the best options to prevent acute ILD exacerbations. For example, in patients with IPF, nintedanib delayed the time to first exacerbation (Richeldi et al. 2014) and pirfenidone reduced the risk of respiratory-related hospitalizations (Ley, B., et al. (2017). Because of a strong association between IPF and GERD, the use of anti-acid therapies may hold promise to prevent exacerbations (Lee et al. 2013). Whether anti-acid medications stabilize progressive IPF and/or prevent acute exacerbations remains controversial.

Unfortunately, randomized controlled trial data does not exist for the management of AE-ILD. However, international guidelines recommend supportive care, oxygen supplementation, and palliation of symptoms (Raghu et al. 2011). These guidelines also provide a weak recommendation for the use of systemic corticosteroids. In patients with scleroderma-related ILD, corticosteroids should be used judiciously because they may precipitate a scleroderma renal crisis (Kolb et al. 2018). If an underlying exposure or medication is suspected, then it is imperative that the exposure be removed and/or the medication be discontinued. Given the high mortality associated with AE-ILD and the difficulty in exclusion of infectious etiologies, empiric use of oseltamivir during flu season is reasonable and broad-spectrum antibiotics are often administered empirically.

As mentioned earlier, exacerbations may cause respiratory failure that under normal circumstances would require invasive mechanical ventilation. However guidelines make a weak recommendation against its use due to high in-hospital mortality rates (Collard et al. 2016, Kolb et al. 2018). Patients do benefit from supplemental oxygen and there are small studies that suggest a benefit from high-flow nasal cannula (Kolb et al. 2018). In addition, non-invasive mechanical ventilation may reduce increased work of breathing. Finally, extracorporeal membrane oxygenation (ECMO) is an emerging modality in AE-ILD because it has the potential to minimize mechanical ventilation induced lung injury and thereby avoid perpetuating the exacerbation. ECMO also has the potential advantage of serving as a bridge to lung transplant in patients who are suitable for transplantation (Kolb et al. 2018).

PROGNOSTIC FACTORS AND FUTURE DIRECTIONS

Several potential prognostic factors have been associated with poor outcomes in acute exacerbations of IPF. For example, reduced baseline pulmonary function (decreased FVC and DLCO), extensive fibrotic changes on CT imaging, and impaired resting oxygenation have all been associated with a worse outcome and mortality in AE-IPF. Blood-based biomarkers hold tremendous potential to assist with diagnosing, monitoring response, and identifying potential causal mechanisms of various AE-ILD/AE-IPF. Some potential targets include: C-reactive protein lactate dehydrogenase, procalcitonin, KL-6, circulating fibrocytes, serum interleukin-17 levels, anti-heat shock protein 70 autoantibodies and syndecan-4. While these biomarkers hold promise, additional studies are needed to validate their clinical utility (Collard et al. 2016, Ley, Collard, and King 2011). It is hoped that additional research will not only validate these potential biomarkers but will develop additional candidates as we move toward a more precision-oriented practice of medicine.

CONCLUSION

Respiratory failure in patients with chronic interstitial lung disease is a potentially life-threatening condition with high morbidity and mortality rates. Respiratory deterioration related to the ILD can present as either progression of the underlying interstitial process or an acute exacerbation of the underlying ILD. Secondary causes of respiratory failure are numerous and should be evaluated with a detailed clinical history, laboratory data, and imaging studies. Respiratory support in addition to other supportive measures are critical to managing acute exacerbations. Several biomarkers may provide prognostic value in patients with IPF however more studies are needed to further explore this area.

REFERENCES

Collard, H. R., C. J. Ryerson, T. J. Corte, G. Jenkins, Y. Kondoh, D. J. Lederer, J. S. Lee, T. M. Maher, A. U. Wells, K. M. Antoniou, J. Behr, K. K. Brown, V. Cottin, K. R. Flaherty, J. Fukuoka, D. M. Hansell, T. Johkoh, N. Kaminski, D. S. Kim, M. Kolb, D. A. Lynch, J. L. Myers, G. Raghu, L. Richeldi, H. Taniguchi, and F. J. Martinez. 2016. "Acute Exacerbation of Idiopathic Pulmonary Fibrosis. An International Working Group Report." *Am J Respir Crit Care Med* 194 (3):265-75. doi: 10.1164/rccm.201604-0801CI.

Collard, H. R., E. Yow, L. Richeldi, K. J. Anstrom, and C. Glazer. 2013. "Suspected acute exacerbation of idiopathic pulmonary fibrosis as an outcome measure in clinical trials." *Respir Res* 14:73. doi: 10.1186/1465-9921-14-73.

Disayabutr, S., C. S. Calfee, H. R. Collard, and P. J. Wolters. 2015. "Interstitial lung diseases in the hospitalized patient." *BMC Med* 13:245. doi: 10.1186/s12916-015-0487-0.

Faverio, P., F. De Giacomi, L. Sardella, G. Fiorentino, M. Carone, F. Salerno, J. Ora, P. Rogliani, G. Pellegrino, G. F. Sferrazza Papa, F. Bini, B. D. Bodini, G. Messinesi, A. Pesci, and A. Esquinas. 2018. "Management of acute respiratory failure in interstitial lung diseases: overview and clinical insights." *BMC Pulm Med* 18 (1):70. doi: 10.1186/s12890-018-0643-3.

Richeldi et al. 2014. "Efficacy and Safety of Nintedanib in Idiopathic Pulmonary Fibrosis." *New England Journal of Medicine* 370 (22):2071-2082. doi: 10.1056/NEJMoa1402584.

Lancaster, L et al. (2019). "Safety and Survival Data in Patient with Idiopathic Pulmonary Fibrosis Treated with Nintedanib: Pooled Data From Six Clinical Trials." *BMJ Open Respir Res* 25/6(1):e000397. doi: 10.1136/bmjresp-2018-000397

Ley, B., et al. (2017). "Pirfenidone Reduces Respiratory-related Hospitalizations in Idiopathic Pulmonary Fibrosis." *Am J Respir Crit Care Med* 196 (6): 756-761.

Hashisako, Mikiko, and Junya Fukuoka. 2016. "Pathology of Idiopathic Interstitial Pneumonias." *Clinical medicine insights. Circulatory, respiratory and pulmonary medicine* 9 (Suppl 1):123-133. doi: 10.4137/CCRPM.S23320.

Kaarteenaho, R., and V. L. Kinnula. 2011. "Diffuse alveolar damage: a common phenomenon in progressive interstitial lung disorders." *Pulm Med* 2011:531302. doi: 10.1155/2011/531302.

Kolb, M., B. Bondue, A. Pesci, Y. Miyazaki, J. W. Song, N. Y. Bhatt, J. T. Huggins, J. M. Oldham, M. L. Padilla, J. Roman, and S. Shapera. 2018. "Acute exacerbations of progressive-fibrosing interstitial lung diseases." *Eur Respir Rev* 27 (150). doi: 10.1183/16000617.0071-2018.

Kouranos, V., J. Jacob, A. Nicholson, and E. Renzoni. 2017. "Fibrotic Hypersensitivity Pneumonitis: Key Issues in Diagnosis and Management." *J Clin Med* 6 (6). doi: 10.3390/jcm6060062.

Lee, J. S., H. R. Collard, K. J. Anstrom, F. J. Martinez, I. Noth, R. S. Roberts, E. Yow, and G. Raghu. 2013. "Anti-acid treatment and disease progression in idiopathic pulmonary fibrosis: an analysis of data from three randomised controlled trials." *Lancet Respir Med* 1 (5):369-76. doi: 10.1016/s2213-2600(13)70105-x.

Leuschner, G., and J. Behr. 2017. "Acute Exacerbation in Interstitial Lung Disease." *Front Med (Lausanne)* 4:176. doi: 10.3389/fmed.2017.00176.

Ley, B., H. R. Collard, and T. E. King, Jr. 2011. "Clinical course and prediction of survival in idiopathic pulmonary fibrosis." *Am J Respir Crit Care Med* 183 (4):431-40. doi: 10.1164/rccm.201006-0894CI.

Marchand, Eric, and Jean-François Cordier. 2006. "Idiopathic chronic eosinophilic pneumonia." *Orphanet journal of rare diseases* 1:11-11. doi: 10.1186/1750-1172-1-11.

Morisset, J., K. A. Johannson, K. D. Jones, P. J. Wolters, H. R. Collard, S. L. F. Walsh, and B. Ley. 2018. "Identification of Diagnostic Criteria for Chronic Hypersensitivity Pneumonitis: An International Modified Delphi Survey." *Am J Respir Crit Care Med* 197 (8):1036-1044. doi: 10.1164/rccm.201710-1986OC.

Natsuizaka, M., H. Chiba, K. Kuronuma, M. Otsuka, K. Kudo, M. Mori, M. Bando, Y. Sugiyama, and H. Takahashi. 2014. "Epidemiologic survey of Japanese patients with idiopathic pulmonary fibrosis and investigation of ethnic differences." *Am J Respir Crit Care Med* 190 (7):773-9. doi: 10.1164/rccm.201403-0566OC.

Noth, I., Y. Zhang, S. F. Ma, C. Flores, M. Barber, Y. Huang, S. M. Broderick, M. S. Wade, P. Hysi, J. Scuirba, T. J. Richards, B. M. Juan-Guardela, R. Vij, M. K. Han, F. J. Martinez, K. Kossen, S. D. Seiwert, J. D. Christie, D. Nicolae, N. Kaminski, and J. G. N. Garcia. 2013. "Genetic variants associated with idiopathic pulmonary fibrosis susceptibility and mortality: a genome-wide association study." *Lancet Respir Med* 1 (4):309-317. doi: 10.1016/s2213-2600(13)70045-6.

Olson, A. L., J. J. Swigris, D. C. Lezotte, J. M. Norris, C. G. Wilson, and K. K. Brown. 2007. "Mortality from pulmonary fibrosis increased in the United States from 1992 to 2003." *Am J Respir Crit Care Med* 176 (3):277-84. doi: 10.1164/rccm.200701-044OC.

King, T. E., Jr., et al. (2014). "A phase 3 trial of pirfenidone in patients with idiopathic pulmonary fibrosis." *N Engl J Med* 370(22): 2083-2092.

Papiris, S. A., E. D. Manali, L. Kolilekas, K. Kagouridis, M. Maniati, G. Filippatos, and D. Bouros. 2016. "Acute Respiratory Events in Connective Tissue Disorders." *Respiration* 91 (3):181-201. doi: 10.1159/000444535.

Raghu, G., H. R. Collard, J. J. Egan, F. J. Martinez, J. Behr, K. K. Brown, T. V. Colby, J. F. Cordier, K. R. Flaherty, J. A. Lasky, D. A. Lynch, J. H. Ryu, J. J. Swigris, A. U. Wells, J. Ancochea, D. Bouros, C. Carvalho, U. Costabel, M. Ebina, D. M. Hansell, T. Johkoh, D. S. Kim, T. E. King, Jr., Y. Kondoh, J. Myers, N. L. Muller, A. G. Nicholson, L. Richeldi, M. Selman, R. F. Dudden, B. S. Griss, S. L. Protzko, and H. J. Schunemann. 2011. "An official ATS/ERS/JRS/ALAT statement: idiopathic pulmonary fibrosis: evidence-based guidelines for diagnosis and management." *Am J Respir Crit Care Med* 183 (6):788-824. doi: 10.1164/rccm.2009-040GL.

Raghu, G., M. Remy-Jardin, J. L. Myers, L. Richeldi, C. J. Ryerson, D. J. Lederer, J. Behr, V. Cottin, S. K. Danoff, F. Morell, K. R. Flaherty, A. Wells, F. J. Martinez, A. Azuma, T. J. Bice, D. Bouros, K. K. Brown, H. R. Collard, A. Duggal, L. Galvin, Y. Inoue, R. G. Jenkins, T. Johkoh, E. A. Kazerooni, M. Kitaichi, S. L. Knight, G. Mansour, A. G. Nicholson, S. N. J. Pipavath, I. Buendia-Roldan, M. Selman, W. D. Travis, S. Walsh, and K. C. Wilson. 2018. "Diagnosis of Idiopathic Pulmonary Fibrosis. An Official ATS/ERS/JRS/ALAT Clinical Practice Guideline." *Am J Respir Crit Care Med* 198 (5):e44-e68. doi: 10.1164/rccm.201807-1255ST.

Riario Sforza, Gian Galeazzo, and Androula Marinou. 2017. "Hypersensitivity pneumonitis: a complex lung disease." *Clinical and Molecular Allergy* 15 (1):6. doi: 10.1186/s12948-017-0062-7.

Sato, Seijiro, Yuki Shimizu, Tatsuya Goto, Akihiko Kitahara, Terumoto Koike, Hiroyuki Ishikawa, Takehiro Watanabe, and Masanori Tsuchida. 2018. "Survival after repeated surgery for lung cancer with idiopathic pulmonary fibrosis: a retrospective study." *BMC Pulmonary Medicine* 18 (1):134. doi: 10.1186/s12890-018-0703-8.

Selman, M., G. Carrillo, A. Estrada, M. Mejia, C. Becerril, J. Cisneros, M. Gaxiola, R. Perez-Padilla, C. Navarro, T. Richards, J. Dauber, T. E. King, Jr., A. Pardo, and N. Kaminski. 2007. "Accelerated variant of idiopathic pulmonary fibrosis: clinical behavior and gene expression pattern." *PLoS One* 2 (5):e482. doi: 10.1371/journal.pone.0000482.

Sharma, O. P., and N. Fujimura. 1995. "Hypersensitivity pneumonitis: a noninfectious granulomatosis." *Semin Respir Infect* 10 (2):96-106.

Sohn, Jang Won. 2013. "Acute eosinophilic pneumonia." *Tuberculosis and respiratory diseases* 74 (2):51-55. doi: 10.4046/trd.2013.74.2.51.

Song, J. W., S. B. Hong, C. M. Lim, Y. Koh, and D. S. Kim. 2011. "Acute exacerbation of idiopathic pulmonary fibrosis: incidence, risk factors and outcome." *Eur Respir J* 37 (2):356-63. doi: 10.1183/09031936.00159709.

In: Respiratory Ventilatory Strategies …
Editor: Antonio M. Esquinas
ISBN: 978-1-53617-847-0
© 2020 Nova Science Publishers, Inc.

Chapter 13

Chronic Respiratory Failure

Mohammed D. AlAhmari*, PhD and Abdullah A. Ghazwani
Respiratory Care Department, Prince Sultan Military College of Health Sciences, Dammam, Kingdom of Saudi Arabia

Abstract

Idiopathic pulmonary fibrosis (IPF) is a form of interstitial lung disease that may be worsened by chronic respiratory failure (CRF) as the disease progresses into advanced stages. Many pathophysiological mechanisms underlying CRF occur with IPF over time, including reduced lung compliance and volume from airway obstruction and capillary surface destruction, resulting in impaired diffusion capacity and ventilation-perfusion mismatch. These complex physiological changes affect all lung functions and compartments and worsen the underlying disease. Consequently, in the majority of these cases, CRF develops as a secondary cause of IPF progression.

Keywords: idiopathic pulmonary fibrosis, chronic respiratory failure, lung function, prognosis

Introduction

Idiopathic pulmonary fibrosis (IPF) is a complex disease that results in development of diffuse lung parenchymal abnormalities that lead to dyspnea, cough, and impaired gas exchange, ultimately leading to rapid progression of respiratory failure and death [1].

* Corresponding Author's E-mails: m.alahmari@psmchs.edu.sa; alahmari87@hotmail.com.

Respiratory failure is a common complication and can be an acute or chronic process in IPF patients.

The natural history of IPF is heterogeneous, ranging from chronic stable symptoms to acute exacerbation to progressive respiratory failure [2]. Research evidence has revealed a pathogenic process where injury to alveolar epithelial cells provokes a dysregulated wound healing response involving fibroblast proliferation that deposits excess extracellular matrix in the interstitium [3]. The process results in deteriorated gas exchange, leading to respiratory failure and increased mortality [4]. This chapter focuses on chronic respiratory failure in IPF.

Pathophysiology of CRF

CRF can be explained by various physiological IPF mechanisms, including restrictive lung, poor gas exchange (ventilation-perfusion mismatch), impaired diffusion capacity, and lung vascular damage. Intermittent exertional hypoxemia is often the initial clinical sign of CRF, which evolves into continuous hypoxemia as IPF progresses. Current evidence supports a pathogenic model in which alveolar epithelial injury provokes a dysregulated wound healing response with fibroblast proliferation and activation resulting in excess extracellular matrix deposition in the interstitium [3]. This impedes gas exchange, leading to respiratory failure and, ultimately, death.

Definition

Respiratory failure is the "inability to maintain either the normal delivery of O_2 to the tissues or the normal removal of carbon dioxide from the tissues [5]," which often results from an imbalance between respiratory workload and ventilator endurance or strength. Respiratory failure criteria based on arterial blood gases were established by Campbell [6], with failure generally defined as arterial partial pressure of oxygen (PaO_2) less than 60 mm Hg (also referred to as hypoxemic or Type I respiratory failure), or alveolar partial pressure of carbon dioxide ($PaCO_2$) greater than 50 mm Hg (hypercapnic or Type II respiratory failure).

Lung Function with CRF

With IPF disease progression, lung function is restricted, reducing forced vital capacity, total lung capacity, and carbon monoxide diffusion capacity [7]. Therefore, assessing lung function assists clinical evaluation and judgment for disease management. Reduced lung function measures of FVC ≥ 10% or DLCO ≥ 15% for a period of six months is an indicator of IPF disease progression [8]. The current primary indicator of lung dysfunction in clinical trials is the rate of decline in FVC [9-11].

In the initial stage, arterial blood gases show reduced gas exchange reflecting moderate hypoxemia only during exercise. Hypercapnia develops at rest in advanced stages [12, 13], eventually progressing into respiratory failure [14, 15]. Advancing lung function impairment over time is associated with the IPF survival rate.

Lung function parameters may reflect fibrotic process; therefore, lung function assessment helps to estimate the degree of functional impairment and the IPF prognosis. Lung function assessment is also helpful to a certain degree for monitoring and evaluating IPF patients' therapeutic plan.

Aetiologies: Chronic Respiratory Failure

CRF is secondary to progression of the underlying IPF that often complicates the clinical course of the disease. Other comorbidities and associated progressive conditions and complications may worsen IPF. Therefore, it is crucial to identify the primary cause of CRF to allow optimal clinical outcomes and proper management selection. The rate of progression in comorbidities and associated complications is a critical factor in assessing CRF in IPF patients.

Causes of CRF in IPF

Clinical outcomes of patients with IPF depend on disease progression over-time. Deterioration associated with CRF varies across patients according to disease stage and/or associated comorbidities. CRF that occurs at a higher rate in earlier IPF stages requires close monitoring and follow-up to identify disease behavior and reduce the mortality rate [16, 17]. Common CRF comorbidities are described in Table 1 [7].

Conclusion

CRF complicates IPF and becomes a management challenge for clinicians as the IPF progresses. Proper prognostic identification of CRF onset in IPF patients will improve clinical outcomes and lead to better management care, especially in the advanced stages.

Table 1. Common CRF comorbidities

Causes of CRF	Description
COPD & emphysema	• Smoking history as a risk factor • Relatively preserved FVC and TLC volumes • Impairment of DLCO
Obstructive sleep apnea	• Presence of risk factors, for example overweight or obesity, snoring, and facial configuration • Excessive daytime sleepiness • Insomnia, reduced attention
Small airway disease	• Small airway obstruction at PFTs • Signs and symptoms of airway obstruction such as wheezing and mucus plug
Congestive heart failure	• Dyspnea • Cancer-related fatigue • Cardiovascular comorbidities, including coronary artery disease and arrhythmias • Cardiovascular symptoms (e.g., angina)
Lung cancer	• Presence of COPD and emphysema overlap • Whole system symptoms such as weight loss and night sweats
Pulmonary hypertension	• Exertional or resting hypoxemia (not due lung injury) • Impairment of V-Q mismatch due to parenchymal damage as evident by low DLCO • Exertional chest pain, syncope or near syncope • Signs of right heart failure • Right atrial enlargement • Right ventricular hypertrophy and/or enlarged pulmonary arteries
Pulmonary embolism	• Presence of risk factors such as inactivity, history of cancer, post-surgery or bone fracture. • Presence of connective tissue disease with prothrombotic effect • Signs and symptoms similar to those present in pulmonary hypertension

FVC: forced vital capacity; TLC: total lung capacity; DLCO: Diffusing capacity of the lungs for carbon monoxide; PFT: pulmonary function test; COPD: chronic obstructive pulmonary disease; V-Q: ventilation/perfusion.

References

[1] Maher, T. M., A. U. Wells, and G. J. Laurent. 2007. "Idiopathic Pulmonary Fibrosis: Multiple Causes And Multiple Mechanisms?". *European Respiratory Journal* 30 (5): 835-839.

[2] Poletti, V., and J. Egan. 2013. "Classification, Natural History and Staging of Idiopathic Pulmonary Fibrosis." *Sarcoidosis Vasculitis and Diffuse Lung Disease* 30 (Suppl 1): 13–20.

[3] Selman, Moisés, and Annie Pardo. 2014. "Revealing the Pathogenic and Aging-Related Mechanisms of the Enigmatic Idiopathic Pulmonary Fibrosis. An Integral Model." *American Journal of Respiratory and Critical Care Medicine* 189 (10): 1161–1172.

[4] Collard, Harold R., Bethany B. Moore, Kevin R. Flaherty, Kevin K. Brown, Robert J. Kaner, Talmadge E. King Jr, Joseph A. Lasky, James E. Loyd, Imre Noth, and Mitchell A. Olman. 2007. "Acute Exacerbations of Idiopathic Pulmonary Fibrosis." *American Journal of Respiratory and Critical Care Medicine* 176 (7): 636–643.

[5] Greene, Kelly E., and Jay I. Peters. 1994. "Pathophysiology of Acute Respiratory Failure." *Clinics in Chest Medicine* 15 (1): 1–12.

[6] Campbell, E. J. M. 1965. "Respiratory Failure." *British Medical Journal* 1 (5448): 1451.

[7] Faverio, Paola, Federica De Giacomi, Giulia Bonaiti, Anna Stainer, Luca Sardella, Giulia Pellegrino, and Giuseppe Francesco Sferrazza Papa et al., 2019. "Management of Chronic Respiratory Failure In Interstitial Lung Diseases: Overview And Clinical Insights". *International Journal of Medical Sciences* 16 (7): 967-980. doi:10.7150/ijms.32752.

[8] Robbie, Hasti, Cécile Daccord, Felix Chua, and Anand Devaraj. 2017. "Evaluating Disease Severity in Idiopathic Pulmonary Fibrosis." *European Respiratory Review* 26 (145): 170051.

[9] King Jr, Talmadge E., Williamson Z. Bradford, Socorro Castro-Bernardini, Elizabeth A. Fagan, Ian Glaspole, Marilyn K. Glassberg, Eduard Gorina, Peter M. Hopkins, David Kardatzke, and Lisa Lancaster. 2014. "A Phase 3 Trial of Pirfenidone in Patients with Idiopathic Pulmonary Fibrosis." *New England Journal of Medicine* 370 (22): 2083–2092.

[10] Parker, Joseph M., Ian N. Glaspole, Lisa H. Lancaster, Tarik J. Haddad, Dewei She, Stephanie L. Roseti, Jon P. Fiening, Ethan P. Grant, Chris M. Kell, and Kevin R. Flaherty. 2018. "A Phase 2 Randomized Controlled Study of Tralokinumab in Subjects with Idiopathic Pulmonary Fibrosis." *American Journal of Respiratory and Critical Care Medicine* 197 (1): 94–103.

[11] Raghu, Ganesh, Fernando J. Martinez, Kevin K. Brown, Ulrich Costabel, Vincent Cottin, Athol U. Wells, Lisa Lancaster, Kevin F. Gibson, Tarik Haddad, and Prasheen Agarwal. 2015. "CC-Chemokine Ligand 2 Inhibition in Idiopathic Pulmonary Fibrosis: A Phase 2 Trial of Carlumab." *European Respiratory Journal* 46 (6): 1740–1750.

[12] Vainshelboim, Baruch. 2016. "Exercise Training in Idiopathic Pulmonary Fibrosis: Is It of Benefit?" *Breathe* 12 (2): 130–138.

[13] Holland, Anne E. 2010. "Exercise Limitation in Interstitial Lung Disease-Mechanisms, Significance and Therapeutic Options." *Chron. Respir. Dis.* 7 (2): 101–11.

[14] Erbes, Reinhard, Tom Schaberg, and Robert Loddenkemper. 1997. "Lung Function Tests in Patients with Idiopathic Pulmonary Fibrosis: Are They Helpful for Predicting Outcome?" *Chest* 111 (1): 51–57.

[15] Cortes-Telles, Arturo, Lutz Forkert, Denis E. O'Donnell, and Onofre Morán-Mendoza. 2014. "Idiopathic Pulmonary Fibrosis: New Insights to Functional Characteristics at Diagnosis." *Canadian Respiratory Journal* 21 (3): e55–e60.

[16] Traila, Daniel, Cristian Oancea, Emanuela Tudorache, Ovidiu Fira Mladinescu, Bogdan Timar, and Voicu Tudorache. 2018. "Clinical Profile of Unclassifiable Interstitial Lung Disease: Comparison with Chronic Fibrosing Idiopathic Interstitial Pneumonias." *Journal of International Medical Research* 46 (1): 448–456.

[17] Ryerson, Christopher J., Eric Vittinghoff, Brett Ley, Joyce S. Lee, Joshua J. Mooney, Kirk D. Jones, Brett M. Elicker, Paul J. Wolters, Laura L. Koth, and Talmadge E. King Jr. 2014. "Predicting Survival across Chronic Interstitial Lung Disease: The ILD-GAP Model." *Chest* 145 (4): 723–728.

In: Respiratory Ventilatory Strategies …
Editor: Antonio M. Esquinas
ISBN: 978-1-53617-847-0
© 2020 Nova Science Publishers, Inc.

Chapter 14

THE DIAGNOSIS AND TREATMENT OF OBSTRUCTIVE SLEEP APNEA IN PATIENTS WITH IDIOPATHIC PULMONARY FIBROSIS

Walter Blake Gribben[1,*], MD and Kimberly Truong[2,3], MD
[1]Division of Pulmonary Diseases and Critical Care Medicine
University of California, Irvine Medical Center Orange, CA, US
[2]Sleep Medicine Clinic, Tibor Rubin Veterans Affairs Medical Center
Long Beach, CA, US
[3]Division of Pulmonary Diseases and Critical Care Medicine
University of California, Irvine Medical Center
Orange, CA, US

ABSTRACT

Idiopathic Pulmonary Fibrosis (IPF) is an incurable condition in which progressive pulmonary fibrosis causes progressive respiratory failure, resulting ultimately in death. Despite the introduction of the first drugs to treat this condition, no agent has been proven yet to reduce mortality. IPF patients commonly have sleep complaints, and obstructive sleep apnea (OSA) has been found to be prevalent among IPF patients.

OSA is a condition that results in significant morbidity, and, with certain patients, increased mortality. OSA was first described in the 1960s using nocturnal polysomnography. It is estimated to occur in anywhere from 4% to 20% of adults, depending on the population, and is most common in age 60 to 69. Unlike IPF, OSA is treatable, resulting in reduced morbidity and mortality in OSA patients. OSA appears to play an important role in quality of life and potentially, mortality in IPF patients. Treatment of OSA in patients with IPF appears to provide patients with better lung

* Corresponding Author's E-mail: wgribben@hs.uci.edu.

function, fewer symptoms, and possibly, improved survival. This raises the possibility of OSA being an important modifiable factor in IPF patients. In this chapter, we discuss physiologic interactions between OSA and IPF as well as the clinical presentation, diagnosis, and treatment of OSA in IPF patients.

INTRODUCTION

Idiopathic Pulmonary Fibrosis (IPF) is an incurable condition in which progressive pulmonary fibrosis causes progressive respiratory failure, resulting ultimately in death. Despite the introduction of the first drugs to treat this condition, no agent has been proven yet to reduce mortality. IPF patients commonly have sleep complaints, and obstructive sleep apnea (OSA) has been found to be prevalent among IPF patients.

OSA is a condition that results in significant morbidity, and, with certain patients, increased mortality. OSA was first described in the 1960s using nocturnal polysomnography. It is estimated to occur in anywhere from 4% to 20% of adults, depending on the population, and is most common in age 60 to 69. Unlike IPF, OSA is treatable, resulting in reduced morbidity and mortality in OSA patients. OSA appears to play an important role in quality of life and potentially, mortality in IPF patients. Treatment of OSA in patients with IPF appears to provide patients with better lung function, fewer symptoms, and possibly, improved survival. This raises the possibility of OSA being an important modifiable factor in IPF patients. In this chapter, we discuss physiologic interactions between OSA and IPF as well as the clinical presentation, diagnosis, and treatment of OSA in IPF patients.

PATHOGENESIS

OSA Pathophysiology

Obstructive sleep apnea is a breathing disorder characterized by partial or complete closure of the upper airway that impairs normal ventilation during sleep (Kapur, 2017). Repetitive upper airway closure during sleep results in intermittent hypoxia, increased sympathetic nervous system activation and oxidative stress, and a resultant systemic inflammatory cascade. Common symptoms include non-refreshing sleep, daytime sleepiness, morning headaches, irritability, difficulty with concentration, and memory loss. Untreated OSA is known to be associated with decreased workplace productivity and increased motor vehicle accidents. OSA is also frequently associated with other comorbidities, including hypertension, insulin resistance, pulmonary artery hypertension, and gastroesophageal reflux disease (Lancaster, 2009).

Anatomic and non-anatomic factors contribute to the development of obstructive sleep apnea. Anatomically, a crowded upper airway is an important and well-established contributor to OSA. A crowded upper airway may be indicated by a long and low-lying soft palate, scalloping of the tongue, thick neck, high Mallampati score, and retrognathia and micrognathia. For most of these reasons, obesity is a significant risk factor to the development of OSA.

Non-anatomic factors also contribute to the development of OSA. These factors include increased upper airway collapsibility, sensitivity to awakening to mild airway narrowing (also referred to as low respiratory arousal threshold), and unstable control of breathing (also referred to as high loop gain). Increased upper airway collapsibility, as defined as a Pcrit value near +5 cmH_2O, is commonly seen in obstructive sleep apnea patients. Pcrit values of -5 cmH_2O, which indicates a stable upper airway, is rarely seen in patients with OSA.

Low threshold for cortical arousals leads to fragmented sleep and prevents maintenance of deeper sleep stages where stable breathing occurs. This perpetuates unstable breathing throughout the night. In addition, about one-third of OSA patients have unstable ventilator drive, referred to as high loop gain. In respiratory physiology, patients with high loop gain tend to have exaggerated responses to small changes in CO_2. This unstable ventilator physiology drives large swings in blood gas and pathogenesis of obstructive sleep apnea.

IPF Pathophysiology

As detailed in earlier book chapters, IPF is a restrictive fibrotic lung disease of unknown etiology. It is associated with hypoxemia, progressing to respiratory failure and, eventually, death. Gastroesophageal Reflux Disease (GERD), a complication of OSA, has been linked to IPF. Until 2014, there were no effective treatments. Although two medications are now available (Esbriet and Ofev), neither have been proven to reduce mortality (Lederer, 2018).

IPF was first formally defined in 2000 in an International consensus statement, which was issued as joint statement of the American Thoracic Society (ATS), and the European Respiratory Society (ERS). Prior to the release of this consensus statement, most studies of sleep-disordered breathing incorporated patients with a wide variety of interstitial lung diseases (ILD). This included patients with other systemic diseases (such as scleroderma or rheumatoid arthritis). These early studies nonetheless were able to show that, in general, ILD patients seemed to have poor sleep quality with less REM sleep and more Type 1 sleep. They also noted that many patients had frequent overnight oxygen desaturation despite the absence of snoring (Schiza, 2015).

The release of consensus guidelines for diagnosing IPF led to the first articles examining sleep disordered breathing in IPF, specifically the 2009 Lancaster study, which was the first prospective study of OSA in patients meeting the 2000 ATS criteria for IPF (Lancaster, 2009). This study made several important observations. First, all groups noted reduced sleep efficiency, slow wave sleep, and REM sleep. Mostly stage 2 sleep was seen in all groups. Second, hypopneas were more common than apneas. Third, 35 of 44 patients with OSA did not require home oxygen, but they did have nocturnal desaturations consistent with sleep-disordered breathing. The mean minimum oxygen desaturation for patients not receiving home O_2 was 79%, whereas their mean baseline awake oxygen saturation was 94% prior to the start of the nocturnal PSG (Lancaster, 2009).

A second study by Kolilekas in 2013 showed that, in IPF patients, intermittent sleep oxygen desaturation exceeded the desaturations seen with maximum exercise. In the study, more oxygen desaturations during both sleep and during exercise were associated with both worsened lung function (as measured by TLC and DLCO) and with worsened survival. When patients wearing CPAP were excluded, AHI correlated inversely with survival. Patients with more sleep oxygen desaturation also had more subjective dyspnea and higher right ventricular systolic pressure (RVSP), as measured by echocardiogram. Therefore, worse sleep apnea seems to be associated with worsened Pulmonary Hypertension, which is another known co-morbidity of IPF. This study implied a link between apnea events and lung damage (Kolilekas, 2013). The IPF guidelines were revised and updated in 2010, with a new consensus statement issued in 2011 by ATS and ERS, now joined by the Japanese Respiratory Society (JRS), and Latin American Thoracic Association (ALAT). At that time, OSA was added to the list of comorbidities of IPF (Schiza, 2015). The guidelines were further revised in 2015, and most recently, 2018 (Raghu, 2018).

OSA Pathogenesis in IPF Patients

The anatomic and non-anatomic factors that contribute to OSA in the healthy population also apply for IPF patients. However, certain alterations in lung mechanics in IPF patients likely predispose this population to the development of OSA. IPF patients tend to have increased arousals, fragmented sleep and more light sleep (N1 stage) throughout the night. The lack of deep sleep prevents IPF patients from reaching stages where stable breathing occurs. This correlates to low threshold for cortical arousals as described previously.

Furthermore, the alterations in IPF lung mechanics are known to cause persistent activation of the central respiratory center (located in medulla and pons). This consequentially leads to an increase in ventilator drive/high loop gain as described in the last paragraph. The pathophysiology of OSA in IPF patients still needs to be further explored in basic science and clinical research.

Sleep hypoventilation is safe in normal patients, but dangerous in patients with chronic respiratory disease. Sleep disturbances play a major role in overall quality of life, as well as morbidity and mortality and IPF (Schiza, 2015). Early studies on ILD, prior to the release of the 2000 ATS IPF diagnostic criteria seemed to show that AHI correlated inversely with forced vital capacity. However, a later study of IPF patients with OSA did not show such a correlation (Lancaster, 2009).

CLINICAL CHARACERISTICS

OSA In IPF Patients

Common symptoms of OSA are non-refreshing sleep, daytime sleepiness, fragmented sleep, morning headaches, irritability, difficulty with concentration and memory loss (Osman, 2018). IPF patients also commonly complain of daytime fatigue, non-refreshing sleep, and fragmented sleep.

Despite the high prevalence of OSA in IPF patients, it can often go unrecognized; although recognition has been improving over the years. Even as late as 2005, only a small minority of patients seen at a tertiary care IPF center were referred for a sleep study (Schiza, 2015). It was not until 2011, over 10 years since the release of the initial ATS guidelines on IPF, that OSA was officially recognized as a comorbidity of IPF in the revised ATS/ERS/ALAT/JRS Guidelines on IPF. The lack of suspicion for OSA in IPF patients may be explained by the fact that OSA usually presents atypically in patients with IPF. Many of the patients do not present with the sleepiness that is typically seen in obstructive sleep apnea. In one study of IPF patients who were later diagnosed with OSA, fewer than half reported snoring, only 22% complained of daytime sleepiness, and only 29% reported witnessed apneas (Mermigkis, 2015). IPF patients with normal BMI are still at risk for OSA. In two different studies, AHI correlated strongly with neck circumference and hip diameter, but not with BMI (Mermigkis, 2015) (Kolilekas, 2013). The use of corticosteroids in IPF patients may cause an increase in fat deposits, particularly in the head and neck area, increasing their risk for OSA (Schiza, 2015).

Screening and Diagnosis

Screening for OSA in IPF Patients

Traditionally used screening tools such as the Epworth sleepiness scale (ESS), Sleep Apnea scale of the Sleep Disorders Questionnaire (SA-SDQ), and STOP-BANG rely on risk factors such as obesity, daytime sleepiness, and snoring to predict the presence of OSA. However, with many of these measures being absent in IPF patients with OSA, screening tools based on these risk factors will likely be unreliable.

In particular, the Epworth Sleepiness Scale has probably the lowest usefulness for screening, as so few IPF/OSA patients report daytime tiredness. In one study, the mean value for all patients with IPF was < 10 (a normal score) for both patients with OSA and those without OSA. In those patients with elevated ESS (> 10), the degree of ESS elevation did not correlate with AHI (Lancaster, 2009). One author hypothesized that because of the persistent fatigue that is reported by nearly all IPF patients, they may not report this at any higher rate than IPF patients without OSA (Mermigkis, 2015).

The SA-SDQ questionnaire performed a little better than the ESS in one study, having a positive predictive value of 88%. However, it performed poorly as a screening tool, yielding a negative predictive value of only 50% (Lancaster, 2009).

The STOP-BANG OSA screening tool may be superior to ESS and SA-SDQ, as it incorporates neck circumference and age. However, it should be noted that the STOP-BANG relies on snoring and daytime tiredness, both of which may be missing in OSA patients with IPF.

The 2017 Clinical Practice Guideline for Diagnostic Testing for Adult Obstructive Sleep Apnea, released by the American Academy of Sleep Medicine recommend that questionnaires and other screening tools be used only for screening purposes, and that only formal sleep testing be used for the diagnosis of OSA (Kapur, 2017).

Diagnosis of OSA in IPF Patients

The presence and severity of OSA has been traditionally defined by the apnea-hypopnea index (AHI). The apnea-hypopnea index represents the number of events per hour of sleep. Mild sleep apnea is defined as 5 to 15 events per hour, moderate as 15 to 30 events per hour, and severe as more than 30 events per hour of sleep (Osman, 2018). Apneas are traditionally defined as a 90% drop in airflow for greater than 10 seconds. Hypopneas are defined as a 50-90% decrease in airflow amplitude and/or oxygen desaturation of greater than 3% or EEG arousal (Lancaster, 2009).

Formal diagnosis of obstructive sleep apnea requires in-lab polysomnography or ambulatory (home) sleep test. Traditional in-lab polysomnogram (PSG) is preferred over home sleep tests (HST) for patients with significant cardiopulmonary disorders. Home sleep studies can underestimate the severity of obstructive sleep apnea as true sleep time and EEG arousals cannot be determined with this type of testing (Kapur, 2017). While the American Academy of Sleep Medicine recommends in-lab polysomnography instead of home sleep testing for patients with “significant cardiopulmonary disease,” there are no clear guidelines for OSA diagnostic testing in the IPF population (Kapur, 2017). However, given the fragmented sleep and risk for hypoventilation seen in IPF patients, we recommend in-lab polysomnography for diagnosis of OSA in IPF. All of the major studies on IPF/OSA patients so far have been done with traditional in-lab PSG. HST has not been tested in the IPF/OSA patient population.

TREATMENT

OSA in IPF Patients

Until 2014, there were no treatments available for idiopathic pulmonary fibrosis. Over the last five years, two different drugs have been introduced to treat IPF. However, neither has yet been proven to reduce mortality (Lederer, 2018). CPAP, however, may reduce mortality in patients with obstructive sleep apnea and idiopathic pulmonary fibrosis. Treatment of obstructive sleep apnea with CPAP has been shown to improve quality of life, enhanced daily activities, and reduced nocturnal oxygen desaturation in patients with idiopathic pulmonary fibrosis and obstructive sleep apnea (Mermigkis, 2015) (Kolilekas, 2013).

Good compliance with CPAP for IPF/OSA patients led to improvement in functional status and energy level. The largest improvement was seen in the Functional Outcomes of Sleep Questionnaire (FOSQ), which is a self-administered 30 question survey on patients’ activity level, vigilance, intimacy, sex, productivity, and social outcomes. Lower scores indicate greater dysfunction. The other large improvement was in the Fatigue Severity Scale (FSS), which is a 9-statement 7-point scale measuring fatigue (Mermigkis, 2015). Since fatigue is the most commonly reported symptom of IPF, this can have a major impact on IPF/OSA patients’ quality of life (Lederer, 2018).

Although data so far is limited, a few studies suggest that treatment of OSA with CPAP in IPF patients may improve mortality (Mermigkis, 2015). Compliance with CPAP is a challenge in patients with IPF. When initiating CPAP therapy, we recommend emphasizing to patients the benefits to quality of life that CPAP can provide to patients with IPF and OSA. CPAP might also help with cough, which is one of the most common symptoms in IPF. We also recommend initiation of CPAP early, when CPAP is more likely to be tolerated (Schiza, 2015).

Patients with OSA and IPF with chronic hypercapnic respiratory failure should be started on bilevel positive airway pressure therapy (commonly known as BiPAP). Patients who have difficulty tolerating CPAP or failed CPAP may benefit from switching to BiPAP. There are no studies that compare the efficacy between BiPAP and CPAP in IPF patients with OSA. Similarly, there are no studies evaluating benefits of mandibular advancement devices for obstructive sleep apnea in the IPF population.

PROGNOSIS

Idiopathic pulmonary fibrosis is an invariably fatal disease. Although two recently introduced drugs have been shown to slow the decline of vital capacity on lung function testing, neither have been proven yet to reduce mortality (Raghu, 2018).

Treatment of obstructive sleep apnea in idiopathic pulmonary fibrosis patients may actually reduce mortality, in addition to improving quality of life (Mermigkis, 2015). In patients with both IPF and OSA, poor compliance with CPAP was associated with worse pain, lower sleep quality, and lower reported quality of life. Further, there was a suggestion in one study that CPAP noncompliance in IPF/OSA patients may be associated with higher mortality. Indeed, out of 55 patients with IPF and moderate/severe OSA, all 37 patients from the compliant group were alive at 24 months follow up. By contrast, 3 patients from the 18 non-compliant patient group had died (Mermigkis, 2015).

PREVENTION

Researchers have been looking at potential triggers for IPF, including environmental exposures, GERD, and OSA. However, no definite cause has been found, and therefore, there is no current way to prevent onset of IPF (Lederer, 2018).

Traditional recommendations for preventing OSA involve weight reduction and lifestyle modification. However, given that OSA is present even in many IPF patients with normal BMI, this alone cannot completely prevent it. However, one study in Greece (with lower BMI patients) had a lower incidence of OSA, while one done in the USA (with higher BMI patients) had a much higher incidence of OSA (Lancaster, 2009).

CONCLUSION

Idiopathic pulmonary fibrosis is a deadly, incurable disease that also has profoundly negative effects on the quality of life of the patients who suffer from it. Obstructive sleep apnea is one of its most common comorbidities, affecting as many as 85% of IPF patients in recent studies. The recurrent oxygen desaturations seen in IPF/OSA patients can be more severe than those seen in even the most strenuous exercise, and lower oxygen desaturations are associated with worsened survival. OSA manifests differently in IPF, with many patients not reporting the symptoms typical of OSA in other populations. This limits the effectiveness of traditional screening tools and reinforces the need for formal sleep studies to make the diagnosis. Consistent with the AASM guidelines, we recommend the use of in-lab polysomnography, as opposed to increasingly common home sleep tests for IPF patients. In IPF patients in whom OSA is diagnosed, we strongly recommend treatment with CPAP. Such treatment has now been proven to improve quality of life for IPF patients and may even reduce their mortality. CPAP treatment may also provide other physiologic benefits, such as lowering right heart pressures and improving lung vital capacity. This relatively simple and low-cost intervention can provide meaningful benefits for patients suffering from this deadly duo of respiratory diseases.

REFERENCES

Kapur, V. K. (2017). Clinical practice guideline for diagnostic testing for adult obstructive sleep apnea: an American Academy of Sleep Medicine clinical practice guideline. *J. Clin. Sleep Med.*, 479-504.

Kolilekas, L. E. (2013). Sleep Oxygen Desaturation Predicts Survival in Idiopathic Pulmonary Fibrosis. *J. Clin. Sleep Med.* 2013, 593-601.

Lancaster, L. H. (2009). Obstructive sleep apnea is common in idiopathic pulmonary fibrosis. *Chest*, 772-778.

Lederer, D. J. (2018). Idiopathic Pulmonary Fibrosis. *N. Engl. J. Med.*, 378, 1811-23.

Mermigkis, C. I. (2015). Obstructive sleep apnea should be treated in patients with idiopathic pulmonary fibrosis. *Sleep Breath*, 385–391.

Osman, A. M. (2018). Obstructive sleep apnea: current perspectives. *Nat. Sci. Sleep.*, 21-34.

Raghu, G. M.-J. (2018). Diagnosis of Idiopathic Pulmonary Fibrosis: An Official ATS/ERS/JRS/ALAT Clinical Practice Guideline. *Am. J. Respir. Crit. Care Med.*, e44-e68.

Schiza, S. C. (2015). Idiopathic pulmonary fibrosis and sleep disorders: no longer strangers in the night. *Eur. Respir. Rev.* 2015, 327–339.

Spicuzza, L. D. (2015). Obstructive sleep apnoea syndrome and its management. *Ther. Adv. Chronic. Dis.*, 273–285.

In: Respiratory Ventilatory Strategies …
Editor: Antonio M. Esquinas
ISBN: 978-1-53617-847-0
© 2020 Nova Science Publishers, Inc.

Chapter 15

INITIAL EVALUATION OF RESPIRATORY FAILURE SEVERITY FOR IDIOPATHIC PULMONARY FIBROSIS: DISEASE SEVERITY STAGING SYSTEM FOR IDIOPATHIC PULMONARY FIBROSIS

Vânia Fernandes**, *MD and Carolina Matos Cabo*†, *MD
Pneumology Unit, Centro Hospitalar e Universitário de Coimbra, Coimbra, Portugal

ABSTRACT

When evaluating respiratory failure severity in Idiopathic Pulmonary Fibrosis (IPF), there are two forms that should be distinguished and analyzed separately. In this chapter we will focus on both acute and chronic respiratory failure.

Chronic respiratory failure and hypoxemia in IPF may be a combination of many mechanisms – mainly ventilation/perfusion mismatch, shunt, and diffusion limitation. Several tests and exams support this assessment, namely pulmonary function tests, 6-minute walk test, cardiopulmonary exercise test and high-resolution chest CT scan.

Acute respiratory failure is linked to acute exacerbations of the disease, often requiring hospital admission. In this chapter we will characterize risk factors for exacerbation, and we will describe a staging system that allows identification of prognostic groups. We will also briefly describe the treatment options in IPF patients with respiratory failure.

* Corresponding Author's E-mail: vania.louro.fernandes@gmail.com.
† Corresponding Author's E-mail: carolinapmatoscabo@gmail.com.

Abbreviations

AE	acute exacerbations.
ARF	acute respiratory failure.
CPAP	continuous positive airway pressure.
CPET	cardiopulmonary exercise test.
CRF	chronic respiratory failure.
DAD	diffuse alveolar damage.
DLCO	diffusing lung capacity for carbon monoxide.
ECMO	extracorporeal membrane oxygenation.
FEV1	forced expiratory volume in 1 second.
FVC	forced vital capacity.
HRCT	high resolution chest tomography.
ICU	intensive care unit.
IMV	invasive mechanical ventilation.
IPF	idiopathic pulmonary fibrosis.
LDH	lactate dehydrogenase.
PEEP	positive end-expiratory pressure.
TLC	total lung capacity.
UIP	usual interstitial pneumonia.
V/Q	ventilation/perfusion.
6MWT	6-minute walk test.

Introduction

Respiratory failure in Idiopathic pulmonary fibrosis (IPF) is very common during the course of the disease, and can be challenging for the clinician in both its acute phase and its chronic advanced state.

When discussing the acute phase, the more accurate term is usually IPF acute exacerbations (AE), where respiratory failure is one of the main complications, frequently leading to death. In this setting, the medical evaluation should be fast, in order to identify the exacerbation so that the best treatment can be initiated; the goal is to optimize lung ventilation in the shortest time. AE is associated with high in-hospital mortality rates, that can reach 55-80%. By providing the best respiratory support, the clinician can reduce patient's discomfort associated with dyspnea, but also mortality.

In chronic phase, respiratory failure represents the natural course of the disease, reflecting progression and severity. Managing chronic respiratory failure with oxygen supplementation, noninvasive ventilation or high-flow nasal cannula aims to improve prognostic, but also contributes to a better quality of life by increasing exercise tolerance and decreasing dyspnea, therefore promoting physical activity and comfort.

Chronic Respiratory Failure on IPF Patients

The mechanisms of chronic respiratory failure (CRF) and hypoxemia in IPF may be a combination of ventilation/perfusion (V/Q) mismatch, shunt, and diffusion limitation; however, V/Q mismatch is the most common cause of hypoxemia both at rest and during exercise.

Increased alveolar-arterial oxygen gradient reflects a gas-exchange impairment. It can be assessed by a defect in diffusion capacity and in ventilation-perfusion ratio. In pulmonary function tests, forced vital capacity (FVC) and total lung capacity (TLC) are reduced, showing a restrictive pattern. Also, diffusing lung capacity for carbon monoxide (DLCO) is reduced. This is linked to a higher respiratory rate, as a compensatory mechanism, which can contribute to hypercapnia in advanced stages. Hypercapnia may develop if forced expiratory volume in 1 second (FEV1) falls below 1.0 L/s.

The increase in respiratory rate is also a consequence of lung compliance reduction (due to deposition of extracellular matrix in the interstitial space) increasing the effort of respiratory muscles and the stimulation of peripheral mechanoreceptors.

Evaluating the Severity of Chronic Respiratory Failure

Many clinical signs, radiological features and functional tests can be evaluated in IPF patients in order to characterize their chronic respiratory failure. In the next points, we explain each one of them, highlighting their interest in this assessment.

Pulmonary Function Tests

In interstitial lung diseases, and particularly in IPF, pulmonary function tests typically present a restrictive pattern, with low lung volumes – low FVC and low TLC. Diffusing lung capacity for carbon monoxide is also frequently decreased, both the absolute value obtained by single breath method, and the alveolar volume adjusted value.

FVC and DLCO are the best studied physiological characteristics to evaluate disease severity, among other aspects, such as progression and response to treatment. FVC decline is a useful prognostic indicator, more than the absolute value itself. When analyzing a period of 6 months, a decrease of more than 10% (both absolutely and relatively to the previous values) in FVC is considered significative for progression, as is a decrease in DLCO of more than 15%. Some authors consider the relative decrease to be the best parameter. However, if the patient's vital capacity is inferior to 1500ml, the

DLCO obtained by single breath method becomes less reliable. Moreover, DLCO is influenced by infection and hemoglobin concentration in the blood. For these reasons, FVC have become a more accurate function parameter.

6-Minute Walk Test

The 6-minute walk test (6MWT) is a reproducible, easy-to-perform tool, requiring only a trained nurse or physiotherapist, a pulse oximeter and a 30-meters corridor. 6MWT evaluates the distance that a patient can quickly walk on a flat, hard surface in a period of 6 minutes. Its simplicity is linked to the fact that it doesn't require any exercise equipment or advanced training for technicians. It evaluates exercise performance in general, not providing specific information about each system – that being possible through the more complex cardiopulmonary exercise test.

The 6MWT is broadly used in chronic lung disease. In IPF, a decline of 50 meters or more in tests performed with a 24-week interval is a significative mortality predictive factor.

Cardiopulmonary Exercise Test

The cardiopulmonary exercise test (CPET) is the gold standard for exercise tolerance evaluation. It is performed in the laboratory, using an electrically braked cycle ergometer or a treadmill. Unlike 6MWT, it provides a comprehensive assessment of the patient's response to exercise, reflecting the influences of the cardiac, respiratory and musculoskeletal systems. Ultimately, it helps to differentiate which of these systems limits exercise capacity and causes exertional dyspnea, and to what extent. It involves measurements of gas exchange, primarily oxygen uptake (i.e., VO2), carbon dioxide output (VCO2), minute ventilation, and anaerobic (lactic acid) threshold.

In interstitial lung diseases, it is useful for differential diagnosis purposes, especially in evaluating characteristics that may suggest pulmonary hypertension. It may also be used as an endpoint for clinical trials, both for pharmacological and non-pharmacological treatments. Regarding prognostic, the evidence is even stronger, and several parameters were linked to survival and transplant-free time.

High Resolution Chest CT Scan

High resolution chest tomography (HRCT) is a fundamental tool in IPF diagnostic evaluation, along with clinical history. The analysis of HRCT classic IPF characteristics – reticular opacities, honeycombing, peripheral traction bronchiectasis – and also its special distribution (typically basal and subpleural-predominant) helps defining a "typical usual interstitial pneumonia (UIP) pattern," as proposed by Fleishner Society, and makes the diagnostic of IPF more reliable. Other patterns were also proposed – "probable UIP pattern," "indeterminate for UIP" and "most consistent with non-IPF diagnosis." Studies suggest that different HRCT classifications and scoring systems can be linked to disease severity and progression, however more studies are needed to provide a solid prognostic tool. The extent of fibrosis on HRCT seems to be the characteristic that correlates the most with mortality.

Staging Systems in IPF

Despite the previously explained prognostic contributors, the use of these characteristics alone is impractical and does not constitute a valid staging system by itself, since it is arbitrary and mainly based on epidemiologic correlations. Some authors have tried to overcome this lack of functionality by setting up IPF staging systems.

In 2012, Ley et al., proposed a GAP score (Table 1) — Gender, Age, Physiology — as a risk prediction model for this disease. It is a multidimensional model, using data from three large cohorts of patients from different geographic locations. They developed a calculator (GAP calculator) that uses a regression model using the baseline variables: gender (G), age (A) and two lung physiology variables (P) (FVC and DLCO). It allows stratification in stages (I, II and III), linked to a 6%, 16% and 39% mortality, respectively; the use of the calculator allows assessment of patient's individual risk, which may facilitate clinical decisions.

Table 1. GAP score system for IPF mortality prediction. Score range 0-8. If the DLCO is not available or was not ordered, the system cannot be applied. Stage I (0-3 points), Stage II (4-5 points), Stage III (6-8 points)

	Predictor	**Points**
Gender	Male	0
	Female	1
Age (years)	≤60	0
	61-65	1
	>65	2
Physiology	FVC (% predicted)	
	>75	0
	50–75	1
	<50	2
	DLCO (% predicted)	
	>55	0
	36–55	1
	≤35	2
	Cannot perform	3

Acute Exacerbation of Idiopathic Pulmonary Fibrosis

Acute respiratory failure is one of the main complications of IPF. A similar entity is present in other forms of chronic interstitial lung diseases but is better characterized in this specific disease. It is associated with worse prognosis and a median survival time of 3 to 4 months.

Definition

The hallmark of AE is the presence of diffuse alveolar damage (DAD), a histopathological pattern. The clinical definition, with less accuracy, has been object of multiple statements and reports. Usually, it is defined as a period of less than 1 month of clinically relevant respiratory deterioration in a patient with a previous diagnosis of IPF, in association with widespread alveolar infiltrates on chest high resolution chest tomography. Many authors have suggested other definitions, being Collard H.R. et al.'s International Group Report one of the most relevant: they define acute exacerbation as any acute respiratory event characterized by new bilateral ground-glass opacification or consolidation not fully explained by cardiac failure or fluid overload. The same group suggests removing the term "idiopathic" from the previous definitions, since there is little clinical or biological support for distinguishing idiopathic from nonidiopathic respiratory events. It appears that neither presence nor absence of a known trigger has an impact on prognosis.

Incidence and Risk Factors

AE-IPF incidence is very variable among studies. Several risk factors have been identified:

1. lower forced vital capacity and diffusion capacity of carbon monoxide
2. reduced walking distance at 6-minute walking test
3. higher dyspnea scores, particularly in never smokers
4. diffuse ground-glass pattern in HRCT (compared to a multifocal or peripheral distribution)
5. presence and extent of honeycombing, consolidation and traction bronchiectasis
6. pulmonary hypertension
7. genetic variants

8. surgical lung biopsy
9. concomitant treatment for lung cancer.

Staging Systems

A staging system was proposed by Kishaba T. et al. They suggest a score consisting of several analytical and radiologic parameters that, if present, represents one point each. The variables are: serum lactate dehydrogenase (LDH) ≥280U/L, sialylated carbohydrate antigen KL-6 ≥ 1000 U/mL, partial pressure of oxygen and fraction of inspiratory oxygen concentration ratio (P/F ratio) <100, and a radiologic score of ground-glass opacity + consolidation ≥20. The sum of these parameters attributes a score to the patient, from 0 to 4. A score of 3 or 4 is associated with extensive disease, having a higher 3-month mortality.

Management of Respiratory Failure

AE-IPF often requires hospital admission and oxygen support, since, in its numerous definitions, it is associated with acute on chronic or *de novo* acute respiratory failure (ARF). ARF is almost invariably the mechanism of death in IPF patients, and its management, associated with the limited available pharmacological treatment, is central in overcoming an AE. Nevertheless, ventilatory support, especially invasive mechanical ventilation (IMV), is associated with a higher risk of ventilator induced lung injury, as well as a higher mortality rate (of as much as 90%). Therefore, introducing IMV is a clinical issue that must take in account the patient wishes and expectations, considering the probability of recovery. The patient's wish should be actively searched; considering the incapacity of many patients to express it during the acute phase, it must be given in a more stable one, by the means of a living will, for example.

Lung transplant is the unique existing definitive treatment for advanced stage IPF. If a patient is enlisted for transplant, intensive care unit (ICU) or high dependency unit admission should be performed, preferably in the local transplant center. Rarely, a patient can be listed after ICU admission, in the form of savage transplant. IMV alone or with extracorporeal membrane oxygenation (ECMO) and noninvasive ventilation have proven to be effective bridge-to-transplant treatments. Recent studies of ambulatory ECMO or non-intubated ECMO show promising results as a bridge to transplant.

Most patients with life-threatening ARF are not listed for transplant. In these patients, the aim is to provide enough oxygen supplementation. There are different delivery systems that allow administration with nasal canula or face mask (with lower oxygen concentration), as well as high concentration flows, with Venturi mask and reservoir mask. Ultimately, high flow nasal cannula is a promising system, that allows high oxygen flow, as well as a continuous positive airway pressure (CPAP) or positive end-expiratory pressure (PEEP) effect. The use of these systems will be explained in more detail in the following chapters.

CONCLUSION

Respiratory failure is a common complication of IPF in both its acute and chronic phase. Several clinical assessments, as well as complementary diagnostic tests should be performed in these patients in order to optimize diagnosis and treatment, but also to predict prognosis. In disease stability, GAP score is a helpful tool that should be accomplished in all patients, providing mortality prediction. More studies and similar tools are needed, especially in acute respiratory failure, in order to identify patients who could benefit from more advanced treatment, such as ICU admission and ECMO.

REFERENCES

[1] Bonini, M., Fiorenzano, G. (2017). Exertional dyspnoea in interstitial lung diseases: the clinical utility of cardiopulmonary exercise testing. *Eur Respir Rev,* 26:160099.

[2] Collard, H. R., Ryerson, C. J., Corte, C. J., et al. (2016). Acute Exacerbation of Idiopathic Pulmonary Fibrosis an International Working Group Report. *Am J Respir Crit Care Med,* 194 (3):265-275.

[3] Faverio, P., De Giacomi, F., Bonaiti, G., et al. (2019). Management of Chronic Respiratory Failure in Interstitial Lung Diseases: Overview and Clinical Insights. *Int J Med Sci,* 16:967-980.

[4] Faverio, P., De Giacomi, F., Sardella, L., et al. (2018). Management of acute respiratory failure in interstitial lung diseases: overview and clinical insights. *BMC Pulm Med,* 18(1):70.

[5] Kishaba, T. (2019) Evaluation and management of Idiopathic Pulmonary Fibrosis. *Respir Investig,* 57(4):300-311.

[6] Kishaba, T., Nei, Y., Momose, M., et al. (2018). Clinical Characteristics Based on the New Criteria of Acute Exacerbation in Patients with Idiopathic Pulmonary Fibrosis. *Eurasian J Med*, 50:6-10.

[7] Kishaba, T., Tamaki, H., Shimaoka, Y. (2014). Staging of Acute Exacerbation in Patients with Idiopathic Pulmonary Fibrosis. *Lung,* 192:141-149.

[8] Kolb, M., Collard, H. R. (2014). Staging of idiopathic pulmonary fibrosis: past, present and future. *Eur Respir Rev,* 23:220-224.

[9] Kondoh, Y., Cottin, V., Brown, K. K. (2017). Recent lessons learned in the management of acute exacerbation of idiopathic pulmonary fibrosis. *Eur Respir Rev,* 26:170050.

[10] Ley, B., Ryerson, C. J., Vittinghoff, E., et al. (2012). A Multidimensional Index and Staging System for Idiopathic Pulmonary Fibrosis. *Ann Intern Med*, 156:684-691.

[11] Raghu, C., Collard, H. R., Egan, J. J., et al. (2011). An Official ATS/ERS/JRS/ALAT Statement: Idiopathic Pulmonary Fibrosis: Evidence-based Guidelines for Diagnosis and Management. *Am J Respir Crit Care Med*, 183:788-824.

[12] Ryerson, C. J., Cottin, V., Brown, K. K. (2015). Acute exacerbation of idiopathic pulmonary fibrosis: shifting the paradigm. *Eur Respir J*, 46:512-520.

In: Respiratory Ventilatory Strategies …
Editor: Antonio M. Esquinas

ISBN: 978-1-53617-847-0
© 2020 Nova Science Publishers, Inc.

Chapter 16

DIAGNOSTIC PROCEDURES TO PERFORM

Tomoo Kishaba*
Department of Respiratory Medicine, Uruma City, Okinawa, Japan

ABSTRACT

Introduction: Purpose of Review

Idiopathic pulmonary fibrosis (IPF) is a relentless progressive parenchymal lung disease [1]. Among the idiopathic interstitial pneumonias (IIPs), IPF is the most common disease and most difficult to manage. Therefore, the purpose of this chapter is to show practical diagnostic approaches for IPF such as serum biomarker, chest radiogragh, chest high resolution computed tomography (HRCT) and broncho-alveolar lavage (BAL).

Keywords: BAL, Biomarker, Chest high resolution computed tomography, fibrosis, volume loss

MAIN FINDINGS

Biomarker

Serum lactate dehydrogenase (LDH) has been identified as a useful biomarker for disease activity and the severity of acute exacerbation (AE) in IPF [2]. LDH is associated with cell apotosis or injury of various organs such as lung, heart, liver, muscle and blood.

* Corresponding Author's E-mail: kishabatomoo@gmail.com.

It is particularly more sensitive for treatment response during acute phase. In addition, serum krebs von den lungen-6 (KL-6) has recently been reported to be a sensitive biomarker for interstitial lung disease (ILD) activity and is associated with fibrosis on chest HRCT as well as future exacerbations [3, 4]. Furthermore, Wakamatsu et al. reported that KL-6 change > 51.8U/ml/year showed poor prognosis in IPF patients [5]. Chronic hypersensitivity pneumonitis (CHP) patients sometime show seasonal variation of serum KL-6 value according to the offending antigen. Therefore, serial measurement of KL-6 is useful for IPF patients. Reduced survival is also associated with other epithelial or macrophage-related proteins such as surfactant protein-A (SP-A), surfactant protein-D(SP-D), chemokine ligand-18, and matrix metalloproteinase-7 [6-9]. SP-A is associated with infection. Therefore, interpretation of elevation of SP-A must be carefully done combined with clinical context. SP-D is often positively associated with the extent of ground glass opacity (GGO) of chest HRCT and negatively associated with the percent predicted FVC (%FVC). However, congestive heart failure (CHF) patient sometimes show elevation of SP-D. Recently, serum periostin have been reported to predict both short-term and long-term survival of IPF patients [10, 11]. Important factors of useful biomarker are less-invasive, reproducible and predictive of mortality and morbidity. The latest international IPF guideline does not recommend measuring serum biomarker for the purpose of distinction IPF from other ILDs [12]. The crucial point of using serum biomarker is to evaluate disease activity and serial measurement of these markers for IPF with adequate clinical context.

Chest Radiograph

Chest radiograph is useful for evaluating disease distribution and serial changes of volume loss in the lower lung field for IPF. Therefore, comparison with previous films is important when deciding to commence treatment. In early phase of IPF patients, bilateral lower lung and peripheral dominant reticular shadow and opacification of costo-phrenic (CP) angle is often seen. IPF patients often develop pulmonary hypertension (PH) in the advanced stage, which can be detected by a change in the cardiothoracic ratio and prominent bilateral hilar shadows with chest radiograph. Furthermore, when IPF patients develop AE, we can distinguish AE from heart failure (HF) partly on the basis of distribution of new shadow. The former usually shows diffuse parenchymal shadow. On the other hand, HF patients demonstrate peri-hilar shadow with pleural effusion such as thickening of inter-lobar fissure or dullness of CP angle.

Chest HRCT

Chest HRCT has occupied the main position for diagnosis of IPF recently. The integration of clinical and imaging information is essential for a definite diagnosis. [13]. Chest HRCT provides useful information about detailed anatomical location of the fibrotic findings in IPF, including reticular opacity, traction bronchi or bronchiolo-ectasis, and honeycombing [14, 15]. Lower lung field and peripheral dominant reticular opacity and linear shadow perpendicular to pleura in upper lung field signifies peri-lobular distribution in early phase of IPF. In addition, spatial heterogeneity is a key issue of IPF. For example, mixed shadow consists of reticular opacity, GGO and normal region within a small area is linked with pathological usual interstitial pneumonia (UIP). Honeycombing appears on HRCT as clustered cystic airspaces with comparable diameters of approximately 3 – 10mm, and is located sub-pleural area and characterized by a well-defined wall [16]. It has recently been proposed that both multilayered clustered cysts and sub-pleural single layered cysts also represent honeycombing [17]. Physician should collect thorough clinical information about the possibility of IPF for secure diagnosis. When we see atypical findings in chest HRCT such as micro nodules, air trapping or head-cheese sign which suggest CHP or extensive GGO and peri-broncho-vascular distribution, which raise possibility of idiopathic non-specific interstitial pneumonitis(iNSIP) or connective tissue disease (CTD) associated ILD, alternative diagnoses must be considered. Furthermore, significant pleural plaques and sub-pleural curvilinear opacity with definite occupational exposure suggest asbestosis, and multifocal peripheral consolidation is associated with organizing pneumonia (OP) [18]. If the pattern is unclear, HRCT can identify the most appropriate site for surgical lung biopsy to provide a definitive diagnosis [19, 20]. Fleischner Society published new diagnostic criteria of HRCT findings for IPF. They divide it into four subgroups such as typical, probable, indeterminate and not consistent UIP pattern [21].

Heterogeneous distribution is one of the key findings for IPF. Smokers who present fibrosis often show similar HRCT findings. However, smoking-related ILD such as airspace enlargement with fibrosis display thinner walls than typical honeycomb cysts. Upper lung distribution, diffuse centri-lobular nodules mosaic attenuation and head cheese sign are important findings for suggestion of CHP. If we see pleural effusion, esophageal dilation, or pericardial abnormality with a UIP pattern, underlying CTD is highly suggestive. On the basis of publication of Fleischner society, the latest international IPF diagnosis guideline was published September 2018 [12]. Concept of both Fleischner society and international IPF guideline is similar.

However, international IPF guideline described findings of early UIP pattern as indeterminate for UIP and detailed other findings such as pleural plaques, dilated esophagus, distal clavicular erosions, extensive lymphnode enlargement and pleural effusion or pleural thickening. This guideline insists upon importance of careful exclusion of CTD. On the other hand, Fleischner society white paper emphasizes on the importance of working diagnosis of IPF in the setting of clinical suspicion of IPF.

BAL

BAL can assist clinician in excluding infection, granulomatous lung disease such as CHP or sarcoidosis and predicting treatment response. It is particularly useful in AE of IPF when bronchoscopy is possible. Furthermore, cellular analysis of the BAL fluid (BALF) provides additional information when evaluating ILD. Standardization of BAL have not been established. In diffuse lung disease, we usually perform BAL in middle lobe or ligula because of its good recovery rate. However, more crucial issue is analysis of different fraction of BALF. First fraction of BALF generally reflects airway information.

On the contrary, third fraction of BALF reflects more distal parts such as alveolar or alveolar wall. In smokers, alveolar macrophage are predominant, whereas cell populations are normal or neutrophil dominant in typical IPF. When there is over 30% lymphocytosis in BALF, CHP, cryptogenic organizing pneumonia (COP) and iNSIP [22-26] as well as sarcoidosis are possible [27-29]. The cluster of differentiation (CD)4/CD8 ratio in BALF usually decreased in acute or subacute hypersensitivity pneumonitis, but elevated in CHP and sarcoidosis. Eosinophilia in BALF is suggestive of eosinophilic pneumonia or drug associated ILD [30-33]. Although there are some limitations to the utility of BAL analysis, BALF biomarkers such as KL-6 and thrombomodulin (TM) in AE of IPF have the potential to predict mortality and treatment response [34]. 2018 international IPF guideline showed conditional recommendation the BAL for distinction eosinophilic pneumonia, COP, sarcoidosis, or infection when we see HRCT pattern of probable UIP, indeterminate, or an alternative diagnosis. However, latest international guideline suggests not performing cellular analysis of their BAL fluid when we suspect of having IPF and an HRCT pattern of UIP [12].

On the other hand, contribution of infection for IPF or AE of IPF have been acknowledged recently. Positive BALF culture such as *Hemophilus influenzae*, *Strepotococcus* and *Staplylococcus* have been reported in stable IPF patients [35, 36]. In AE of IPF patients, increase of *Campylobacter* and *Stenotrophomonas* and decreased *Veillonella* of BALF have been described [37].

Conclusion

IPF have heterogeneous clinical course. Therefore, we can make provisional or definite diagnosis based on multiple information such as useful biomarker, chest HRCT and wise use of BAL.

References

[1] American Thoracic Society, European Respiratory Society. American Thoracic Society/European Respiratory Society international multidisciplinary consensus classification of the idiopathic interstitial pneumonias. *Am. J. Respir. Crit. Care Med.,* 2002 Jan. 15; 165(2): 277 - 304.

[2] Kishaba, T., Tamaki, H., Shimaoka, Y., Fukuyama, H., Yamashiro, S. Staging of acute exacerbation in patients with idiopathic pulmonary fibrosis. *Lung,* 2014 Feb.; 192(1): 141 - 9.

[3] Fujimoto, K., Taniguchi, H., Johkoh, T., Kondoh, Y., Ichikado, K., Sumikawa, H., Ogura, T., Kataoka, K., Endo, T., Kawaguchi, A., Müller, N. L. Acute exacerbation of idiopathic pulmonary fibrosis: high-resolution CT scores predict mortality. *Eur. Radiol.,* 2012 Jan.; 22(1): 83 - 92.

[4] Satoh, H., Kurishima, K., Ishikawa, H., Ohtsuka, M. Increased levels of KL-6 and subsequent mortality in patients with interstitial lung diseases. *J. Intern. Med.,* 2006 Nov.; 260(5):429 - 34.

[5] Wakamatsu, K., Nagata, N., Kumazoe, H., Oda, K., Ishimoto, H., Yoshimi, M., Takata, S., Hamada, M., Koreeda, Y., Takakura, K., Ishizu, M., Hara, M., Ise, S., Izumi, M., Akasaki, T., Maki, S., Kawabata, M., Mukae, H., Kawasaki, M. Prognostic value of serial serum KL-6 measurements in patients with idiopathic pulmonary fibrosis. *Respir. Investig.,* 2017 Jan.; 55(1):16 - 23.

[6] Barlo, N. P., van Moorsel, C. H. M., Ruven, H. J. T., Zanen, P., van den Bosch, J. M. M., Grutters, J. C. Surfactant protein-D predicts survival in patients with idiopathic pulmonary fibrosis. *Sarcoidosis Vasc. Diffuse Lung Dis.,* 2009 Jul.; 26(2):155 - 61.

[7] Kinder, B. W., Brown, K. K., McCormack, F. X., Ix, J. H., Kervitsky, A., Schwarz, M. I., King, T. E. Jr. Serum surfactant protein-A is a strong predictor of early mortality in idiopathic pulmonary fibrosis. *Chest,* 2009 Jun.; 135(6):1557 - 1563.

[8] Prasse, A., Probst, C., Bargagli, E., Zissel, G., Toews, G. B., Flaherty, K. R., Olschewski, M., Rottoli, P., Müller-Quernheim, J. Serum CC-chemokine ligand 18 concentration predicts outcome in idiopathic pulmonaryfibrosis. *Am. J. Respir. Crit. Care Med.,* 2009 Apr. 15; 179(8):717 - 23.

[9] Prasse, A., Pechkovsky, D. V., Toews, G. B., Schäfer, M., Eggeling, S., Ludwig, C., Germann, M., Kollert, F., Zissel, G., Müller-Quernheim, J. CCL18 as an indicator of pulmonary fibrotic activity in idiopathic interstitial pneumonias and systemic sclerosis. *Arthritis Rheum.,* 2007 May; 56(5):1685 - 93.

[10] Tajiri, M., Okamoto, M., Fujimoto, K., Johkoh, T., Ono, J., Tominaga, M., Azuma, K., Kawayama, T., Ohta, S., Izuhara, K., Hoshino, T. Serum level of periostin can predict long-term outcome of idiopathic pulmonary fibrosis. *Respir. Investig.,* 2015 Mar.; 53(2): 73 - 81.

[11] Ohta, S., Okamoto, M., Fujimoto, K., Sakamoto, N., Takahashi, K., Yamamoto, H., Kushima, H., Ishii, H., Akasaka, K., Ono, J., Kamei, A., Azuma, Y., Matsumoto, H., Yamaguchi, Y., Aihara, M., Johkoh, T., Kawaguchi, A., Ichiki, M., Sagara, H., Kadota, J. I., Hanaoka, M., Hayashi, S. I., Kohno, S., Hoshino, T., Izuhara, K.; Consortium for Development of Diagnostics for Pulmonary Fibrosis Patients (CoDD-PF). The usefulness of monomeric periostin as a biomarker for idiopathic pulmonary fibrosis. *PLoS One,* 2017 Mar. 29; 12(3):e0174547.

[12] Raghu, G., Remy-Jardin, M., Myers, J. L., Richeldi, L., Ryerson, C. J., Lederer, D. J., Behr, J., Cottin, V., Danoff, S. K., Morell, F., Flaherty, K. R., Wells, A., Martinez, F. J., Azuma, A., Bice, T. J., Bouros, D., Brown, K. K., Collard, H. R., Duggal, A., Galvin, L., Inoue, Y., Jenkins, R. G., Johkoh, T., Kazerooni, E. A., Kitaichi, M., Knight, S. L., Mansour, G., Nicholson, A. G., Pipavath, S. N. J., Buendía-Roldán, I., Selman, M., Travis, W. D., Walsh, S., Wilson, K. C.; American Thoracic Society, European Respiratory Society, Japanese Respiratory Society, and Latin American Thoracic Society. Diagnosis of Idiopathic Pulmonary Fibrosis. An Official ATS/ERS/JRS/ALAT Clinical Practice Guideline. *Am. J. Respir. Crit. Care Med.,* 2018 Sep. 1; 198(5): e44 - e68.

[13] Nishimura, K., Kitaichi, M., Izumi, T., Nagai, S., Kanaoka, M., Itoh, H. Usual interstitial pneumonia: histologic correlation with high-resolution CT. *Radiology,* 1992 Feb.; 182 (2):337 - 42.

[14] Kishaba, T. Integration of Clinical Findings and Physiology in Respiratory Disease. *J. of Respir. Res.,* 2015; 1(1): 1 - 4.

[15] Johkoh, T., Muller, N. L., Cartier, Y., Kavanagh, P. V., Hartman, T. E., Akira, M., Ichikado, K., Ando, M., Nakamura, H. Idiopathic interstitial pneumonias: diagnostic accuracy of thin-section CT in 129 patients. *Radiology,* 1999 May; 211(2): 555 - 60.

[16] Hansell, D. M., Bankier, A. A., Macmahon, H., McLoud, T. C., Muller, N. L., Remy, J. Fleischner Society: Glossary of terms for thoracic imaging. *Radiology,* 2008 Mar.; 246(3):697 - 722.

[17] Johkoh, T., Sakai, F., Noma, S., Akira, M., Fujimoto, K., Watadani, T., Sugiyama, Y. Honeycombing on CT; its definition, pathologic correlation, and future direction of its diagnosis. *Eur. J. Radiol.,* 2014 Jan.; 83(1): 27 - 31.

[18] Hwang, J. H., Misumi, S., Sahin, H., Brown, K. K., Newell, J. D., Lynch, D. A. Computed tomographic features of idiopathic fibrosing interstitial pneumonia: comparison with pulmonary fibrosis related to collagen vascular disease. *J. Comput. Assist. Tomogr.,* 2009 May-Jun.; 33(3):410 - 5.

[19] Luo, Q., Han, Q., Chen, X., Xie, J., Wu, L., Chen, R. The diagnosis efficacy and safety of video-assisted thoracoscopy surgery (VATS) in undefined interstitial lung diseases: a retrospective study. *J. Thorac. Dis.,* 2013 Jun.; 5(3):283 - 8.

[20] Wang, Z. X., Li, L., Zhang, Z., Wang, G. H., Kong, D. M., Wang, X. D., Wang, F. High-resolution computed tomography features and CT-guided microcoil localization of subcentimeter pulmonary ground-glass opacities: radiological processing prior to video-assisted thoracoscopic surgery. *J. Thorac. Dis.,* 2018 May; 10(5):2676 - 2684.

[21] Lynch, D. A., Sverzellati, N., Travis, W. D., Brown, K. K., Colby, T. V., Galvin, J. R., Goldin, J. G., Hansell, D. M., Inoue, Y., Johkoh, T., Nicholson, A. G., Knight, S. L., Raoof, S., Richeldi, L., Ryerson, C. J., Ryu, J. H., Wells, A. U. Diagnostic criteria for idiopathic pulmonary fibrosis: a Fleischner Society White Paper. *Lancet Respir. Med.,* 2018 Feb.; 6(2):138 - 153.

[22] Costabel, U., Bonella, F., Guzman, J. Chronic hypersensitivity pneumonitis. *Clin. Chest Med.,* 2012 Mar.; 33(1):151 - 63.

[23] Ohshimo, S., Bonella, F., Cui, A., Beume, M., Kohno, N., Guzman, J., Costabel, U. Significance of bronchoalveolar lavage for the diagnosis of idiopathic pulmonary fibrosis. *Am. J. Respir. Crit. Care Med.,* 2009; 179: 1043 - 47.

[24] Yoshizawa, Y., Ohtani, Y., Hayakawa, H., Sato, A., Suga, M., Ando, M. Chronic hypersensitivity pneumonitis in Japan: a nationwide epidemiologic survey. *J. Allergy Clin. Immunol.,* 1999 Feb.; 103(2 Pt 1): 315 - 20.

[25] Pardo, A., Smith, K. M., Abrams, J., Coffman, R., Bustos, M., McClanahan, T. K., Grein, J., Murphy, E. E., Zlotnik, A., Selman, M. CCL18/DC-CK-1/PARC up-regulation in hypersensitivity pneumonitis. *J. Leukoc. Biol.,* 2001 Oct.; 70(4): 610 - 6.

[26] Ratjen, F., Costabel, U., Griese, M., Paul, K. Bronchoalveolar lavage fluid findings in children with hypersensitivity pneumonitis. *Eur. Respir. J.,* 2003 Jan.; 21(1): 144 - 8.

[27] Keogh, B. A., Hunninghake, G. W., Line, B. R., Crystal, R. G. The alveolitis of pulmonary sarcoidosis: evaluation of natural history and alveolitis-dependent changes in lung function. *Am. Rev. Respir. Dis.,* 1983 Aug.; 128(2): 256 - 65.

[28] Poulter, L. W., Rossi, G. A., Bjermer, L., Costabel, U., Israel-Biet, D., Klech, H., Pohl, W., Velluti, G. The value of bronchoalveolar lavage in the diagnosis and prognosis of sarcoidosis. *Eur. Respir. J.,* 1990 Sep.; 3(8): 943 - 4.

[29] Winterbauer, R. H., Lammert, J., Selland, M., Wu, R., Corley, D., Springmeyer, S. C. Bronchoalveolar lavage cell populations in the diagnosis of sarcoidosis. *Chest,* 1993 Aug.; 104(2): 352 - 61.

[30] Allen, J. N., Davis, W. B., Pacht, E. R. Diagnostic significance of increased bronchoalveolar lavage fluid eosinophils. *Am. Rev. Respir. Dis.,* 1990 Sep.; 142(3): 642 - 7.

[31] Pope-Harman, A. L., Davis, W. B., Allen, E. D., Christoforidis, A. J., Allen, J. N. Acute eosinophilic pneumonia: a summary of 15 cases and review of the literature. *Medicine,* (Baltimore). 1996 Nov.; 75(6): 334 - 42.

[32] Sitbon, O., Bidel, N., Dussopt, C., Azarian, R., Braud, M. L., Lebargy, F., Fourme, T., de Blay, F., Piard, F., Camus, P. Minocycline pneumonitis and eosinophilia: a report on eight patients. *Arch. Intern. Med.,* 1994 Jul. 25; 154•14):1633 - 40.

[33] Costabel, U., Uzaslan, E., Guzman, J. Bronchoalveolar lavage in drug-induced lung disease. *Clin. Chest Med.,* 2004 Mar.; 25(1): 25 - 35.

[34] Meyer, K. C., Raghu, G., Baughman, R. P., Brown, K. K., Costabel, U., du Bois, R. M., Drent, M., Haslam, P. L., Kim, D. S., Nagai, S., Rottoli, P., Saltini, C., Selman, M., Strange, C., Wood, B.; American Thoracic Society Committee on BAL in Interstitial Lung Disease. An Official American Thoracic Society Clinical Practice Guideline: The Clinical Utility of Bronchoalveolar Lavage Cellular Analysis in Interstitial Lung Disease. *Am. J. Respir. Crit. Care Med.,* 2012 May 1; 185(9): 1004 - 14.

[35] Richter, A. G., Stockley, R. A., Harper, L. et al. Pulmonary infection in Wegener granulomatosis and idiopathic pulmonary fibrosis. *Thorax,* 2009; 64: 692 - 697.

[36] Knippenberg, S., Ueberberg, B., Maus, R. et al. Streptococcus pneumoniae triggers progression of pulmonary fibrosis through pneumolysin. *Thorax,* 2015; 70: 636 - 646.

[37] Molyneaux, P. L., Cox, M. J., Wells, A. U. et al. Changes in the respiratory microbiome during acute exacerbations of idiopathic pulmonary fibrosis. *Respir. Res.*, 2017; 18: 29.

In: Respiratory Ventilatory Strategies …
Editor: Antonio M. Esquinas
ISBN: 978-1-53617-847-0
© 2020 Nova Science Publishers, Inc.

Chapter 17

DIAGNOSTIC PROCEDURES IN IDIOPATHIC PULMONARY FIBROSIS: BRONCHOSCOPY AND OTHER PROCEDURES

Bahman Saatian[1,2,*], MD and Monique Patel[2], MD
[1]Department of Medicine, Pulmonary and Critical Care Section, Veterans Affairs Long Beach Healthcare System, Long Beach, CA, US
[2]Department of Medicine, UC Irvine, Irvine, CA, US

ABSTRACT

Idiopathic pulmonary fibrosis (IPF) is a progressive form of interstitial lung disease of unknown cause. Comprehensive history, physical examination and noninvasive diagnostic testing are required to exclude other causes of interstitial lung diseases. Diagnosis of IPF may be established based on usual interstitial pneumonia (UIP) characteristic findings on high-resolution CT scan and compatible clinical history. Lung biopsy is required to establish a diagnosis when HRCT pattern is suggestive of probable UIP, indeterminate for UIP or an alternative diagnosis. The potential values of establishing the diagnosis of IPF include discontinuation of harmful medications such as systemic steroid, starting recently Food and Drug Administration (FDA) approved medications and timely referral to lung transplant centers. It also has prognostic value given the average life expectancy is similar to many advanced cancers. Bronchoscopic transbronchial lung biopsy using forceps and / or cryoprobe and surgical lung biopsy are the main modalities for obtaining lung tissues for the diagnosis of IPF.

---

* Corresponding Author's E-mail: bsaatian@uci.edu.

Keywords: idiopathic pulmonary fibrosis, high resolution CT scan, usual interstitial pneumonia, transbronchial lung biopsy, surgical lung biopsy

INTRODUCTION

Idiopathic pulmonary fibrosis (IPF) is a chronic progressive form of interstitial lung disease of unknown cause. Diagnosis of IPF requires a detailed history of medications, environmental exposure and underlying rheumatologic disorders to exclude other causes of interstitial lung disease (ILD). Current diagnostic criteria for interstitial lung disease can rely on clinical evaluation, pulmonary function testing, and high-resolution CT (HRCT). The results of these tests guide the decision of whether bronchoscopic, thoracoscopic, or surgical lung biopsy is required to provide additional diagnostic or prognostic value.

Pattern of high-resolution CT scan of chest may suggest definite unusual interstitial pneumonia (UIP), probable UIP, indeterminate for UIP or an alternative diagnosis [1]. The new diagnostic criteria for radiology and histopathology are more precise than previously and now include three radiographic categories and four histological categories, namely 1) UIP, 2) possible UIP and 3) inconsistent with UIP for HRCT, and 1) UIP, 2) probable UIP, 3) possible UIP and 4) not UIP for histopathology.

American Thoracic Society (ATS) / European Thoracic Society (ERS) /Japanese Respiratory Society (JRS) / Latin American Thoracic Association (ALAT) practice guidelines recommended flexible bronchoscopy and bronchioalveolar lavage (BAL) and surgical lung biopsy to establish a diagnosis when high resolution CT scan (HRCT) pattern is suggestive of probable UIP, indeterminate for UIP or an alternative diagnosis [1]. ATS did not make recommendation for or against transbronchial lung biopsy (TBBX) or lung cryobiopsy. No diagnostic procedures were suggested by ATS/ERS/JRP/ALAT for patients with IPF who have HRCT pattern of UIP.

DIAGNOSTIC PROCEDURES

Bronchoscopy and Bronchoalveolar Lavage (BAL)

In evaluation of patients with possible IPF, cellular analysis of bronchoalveolar lavage is routinely recommended for exclusion of infection and other interstitial lung diseases such as chronic hypersensitivity pneumonitis (HP), nonspecific interstitial pneumonia (NSIP) and connective tissue disease-interstital lung disease (CTD-ILD) [1,3]. The disgnostic value of BAL lies in presence or absence of lymphocytosis. In large series of patients, Walker and colleagues demonstrated a BAL lymphocyte count of < 30% was associated with 90% reduction in the likelihood of HP [2]. In a retrospective study, Ohshimo et al., showed that six of 74 patients (8%) with high resolution CT scan UIP pattern had lymphocytosis of 30% or greater in BAL [3]. The final diagnoses of HP or NSAIP were made on further evaluation [3]. The 2011 ATS / ERS guidelines recommended BAL cellular analysis should not be performed in most patients given it is unclear BAL has a significant diagnostic value in the right clinical setting [1].

Lung Biopsy

There are two main biopsy modalities for diagnosis of IPF: bronchoscopic transbronchial lung biopsy (TBLB) and surgical lung biopsy (SLB). Recently, transbronchial lung biopsy with a cryoprobe (TBLC) has attracted attention. TBLC is a novel technique that allows obtaining larger samples with fewer artifacts as compared to conventional TBLB [4].

Indications

Lung biopsies should be considered in the setting of atypical features [5]. These atypical features include age < 50 years, fever, weight loss, or hemoptysis, which may confound diagnosis. Lung biopsy may also be required for evaluation of atypical or rapidly changing HRCT findings, unexplained extrapulmonary manifestations or pulmonary vascular disease of unclear origin, and probable or possible UIP. Lung biopsy may be indicated to exclude neoplastic and infectious processes that may mimic ILD [6]. It may also be indicated to identify a more treatable process than originally suspected, for instance differentiating hypersensitivity pneumonitis from idiopathic pulmonary fibrosis. It can aid in predicting the likelihood of response to therapies, particularly for therapies with serious side effects [7]. Rarely, it can be used to diagnose ILD in patients with hypoxemia and pulmonary function tests (PFT) suggestive of ILD, with a normal HRCT. The decision to pursue biopsy also involves patient preference. Some patients may prefer initial observation over several months with reevaluation with repeat pulmonary function tests and HRCT before proceeding to biopsy.

Contraindications

Relative contraindications have been implicated in all types of biopsies. One relative contraindication includes diffuse end-stage disease seen on HRCT, since biopsy of end-stage fibrosis is unlikely to reveal an etiology. Extensive pleural disease or emphysema also increases the risk of biopsy and decisions in these cases must be on case-by-case basis. Severe pulmonary dysfunction evidenced by DLCO < 35% predicted, severe hypoxemia or mechanical ventilation are also relative contraindications [9]. Patients with these relative contraindications may undergo transbronchial lung biopsy as opposed to surgical lung biopsy.

Transbronchial Lung Biopsy (TBLB)

TBLB has a potential role in guiding diagnosis and may be indicated when clinical and HRCT data are suggestive, but not diagnostic of UIP. It can increase clinician confidence in IPF diagnosis or the need for further biopsy. Additionally, it is generally the preferred procedure when ILD is suspected to have a centrilobular location; this gives TBLB a higher likelihood of diagnostic success. Centrilobular diseases include sarcoidosis, hypersensitivity pneumonitis, lymphangitic carcinomatosis, eosinophilic pneumonia, and pulmonary alveolar proteinosis. TBLB is also preferred when small samples of lung tissue can be used to make diagnosis. In patients with sarcoidosis, TBLB has a 70% diagnostic rate. In a recent case series by Sheth et al, TBLB in addition to a possible UIP pattern on HRCT resulted in a confident IPF diagnosis [7].

Diagnostic Limitations

Biopsy results from TBLB are usually around 1-3mm in size and are therefore subject to crush artifact. There are also limitations when disease is patchy given small biopsy size and when whole pulmonary acini is needed for diagnosis. Additionally, areas of more diffuse fibrotic nonspecific interstitial pneumonia-like fibrosis cannot be seen on transbronchial biopsy.

Diagnosis of UIP requires features of repetitive combination of fibrosis, fibroblastic foci and microscopic honeycombing with intervening normal lunch parenchyma. This pathology requires low power visualization of gross architectural features which is difficult to attain from small transbronchial samples [8].

Safety

TBLB is minimally invasive with estimated mortality < 0.05%. Pneumothorax is estimated to occur in 0.7-2%. Bilateral TBLB are not recommended during single procedure due to high risk of bilateral iatrogenic pneumothorax [9].

Diagnostic Yield

The diagnostic yield for TBLB is variable and influenced by size and risk of crush artifact. The number of specimens is based on patient's tolerance of procedure. Few case series have shown that average of 5-6 biopsies per patient gave overall diagnostic yield of 50% [8]. Compared to prior studies, Sheth et al. showed 18% of TBLB specimens were inadequate, mostly due to crush artifact [7]. Additional testing can be performed during the TBLB to either aid diagnosis or provide evidence against a diagnosis. Endobronchial biopsies are helpful in patients suspected of having sarcoidosis or chronic beryllium disease. Endobronchial ultrasound-guided transbronchial needle aspiration (EBUS-TBNA) is used for evaluation of hilar and mediastinal lymph nodes.

Transbronchial Lung Cryobiopsy (TBLC)

Transbronchial lung cryobiopsy has focused on the diagnosis of diffuse parenchymal lung diseases since traditional forceps cause crush artifact and provide small sample sizes. The use of cryobiopsy in patients with central and peribronchial interstitial processes is gaining acceptance. It is difficult to draw any clear conclusions about procedural technique, safety, and yield due to lack of consistency in methodology, uniform reporting on yield and complications and lack of direct comparison to surgical lung biopsy in the available studies [10].

Procedure

Transbronchial lung cryobiopsy is a relatively new procedure for lung biopsy. Authors recommend patients to be intubated with a rigid tracheoscope [11] or a large endotracheal tube [4] given the risk of significant bleeding although it can be performed under moderate sedation and using a flexible bronchoscopy and cryoprobe [10]. The cryoprobe is advanced through the working channel of the flexible bronchoscope. The tip of the probe is applied to the area of interest. The optimal area is considered a distance < 10 mm from pleura. Within seconds, nitrous oxide or carbon dioxide rapidly cools tip of cryoprobe to -79C or -89C respectively under fluoroscopy guidance. The adjacent tissue is frozen for 3-5 seconds which is then removed *en-bloc* with the bronchoscope, since the sample is larger than the working channel [7]. The efferent channel allows the gas to escape down and vent to the atmosphere. It is recommended to place a Fogarty balloon or endobronchial blocker prophylactically in proximity of biopsy segment to minimize the bleeding [11].

Diagnostic Yield

Transbronchial cryobiopsy provides biopsy samples larger and with better quality than forceps biopsy samples. The samples are typically 7-10mm in size. Given the larger biopsy size and better quality, the optimum number of biopsies for best diagnostic yield is around 4 samples. However, there is little consistency in technique between studies, making information regarding safety and diagnostic yield unclear. In a randomized control trial by Pajares et al, cryobiopsy showed a diagnostic yield of 74% compared to 34.1% with TBLB [18]. Although overall complications were similar, the incidence of moderate bleeding was higher in the cryobiopsy group compared to TBLB group (56.4% vs 34.2%). When comparing surgical lung biopsy, data is limited to diffuse pulmonary parenchymal lung disease (DPLD). An intriguing cross-sectional study by Tomassetti and colleagues compared TLCB with SLB and evaluated the impact of these two biopsy modalities on the diagnostic confidence for IPF in the multidisciplinary group discussion [18]. Biopsy data in providing definitive diagnosis was not significantly different between cryobiopsy and surgical lung biopsy. Ravaglia et al., compared the diagnostic yield and safety of TBLC and SLB in a met-analysis of including 447 cases with ILD [11]. The diagnostic yield was higher for SLB at 98.7% compared to cryobiopsy at 82.8%. Interestingly, diagnostic yield from diagnostic confidence was not significantly improved between two groups (29% to 63% with TBLC and 30% to 65% with SLB) when biopsy data were provided. Length of hospital stay, and mortality were lower in TBLC group (2.6 days, 0.3% vs 6.9 days, 2.7%) [10]. Met-analysis of 11 studies by Johnson et al. including 731 patients demonstrated 78% (74-98%) diagnostic yield with cryobiopsy when used in isolation and 86% (51-98%) when discussed in multidisciplinary group setting [12]. Dhooria et al. reported diagnostic yield for TBLC was 76.9-85.9% in met analysis of 14 studies [13].

Safety

The procedure is generally safe; however, pneumothorax, moderate to severe bleeding and rarely death have been reported. Due to its larger sample size, cryobiopsy has the potential to cause greater pleural or vascular disruption and therefore, the complication rate of pneumothorax or hemorrhage, may be higher. Moderate bleeding was noted to be 56.4% in cryobiopsy group compared to 34.2% in TBLB [10]. A recent prospective randomized, multicenter, cross-over study showed significantly greater risk of moderate and severe bleeding in cryobiopsy group compared to TBLB group (moderate 15% / 4.2% and severe 1.2% / 0%) [20]. Several methods to limit airway bleeding are being adopted. The use of bronchial blockers placed proximal to biopsied segment controls emergent hemorrhage, while bronchoscopic techniques through scope tamponade or iced saline can manage milder bleeds. Additionally, compared to surgical lung biopsy, one study with Ravaglia et al., showed decreased length of hospital stay and mortality in patients who underwent cryobiopsy compared to surgical lung biopsy [11]. However, persistent fever, prolong air leak and acute exacerbation of ILD was higher in SLB cases [10]. The mean rate of pneumothorax and bleeding were 8.8% (0-25.9%) and 26.6% (0-78%) respectively in met analysis by Johnson et al., [12]. A larger met analysis reporting on 1183 patients showed complications included pneumothorax (6.8%), severe bleeding (0.3%) and death (0.1%) [13].

Surgical Lung Biopsy (SLB)

Historically, surgical lung biopsy has been considered gold standard in diagnosis of IPF. The new guidelines and statements have recommended a multidisciplinary approach for the ultimate diagnosis. SLB is currently considered for the patients with non-typical IPF who do not fulfill criteria for UIP pattern on HRCT. For a "probable" UIP pattern, the decision to pursue biopsy should be based on pre-test probability for IPF, the confidence in the HRCT diagnosis, and the risks of perioperative mortality. For an indeterminate UIP radiographic pattern or radiographic findings suggesting an "alternative diagnosis," a surgical lung biopsy should be considered to evaluate for non-IPF diagnoses [1].

There are two subpopulations in which surgical lung biopsy is not necessary since biopsy adds little diagnostic or prognostic information; systemic rheumatic disease and undiagnosed ILD in setting of respiratory failure. In patients with systemic rheumatic disease, HRCT provides specificity and PPV of 96% and 95% respectively [14]. For patients with acute respiratory failure in setting of new interstitial lung disease, surgical biopsy does not lead to a better outcome since the severity of disease limits diagnosis and therapeutic options. Additionally, there is increase perioperative mortality with surgical lung biopsy in these patients [15].

Procedure

Surgical specimens are obtained by video assisted thoracoscopic surgery (VATS) or thoracotomy. VATS is minimally invasive, and incisions are typically small. One lung ventilation is performed during surgery to allow the target lung to be deflated and easily biopsied. Thoracotomy involves a larger incision and one lung ventilation is not required [16]. VATS is associated with less morbidity; however, this may be skewed since thoracotomies are necessary in the setting of severe pleural disease, bleeding diathesis or in patients with severe hypoxemia. In these settings, one lung ventilation is not recommended, and these more critical patients require thoracotomy [16].

Diagnostic Yield

Diagnostic yield can range from 85-92% with the appropriate samples [5]. An adequate sample size of at least 3x2x1 cm^3 and at least two specimens from separate lobes allow for greater diagnostic yield. Surgical lung biopsies are substantially larger (several centimeters in diameter) than those obtained by other types of biopsy. For diffuse parenchymal lung disease suspected on HRCT, surgical lung biopsy has a diagnostic yield of approximately 90%, as compared to 20-30% with TBLB. Samples from VATS and thoracotomies have similar diagnostic yields [17]. It is ideal if surgical lung biopsies can be performed prior to initiation of systemic glucocorticoids or other immunosuppressive therapy for improved yield.

Safety

In patients undergoing elective SLB, in-hospital mortality was found to be 1.7%, and overall complication rate (including pneumothorax, pneumonia, and respiratory failure) was 30% [16]. In-hospital mortality rate for non-elective biopsies was 16%. High risk factors for increased mortality include preoperative hypoxemia and acute exacerbation of ILD. The presence of hypoxemia preoperatively correlated with worse outcomes [10]. Additionally, patients on single lung ventilation are at higher risk of developing postoperative non-cardiogenic pulmonary edema in the lung contralateral to the biopsied lung [15]. Therefore, lung protective ventilation is commonly practiced when performing thoracotomies. Surgical lung biopsies have been less common for ILD due to noninvasive definitive diagnosis of IPF and adoption of multidisciplinary discussion as the preferred approach to diagnosis.

Conclusion

Accurate diagnosis of IPF involves a multifactorial evaluation and multidisciplinary team, involving pulmonologists, radiologists and pathologists. The process requires comprehensive clinical evaluation, pulmonary function tests, and chest imaging. Further investigation with bronchoscopy with biopsy and/or surgical lung biopsy is necessary if initial investigations are unable to provide a confident diagnosis. Traditional transbronchial lung biopsy, transbronchial cryobiopsy and surgical lung biopsy have varying roles in aiding diagnosis, and which modality is best suited for the patient depends on each case individually. ATS/ERS/JRS/ALAT guidelines recommend patients with suspected ILD and HRCT with probable UIP, indeterminate of UIP or alternative diagnosis undergo BAL or surgical lung biopsy for diagnosis. Given the lack of evidence, recommendations were not made regarding cryobiopsy or transbronchial biopsy. However, transbronchial biopsies should be considered for central or peribronchial diseases such as sarcoidosis, berylliosis, pulmonary alveolar proteinosis or lymphangitic carcinomatosis. Many IPF patients are older and have multiple comorbidities, making SLB a higher risk procedure. While there are limitations to TBLB and cryopbiopsy, these new diagnostic tools may have fewer risks, make diagnosing ILD more accurate and safer.

REFERENCES

[1] Raghu, G., Collard, Harold R., Egan, Jim J., Martinez, Fernando J., Behr, J., Brown, Kevin K., Colby, Thomas V., Cordier, JF., Flaherty, Kevin R., Lasky, Joseph A., Lynch, David A., Ryu, Jay H., Swigris, Jeffrey J., Wells, Athol U., Ancochea, J., Bouros, D., Carvalho, C., Costabel, U., Ebina, M., Hansell, David M., Johkoh, T., Kim, Dong S., King Jr, Talmadge E., Kondoh, Y., Myers, J., Muller, Nestor L., Nicholson, Andrew G., Richeldi, L., Selman, M., Dudden, Rosalind F., Griss, Barbara S., Protzko, Shandra L., Schunemann, Holger J. (2011). An official ATS/ERS/JRS/ALAT statement: Idiopathic pulmonary fibrosis: Evidence-bases guidelines for diagnosis and management. *Am. J. Respir. Crit. Care Med.* Vol 183. Pp 788-824.

[2] Welker, L, Jorres, RA, Costabel U, Magnussen, H. (2004). Predictive value of BAL cell differentials in the diagnosis of interstitial lung diseases. *Eur. Respir. J.* 24:1000-1006.

[3] Ohshimo, S, Bonella F, Cui A, Beume M., Kohno N., Guzman J., Costabel U. (2009). Significance of bronchoalveolar lavage for the diagnosis of idiopathic pulmonary fibrosis. *Am. J. Respir. Crit. Care Med.* 179:1043–1047.

[4] Lentz, RJ., Taylor Trevor M., Kropski, Jonathan A., et al., (2018). Utility of flexible cryobiopsy for diagnosis of diffuse parenchymal lung diseases. *J. Bronchology Interv. Pulmonol.* 25(2): 88-96.

[5] Raj, R., Raparia, K., Lynch, David A., Brown, Kevin K. (2017). Surgical lung biopsy for interstitial lung diseases. *CHEST.* 151.5: 1131-1140.

[6] Nicholson, Andrew G., Fulford Laura G., Colby, Thomas V., du Bios, Ronald M., Hansell, David M., Wells, Athol U. (2002). The relationship between individual

histologic features and disease progression in idiopathic pulmonary fibrosis. *American Journal of Respiratory and Critical Care medicine*. 166.2: 173-177.

[7] Sheth, Jamie S., Belperio, John A., Fishbein, Michael C., Kazerooni, Ella A., Lagstein, A., Murray, S., Myers, Jeff L., Simon, Richard H., Sisson, Thomas H., Sundaram B., White, Eric S., Xia, M., Zisman, D., Flaherty, Kevin R. (2017). Utility of transbronchial vs surgical lung biopsy in the diagnosis of suspected fibrotic interstitial lung disease. *CHEST*. 151.2: 389-399.

[8] Wall, CP., Gaensler, EA., Carrington, CB., and Hayes, KA. (1981). Comparison of transbronchial and open biopsies in chronic infiltrative lung diseases. *American Review of Respiratory Disease* 123.3: 280-285.

[9] Kebbe, J., and Abdo, T. (2017). Interstitial lung disease: the diagnostic role of bronchoscopy. *Journal of thoracic disease* 9. Suppl 10 S996.

[10] Lentz, RJ., Argento AC., Colby TV., Rickman OB., Maldonado F. (2017). Transbronchial cryobiopsy for diffuse parenchymal lung disease: a state-of-art review of procedural techniques, current evidence, and future challenges. *Journal of Thoracic Disease*. 9(7):2186-2203.

[11] Ravaglia, C., Wells, Athol U., Tomassetti, S., Gurioli, C., Gurioli Ch., Dubini, A., Cavazza, A., Colby, Thomas V., Piciucchi, S., Puglisi, S., Bosi, M., Poletti, V. (2019). Diagnostic yield and risk/benefit analysis of trans-bronchial lung cryobiopsy in diffuse parenchymal lung diseases: a large cohort of 699 patients. *BMC Pulmonary Medicine.* 19.1: 16.

[12] Johnson, KA, Marcoux VS, Ronksley PE, et al., (2016). Diagnostic yield and complications of transbronchial lung cryobiosy for interstitial lung disease. A systematic review and metanalysis. *Ann, Am, Thorac, Soc.* 13:1828-38.

[13] Dhooria, S, Sehgal IS, Aggarwal AN, et al., (2016). Diagnostic yield and safety of cryoprobe transbronchial lung biopsy in diffuse parenchymal lung diseases: Systematic review and metanalysis. *Respir. Care.* 61:700-12.

[14] Kim, EJ., Collard, H., and King Jr, TE., (2009). Rheumatoid arthritis-associated interstitial lung disease: the relevance of histopathologic and radiographic pattern. *CHEST*. 136.5: 1397-1405.

[15] Chuang, ML., Lin, IF., Tsai, YH., and Pang, LC. (2003). The utility of open lung biopsy in patients with diffuse pulmonary infiltrates as related to respiratory distress, its impact on decision making by urgent intervention, and the diagnostic accuracy based on the biopsy location. *Journal of intensive care medicine* 18.1: 21-28.

[16] Ayed, A. K., and R. Raghunathan. (2000). Thoracoscopy versus open lung biopsy in the diagnosis of interstitial lung disease: a randomised controlled trial. *Journal of the Royal College of Surgeons of Edinburgh*. 45.3: 159-163.

[17] Ravini, M., Ferraro, G., Barbieri, B., Colombo, P., and Rizzato, G.(1998). Changing strategies of lung biopsies in diffuse lung diseases: the impact of video-assisted thoracoscopy. *European Respiratory Journal.* 11.1: 99-103.

[18] Pajares, V., Puzo, C., Castillo, D., Lerma, E., Montero, M. A., Ramos-Barbon, D., Armor-Carro, O., Gil de Bernabe, A., Franquet, T., Plaza, V., Hetzel, J., Sanchis, J., Torrego, A. (2014). Diagnostic yield of transbronchial cryobiopsy in interstitial lung disease: A randomized trial: Transbronchial cryobiosy. *Respirology.* 19:900-6.

[19] Tomassetti, S., Wells, AU., Costabel, U., Cavazza, A., Colby, TV., Rossi, G., Sverzellati, N., Carloni, A., Carretta, E., Buccioli, M., Tantalocco, P., Ravaglia, C., Gurioli, C., Dubini, A., Piciucchi, S., Ryu, JH., Poletti, V. (2016). Bronchoscopic Lung Cryobiopsy Increases Diagnostic Confidence in the Multidisciplinary Diagnosis of Idiopathic Pulmonary Fibrosis. *Am. J. Respir. Crit. Care Med.* 1;193(7):745-52.

[20] Hetzel, j., Eberhardt, R., Petermann, C., Gesierich, W., Darwiche, K., Hagmeyer, L., Muche, R., Kreuter, M., Lewis, R., Ehab, A., Boeckeler, M., Haentschel, (2019). M. Bleeding risk of transbronchial cryobiopsy compared to transbronchial forceps biopsy in interstitial lung disease- a prospective, randomized, multicenter cross-over trial. *Respiratory Research.* 20:140.

In: Respiratory Ventilatory Strategies …
Editor: Antonio M. Esquinas
ISBN: 978-1-53617-847-0
© 2020 Nova Science Publishers, Inc.

Chapter 18

OXYGEN THERAPY IN PATIENTS WITH FIBROTIC INTERSTITIAL LUNG DISEASE

Giuseppe Fiorentino[1], MD, Anna Annunziata[2], MD and Maurizia Lanza[2], MD
[1]Head of Unit of Respiratory Physiopathology, Monaldi Hospital, Naples, Italy
[2]Unit of Respiratory Physiopathology, Monaldi Hospital, Naples, Italy

ABSTRACT

Patients with Fibrotic Interstitial Lung Disease have a poor prognosis and have symptoms that destroy quality of life. Patients usually develop hypoxemia due to multiplied physiologic derangements, including diffusion limitation, ventilation-perfusion mismatching, and abnormalities of the pulmonary vasculature. Many patients will require supplemental oxygen at some point in the course of their disease, and although it can increase blood oxygen and symptoms, it also creates physical and emotional challenges for patients and their cherished ones. Oxygen supplementation is typically use in patients with advanced lung disease with resting hypoxemia; however, there is a paucity of evidence guiding the use of supplemental oxygen in ILD, and significant heterogeneity in clinical practice. It rests unclear whether supplemental oxygen improves clinically significant outcomes, and the role of ambulatory oxygen supplementation in isolated exertional hypoxemia is not yet explicit today.

Keywords: interstitial lung disease, idiopatic pulmonary fibrosis, oxygen therapy, quality of life

ABBREVIATIONS

Chronic obstructive pulmonary disease	COPD
Idiopatic pulmonary fibrosis	IPF
Interstitial lung disease	ILD
Long-term oxygen therapy	LTOT
Medical Research Council	MRC
Nocturnal Oxygen Therapy Trial	NOTT
Oxygen therapy	O2 therapy

INTRODUCTION

Interstitial lung disease (ILD) is an area of increasing interest in respiratory medicine. People with ILD show a range of specific acute or chronic progressive parenchymal alterations in their lung structure. These conditions are marked by changing levels of pulmonary inflammation and fibrosis. While some ILDs can be quickly reversible, a large proportion results in unchangeable fibrosis, which appears in the impairment of gas exchange and respiratory volumes due to alveolar damage or loss. This directs to hypoxaemia in some individuals, both on exertion and at rest. The usual common ILD is idiopathic pulmonary fibrosis (IPF). The incidence of IPF appears to be higher in North America and Europe (3 to 9 cases per 100,000 person-years) than in South America and East Asia (fewer than 4 cases per 100,000 person-years). IPF is a fatal disease with a median survival of three years, which is more severe than that of many cancers. Dyspnoea is controlled with drugs and supportive therapies, together with assistance from palliative care specialists. Unfortunately, there is not adequate data to indicate the most accurate management for these events. Over the past five years, strategies have become available for a number of ILDs, particularly IPF, and there is some clear evidence that disease improvement can be achieved and fibrosis lessened with these interventions. But most people with IPF and several others with ILD will get worse over time. This leads to continuous hypoxemia, limitation of exercise, pulmonary heart and ultimately death. The number of interventions targeted at manifestation relief that have a strong data base in ILD is quite low. Despite the current approaches to pharmacotherapy, many patients with ILD have limited treatment options [1]. Long-term oxygen therapy (LTOT) is used for people with resting hypoxemia, while a range of antitussive agents can be provided for cough treatment [1]. Oxygen therapy is usually prescribed for people with ILD, to reduce breathlessness and increase physical capacity through increased gas exchange. Despite its regular use, there is a lack of data to support the efficacy of oxygen therapy in ILD. A previous systematic review included only one small study long-term on oxygen therapy

(LTOT) is left unprinted and assumed that there was no impact on survival. Although, there is an association well accepted in the use of LTOT and an increase in health outcomes in people with chronic obstructive pulmonary disease (COPD), suggesting the possibility that LTOT may have comparable effects nell'ILD. A recent review of walking oxygen therapy in the ILD eliminated several studies that examined the results of oxygen when measuring exercise in the ILD, so that no results could be expressed on your impression of symptoms or performance [2]. This Cochrane review comprised three randomized controlled trials (RCTs) that examined supplemental (ambulatory) oxygen to medical air in patients with interstitial lung disease (ILD), and all only selected patients with idiopathic pulmonary fibrosis (IPF). The ambulatory oxygen has not appeared in a better exercise capacity or dyspnea in two studies combined. However, none of these studies require adequate oxygen titration for the exact desaturation of stress, which may have altered the results. The resting included study did show an increase in resistance time at regular load cycle ergometry with oxygen and also expressed that the intervention had increased oxygen saturations during the test. Moreover, none of these studies has estimated the reproducibility of recognition supplemental oxygen [2].

Why Use Oxygen Therapy in ILD

The subjects with advanced ILD usually reveal hypoxemia due to multiplied physiological disorders, including lack of diffusion, ventilation-perfusion mismatch and aberrations of the pulmonary vascular system. Exercise desaturation can be serious in some patients with ILD, causing exertional dyspnea which is distressing and related to sadness, impaired work and reduced quality of life [3]. Hypoxemia during training reduces the maximum workload and resistance point, mitigating the benefits obtained from pulmonary rehabilitation [4]. This is the largest RCT of nell'ILD exercise and the first to confirm the impact of the etiology and severity of the disease on response to training. We confirmed clinically important increases in 6MWD, symptoms and HRQoL following year, confirming previous results and producing compelling evidence for the workout to be taken as prescribed treatment for all patients with ILD. This study determined that people with asbestosis and IPF, and to a lesser extent CTD-ILD, receive clinically essential benefits and that the severity of the disease requires long-term benefits with continuous therapeutic effects that favor the milder disease. A further choice for the story was that successfully combining exercise progression maximizes benefits. Limited changes in dyspnea, strength, anxiety and depression have been observed. The diversity of strength may not have been significant enough to overcome the change in determination between the two assessors or the resistance training may not have been delivered with adequate intensity to produce significant changes in strength. The limited change in anxiety and depression was likely attributed to the low numbers of participants with clinically significant anxiety and depression at baseline. Although this study may not have been sufficiently powered to see an effect on MMRC dyspnoea, or this measure may not be sensitive enough to detect changes following exercise [4]. Hypoxemia can also provide progress of pulmonary hypertension, a significant prognostic comorbidity point of view without a proven cure ILD. Supplemental oxygen can correct many of these inopportune changes; but, there is no agreement on the defined threshold below which the integration of oxygen is justified because of inadequate data and discrepant. Despite the lack of data, the additional clinical oxygen is used dall'11-28% of patients with idiopathic pulmonary fibrosis mild to moderate at the time of enrollment in the clinical trial [5]. The management of continuous supplemental oxygen for resting hypoxemia in ILD is first extrapolated from data in patients with chronic obstructive pulmonary disease (COPD) that were declared over 35 years ago. The Nocturnal Oxygen Therapy Trial (NOTT) and Medical Research Council (MRC) studies were randomized controlled analyses that showed a death benefit of supplemental oxygen in COPD patients with unmanageable resting hypoxemia, demonstrated survival benefits of providing long-term oxygen therapy to patients with resting arterial partial pressure of oxygen consistently less than 55 mmHg [6]. Furthermore inadequate studies have since confirmed that supplemental oxygen increases oxygen transfer, cardiac output, arterial oxygen content, minute ventilation, exertional dyspnea and exercise tolerance in patients with COPD with hypoxemia. Extrapolating these data, IPF clinical practice guidelines make a powerful support for the use of oxygen in sufferers with resting oxygen saturations under 88% [7], despite no direct indication of advantage in this clinical setting. Supported by the Research for Patient Benefit Program of the National Institute for Health Research, the Ambulatory oxygen in fibrotic lung disease (Ambox) was a multicenter, randomized, controlled, crossover controlled trials (RCTs). The study examines the ambulatory oxygen used during daily activities without ambulatory oxygen in patients with fibrotic lung disease whose oxygen saturation (SaO2) is ≥94% at rest, but it comes down to ≤88% in a walk test of six minutes. The randomized controlled trial (RCT) estimate the effects on health status (measured by the King's Brief ILD Questionnaire: K-BILD) of ambulatory oxygen used at home, at an optimal flux rate defined by titration at the screening visit, and administered for two weeks, compared to 2 weeks off oxygen. Key secondary outcomes incorporate breathlessness on activity scores as measured by the University of California San Diego Shortness of Breath Questionnaire, global patient assessment of change scores, as well as quality of life scores (St George's Respiratory Questionnaire), anxiety and depression scores (Hospital Anxiety and Depression Scale), activity markers regulated by SenseWear Armbands, pulse oximetry measures, patient-reported daily activities, patient- and oxygen company-reported oxygen cylinder use. The study also includes a qualitative element in interviews and explore patients' realities of the use of a portable oxygen supply and trial participation in a subgroup of 20 patients and carers [7]. This study is the first to prospectively assess the influence of oxygen in ambulatory patients with fibrotic ILD and to explore the results for which it is most effective, the advantage predictors and patient variables/features related to the lack of response. This study makes a necessary precursor to the development of ILD-specific guidelines on ambulatory oxygen use. Ultimately, if proven to be practical and inexpensive, the appropriate prescription and use of ambulatory oxygen should lead to prolonged patient independence and mobility, allowing the maintenance of fitness levels and active roles in daily life, with a greater psychological and physical well-being, such as potentially related health-related costs [7]. No high-quality studies are evaluating the utility of supplemental oxygen in ILD subjects who desaturate exclusively with exertion. A current study of cases of stationary COPD with hypoxemia to moderate rest or exercise-induced hypoxemia average has not observed any influence on the working capacity of supplemental oxygen, on quality of life, on the need for hospitalization or death. Patients with severe ILD usually have more accelerated and also critical exertional hypoxemia matched to COPD, proposing that it is probable inapt to extrapolate these data to ILD. Observational research of 133 IPF cases with moderate exertional hypoxemia notified no death advantage of supplemental oxygen; despite, however, the study was underpowered to identify a key benefit. Double-blind placebo-controlled crossover research of 20 IPF patients with exertional desaturation affirmed that breathing 4 liters per minute of supplemental nasal oxygen spikes did not improve 6-minute walk distance compared to breathing room air. Diversity, some small investigations in cases with ILD confirm that breathing supplemental oxygen or hyperoxia during exercise period increases endurance, walk distance, dyspnea, maximal oxygen uptake, and maximal workload [8]. These studies have significant limitations, including small reproduction sizes, usually retrospective study, loss of blinding pretext with oxygen, and contradictory evidence of possible confounders such as condition or severity of pulmonary hypertension. It is more unclear whether some conclusions regard to subjects with resting or exertional hypoxemia, and what range of hypoxemia refusal must be achieved in sequence to obtain the clinical benefit. Besides, there are no studies that have adequately measured the volume of longer-term ambulatory oxygen supplementation in the patient group, and no studies have evaluated the quality of life. An open-ended randomized controlled trial will discuss some of certain restrictions by exploring possible practical and symptomatic advantages of supplemental oxygen during an 8-week exercise performance in patients with IPF who do not change for resting oxygen supplementation (ClinicalTrials.gov Identifier: NCT02551068) [9]. A supplementary randomized controlled crossover trial of walking oxygen will evaluate the longer-term role of supplemental oxygen for the practice of isolated exertional hypoxemia in patients with ILD (ClinicalTrials.gov Identifier NCT02286063) [7]. It is unclear whether oxygen supplementation may on the contrary be correlated with an improvement in the risk of serious exacerbation of ILD or other adverse effects. Although acute aggravations of IPF are added prevalent in patients with advanced illness, including common on oxygen supplementation, there are no results recommending toxicity of supplemental oxygen for stationary ILD subjects with resting or exertional hypoxemia. Severe exacerbations in patients with IPF receiving high amounts of oxygen occurred primarily in mechanically ventilated patients during surgical procedures and are not immediately applicable to an outpatient community. One small crossover study of IPF subjects obtained no difference in biomarkers of oxidative stress after activity while breathing supplemental oxygen matched to medical air, suggesting that oxygen is likely a secure intervention at least in the short-term. This study shows that oxygen increases exercise tolerance, exercise-induced hypoxaemia relieves and decreases exertional dyspnoea in patients with IPF. The supplemental oxygen can promote an increase in skeletal muscle metabolism through an increased release of oxygen. Supplemental oxygen may consequently be a beneficial adjunct to exercise training in IPF, optimizing physiological changes through increased endurance training time [10]. However, there persists a necessary for prospective studies to estimate the possible toxicity of oxygen in subjects with ILD.

References for Oxygen Supplementation in ILD

The 2011 IPF guideline, underwritten by different respiratory societies, supported that IPF patients with resting oxygen saturation <88% should be treated with supplemental oxygen; despite, specific criteria for patients by confined exertional hypoxemia were not afforded. A 2008 multi-Society guideline recommended that walking oxygen considered for IPF patients who are breathless, transportable, and who desaturate with exercise (oxygen saturation <90%), performed there is also improvement in exercise ability and breathlessness with supplemental oxygen. Guideline from the British Thoracic Society explains that long-term oxygen therapy may increase tissue oxygenation and survival in ILD subjects with chronic resting hypoxemia, while blocking complexities such as pulmonary hypertension, and recommends that ILD patients with intractable breathlessness could considered for palliative oxygen therapy [11]. Though, this additional guideline states that ambulatory oxygen should not be routinely administered to patients out chronic hypoxemia at rest (Grade B recommendation). The references presented in these guidelines are based principally on the expert conclusion given the scarcity of direct and robust evidence. The poor data and inadequacy of any cost report has likewise led to opinion-based local funding measures in many health areas; despite, these measures are frequently more limiting than current guideline references. The mutable funding criteria across health areas and their frequent misunderstandings with guideline recommendations have provided to the confusion among subjects and health care providers, mentioning the need for recommendations modernized guidelines sponsored by the main international community [11].

CRITERIA FOR OXYGEN SUPPLEMENTATION

Local models for the funding of supplemental oxygen are mixed with each supervisory agency that authorizes the policy for their local community and some agencies do not support all the oxygen for exertional hypoxemia. Standards for resting oxygen supplementation are typically compatible with the NOTT and MRC trials, including severe resting hypoxemia (PaO2 < 55 mmHg) or moderately severe resting hypoxemia (PaO2 < 60 mmHg) with complexities of chronic hypoxemia (e.g., cor pulmonale, polycythemia). Funding to ambulatory oxygen usually needs a mixture of exertional hypoxemia that is reversed by oxygen supplementation, with additional necessary in any areas of a tangible increase in both walk distance or dyspnea. Some regulatory actions support oxygen alone with desaturation at <80%, while others provide funding for ambulatory saturation <88% [11]. Some companies require also that particular criteria be met on tests taken out over various days, while others have complex pre-testing algorithms that requirement be met before patients are even available for trial and an increase in walk distance is required in some regions (e.g., improvement in walk distance of 30 meters and 20-25% matched to the walk distance completed on room air). Nevertheless, subjects with chronic lung disease can tolerate from important deconditioning that may impede important benefit of oxygen supplementation, intimating that a single test may not implement an adequate evaluation of potential benefit from longer-term oxygen supplementation. The United States' Centers for Medicare and Medicaid do not have a 'distance' criterion for oxygen funding; but, these criteria are likewise not evidence-based but preferably appear to rely on expert evaluation. Supplementary criteria exist inside specific areas and patient populations. Some administrative agencies demand that candidates for ambulatory oxygen supplementation first match criteria for 'severe lung disease'; though, the presented definition of 'severe lung disease' is extrapolated from fatality prediction criteria in IPF that have not been approved to predict benefit from supplemental oxygen in ILD or any other chronic lung disease [12]. Obviously, oxygen eligibility criteria for funding must be established, but the large variability in particular criteria that highlights the optimal metrics of evaluation and requirement for continuous ambulatory oxygen unclear.

ACCOMMODATION TO OXYGEN USE

Oxygen is a costly therapy that is not confirmed for some patients who appear to receive significant benefits. Some groups and areas have no funding for supplemental oxygen in samples of confined exertional hypoxemia, while any problems have substantial out-of-pocket expenses before coverage interests. This limited access to funding needs many patients to decide within significant personal investments or to proportion their oxygen use. There are many additional requests to the application of supplemental oxygen. Some subjects find disturbing oxygen and it makes them perceive that seem old and frail [13], leading to the use of oxygen only in the context of significant practical limitation and breathlessness. Providers may encourage patients to just use oxygen during exercise; nevertheless, this may cause uncertainty as to what extent of exertion approves its use and what flow rates to use. It can additionally be challenging to justify the use of oxygen to patients who are moderately symptomatic despite substantial desaturation, including patients who have progressed symptomatic tolerance to chronic hypoxemia. Conversely, oxygen may contribute comparatively little characteristic relief in some patients who refuse thus oxygen as an ineffective therapy despite other potential physiological advantages [14]. There are additional practical problems related to oxygen tubes, tanks and other equipment that may affect compliance in patients who are often fragile. Importantly, patients with advanced ILD may require high oxygen flow rates that exceed the capacity of portable or compact systems, resulting in limited mobility and hindering their ability to leave home. These natural barriers to oxygen use highlight the complexity of specific needs and expectations that must be acknowledged when explaining an approach to oxygen therapy.

CONSIDERATION TO OXYGEN USE IN ILD

Oxygen treatment is the most generally used procedure for patients with ILD and IPF to treat hypoxemia and halt improvement or prevent evolution of hypoxia-induced pulmonary hypertension, cardiovascular morbidity, or cognitive dysfunction [11]. One study had investigated the impact of carrying O2 on symptoms and functional capacity in patients with ILD and had seen that when subjects carried O2 (or for subjects who did not need O2, when they carried a weighted backpack), they experienced more significant dyspnea and included less distance during a timed walk test matched to when they did not carry the backpack. Among subjects with ILD, carrying O2 leads to increased dyspnea and shorter length covered during a time walked test, effects that appear to be increased in subjects who are more functionally impaired at baseline. Future research should look to confirm and extend these findings in ILD subjects with low and shallow physical functional capacity and to identify practical, non-constraining ways in which ILD patients can take O2 [14]. In one study, exertional hypoxemia was determined to be more critical for patients with fibrotic lung disease than those subjects with COPD. This group matched results of a 6-min walk test (6MW) completed on room air in 134 patients with ILD and 247 patients with COPD. Diffusing capacity (DLco) was the most potent predictor of desaturation in both cohorts with ILD subjects confronting more significant oxygen desaturation during the 6MW matched to patients with COPD. Supplemental oxygen has conceded patients who differently would be homebound to be added mobile, work, exercise or attend pulmonary rehabilitation, travel, care for family members, moreover, also experience improvement in their symptoms, including dyspnea, eventually improving their state of life. Patients who need supplemental oxygen, particularly those with ILD, experience various and different problems with receiving sufficient manageable systems to meet their dose requirement. Oxygen equipment is bulky, and options are limited as oxygen increases dose. In a study of 30 clinically stable ILD patients with differing disease severity, providing portable oxygen versus using oxygen from a stationary concentrator resulted in dyspnea significantly greater and shorter distances in timed testing [15]. Compact systems can deliver continuously flow (CF) and alternating flow (IF), and while IF devices are safe and effective in improving hypoxemia generally, there is variability in delivery and patient response, and therefore, patients need to be tested on these devices [16]. Use of a pulse an oximeter is suggested to allow patients to adjust their oxygen flow to support saturations >89% at all times [16]. In a contemporary ATS survey of 1926 patients with lung disease who used oxygen, individuals with IPF were unusually on oxygen more than five years, but frequently used oxygen >5LPM. Patients who received oxygen education had less health care utilization, including emergency appointments and hospitalizations [16]. Use of "a detailed proposal that incorporates an educational overview of oxygen, recommendations for how to use oxygen correctly, and revealing of what difficulties and benefits the patient (and their caregiver) strength expect from oxygen" is endorsed for patients designated oxygen therapy. The oxygen prescription process can increase providing patients with the most accurate and reliable educational resources expectations.

CONCLUSION

Supplemental oxygen is usually prescribed to patients with advanced ILD; though there is a paucity of accurate data encouraging its use, and there are significant limitations to accessing this therapy in many areas. ILD patients with resting hypoxemia are typically administered supplemental oxygen; however, there is a crucial necessity for a consistent procedure towards oxygen therapy for ILD patients, particularly those with isolated exertional hypoxemia. The current shortage of evidence may result in over-prescription of oxygen in some provinces, while in our practice, it has produced complex barriers to accessing this therapy. Prospective randomized controlled trials of ambulatory oxygen treatment in ILD patients with exertional hypoxemia are needed to assess clinically meaningful outcomes. Until such data become available, our subjects will acceptable continue to have poor access to an intervention that may significantly impact symptoms, patient autonomy, and improve quality of life.

References

[1] Raghu G, Rochwerg B, Zhang Y, et al. An official ATS/ERS/JRS/ALAT clinical practice guideline: treatment of idiopathic pulmonary fibrosis. An update of the 2011 clinical practice guideline. *Am. J. Respir. Crit. Care Med.* 2015; 192: e3-e19.

[2] Sharp C, Adamali H, Millar AB. Ambulatory and short-burst oxygen for interstitial lung disease. *Cochrane Database Syst. Rev.* 2016; 7: CD011716.

[3] Nishiyama O, Taniguchi H, Kondoh Y, Kimura T, Ogawa T, Watanabe F, Nishimura K. Health-related quality of life in patients with idiopathic pulmonary fibrosis: what is the main contributing factor? *Respir. Med.* 2005; 99:408-414.

[4] Dowman LM, McDonald CF, Hill CJ, Lee AL, Barker K, Boote C, Glaspole I, Goh NSL, Southcott AM, Burge AT, et al. The evidence of benefits of exercise training in interstitial lung disease: a randomised controlled trial. *Thorax* 2017;72:610-619.

[5] King TE Jr, Bradford WZ, Castro-Bernardini S, Fagan EA, Glaspole I, Glassberg MK, Gorina E, Hopkins PM, Kardatzke D, Lancaster L, et al. ASCEND Study Group. A phase 3 trial of pirfenidone in patients with idiopathic pulmonary fibrosis. *N. Engl. J. Med.* 2014;370: 2083-2092.

[6] Swigris J. Caution against extrapolating results from the trial of longterm oxygen for chronic obstructive pulmonary disease. Ann. Am. Thorac. Soc. 2017;14:296.

[7] Visca D, Tsipouri V, Mori L, Firouzi A, Fleming S, Farquhar M, Leung E, Maher TM, Cullinan P, Hopkinson N, et al. Ambulatory oxygen in fibrotic lung disease (AmbOx): study protocol for a randomised controlled trial. *Trials* 2017;18:201.

[8] Schaeffer MR, Ryerson CJ, Ramsook AH, Molgat-Seon Y, Wilkie SS, Dhillon SS, Mitchell RA, Sheel AW, Khalil N, Camp PG, et al. Effects of hyperoxia on dyspnoea and exercise endurance in fibrotic interstitial lung disease. *Eur. Respir. J.* 2017;1602494.

[9] Ryerson CJ, Camp PG, Eves ND, Schaeffer M, Syed N, Dhillon S, Jensen D, Maltais F, O'Donnell DE, Raghavan N, et al. High oxygen delivery to preserve exercise capacity in patients with idiopathic pulmonary fibrosis treated with nintedanib: methodology of the HOPE-IPF Study. *Ann. Am. Thorac. Soc.* 2016:1640-1647.

[10] Dowman LM, McDonald CF, Bozinovski S, Vlahos R, Gillies R, Pouniotis D, Hill CJ, Goh NSL, Holland AE. Greater endurance capacity and improved dyspnoea with acute oxygen supplementation in idiopathic pulmonary fibrosis patients without resting hypoxaemia. *Respirology* 2017; 22:957-964.

[11] Hardinge M, Annandale J, Bourne S, Cooper B, Evans A, Freeman D, Green A, Hippolyte S, Knowles V, MacNee W, et al. British Thoracic Society Home

Oxygen Guideline Development Group; British Thoracic Society Standards of Care Committee. British Thoracic Society guidelines for home oxygen use in adults. *Thorax* 2015;70: i1-i43.

[12] Ley B, Bradford WZ, Weycker D, Vittinghoff E, du Bois RM, Collard HR. Unified baseline and longitudinal mortality prediction in idiopathic pulmonary fibrosis. *Eur. Respir. J.* 2015;45:1374-1381.

[13] Khor YH, Goh NSL, McDonald CF, Holland AE. Oxygen thera for interstitial lung disease: a mismatch between patient expectations and experiences. *Ann. Am. Thorac. Soc.* 2017;14: 888-895.

[14] Ramadurai D, Riordan M, Graney B, Churney T, Olson AL, Swigris JJ. The impact of carrying supplemental oxygen on exercise capacity and dyspnea in patients with interstitial lung disease. *Respir. Med.* 2018;138:32-7.

[15] Swigris J. Supplemental oxygen for patients with interstitial lung disease: managing expectations. *Ann. Am. Thorac. Soc.* 2017;14: 831-2.

[16] Graney BA, Wamboldt FS, Baird S, Churney T, Fier K, Korn M, et al. Looking ahead and behind at supplemental oxygen: a qualitative study of patients with pulmonary fibrosis. *Heart Lung*. 2017;46(5):387-93.

In: Respiratory Ventilatory Strategies …
Editor: Antonio M. Esquinas
ISBN: 978-1-53617-847-0
© 2020 Nova Science Publishers, Inc.

Chapter 19

OXYGEN THERAPY AND HIGH-FLOW NASAL CANNULA

Ricardo Estêvão Gomes[1,*], MD and Vasco Salgado da Costa[2,†], MD
[1]Pulmonology Department, Hospital Garcia de Orta, Almada, Setúbal, Portugal
[2]Intensive Care Unit, Centro Hospitalar Lisboa Ocidental, Lisboa, Portugal

ABSTRACT

Interstitial lung diseases (ILD) comprise a group of pulmonary diseases characterized by inflammation and fibrosis of the lung parenchyma. Associated with respiratory failure and dyspnoea, these are chronically evolving entities marked by acute exacerbations (AE-ILD) with further decreases in pulmonary function, hypoxemia and ultimately, higher mortality. The mainstay of treatment for AE-ILD consist of oxygen therapy, which mainly included invasive mechanical ventilation, non-invasive ventilation and conventional oxygen therapy. The first two options have not shown clinical benefit, being the latter the recommended initial approach. In the last few years, another focus has been placed on the high-flow nasal cannula oxygen therapy (HFNC), a non-invasive method that provides heated and humidified air-oxygen mixture with flow rates up to 70 L/min. HFNC enables the correction of more severe degrees of hypoxemia, better mucociliary clearance, washout of anatomic dead space gasses, creating a PEEP effect, but most importantly, leading to improving patient comfort and tolerance to treatment. When compared to previous methods, HFNC also reduced mortality risk and need for intubation in cases of acute respiratory failure. Consequently, HFNC can be regarded as an excellent option for AE-ILD refractory to low-flow conventional oxygen therapy.

Keywords: oxygen therapy, high-flow nasal cannula, acute exacerbation, interstitial lung disease

---

* Corresponding Author's E-mail: ricardoegomes@gmail.com.
† Corresponding Author's E-mail: Vasco_costa@hotmail.com.

Key Messages

- Acute exacerbations of ILD present with hypoxemia, decrease in pulmonary function and increased risk of mortality;
- No best treatment for AE-ILD is currently established;
- HFNC provides high flow-rates (up to 70 L/min) and FiO_2 1.0;
- HNFC improves hypoxemia refractory to conventional oxygen therapy, reduction of respiratory rate, and increased tolerance to treatment.

Introduction

Interstitial lung diseases are a group of more than 200 diseases characterized by widespread inflammatory or fibrotic abnormalities of the lung parenchyma.

In a general way, this group of diseases tend to have a long-term progression that is associated with the development of respiratory failure and shortness of breath, having a great impact on quality of life for patients and affecting their ability to carry out daily activities. In addition, the chronic course of ILDs may also complicate with acute episodes of symptomatic and lung function deterioration. Those episodes are referred as AE-ILD and are defined as a clinical significant deterioration, with less than 1 month in duration, accompanied with new computerised tomography bilateral ground glass opacities and/or consolidation in the context of a known, diagnosed, ILD [1]. Alternative diagnosis that would give similar presentation and radiological appearance must be excluded.

Acute exacerbations of ILD share several clinical features with acute respiratory distress syndrome and have great impact on disease's prognosis with high mortality rates [1]. These patients generally have a high degree of V/Q mismatch, tend to be severely hypoxemic and require respiratory support with high oxygen concentrations to achieve satisfactory oxygenation. The risk of CO_2 retention is minimal and limited at the end stages.

The optimal strategy for respiratory support management in AE-ILD is not set. The benefits of invasive mechanical ventilation are questionable because it does not improve clinical outcome. As for non-invasive ventilation (NIV), although some small retrospective studies suggest benefits, others report NIV failure. Recent statements and clinical trials have described and studied the use of high-flow nasal cannula oxygen therapy (HFNC) in managing ILD patients admitted to the hospital due to AE-ILD. Although the prognosis of these patients is extremely poor, despite respiratory support, HFNC has shown to be effective in correcting hypoxemia, dyspnoea and increasing patient's comfort [2]. The use of HFNC must be considered when conventional oxygen therapy fails to improve patient condition and may be an effective treatment in preventing mechanical ventilation initiation.

In this chapter we will focus on oxygen therapy in ARF management originated by an AE-ILD, with particular emphasis on HFNC.

Conventional Oxygen Therapy in AE-ILD

Conventional oxygen therapy may be administered through low flow nasal cannula (LFNC), simple facemask, Venturi mask and non-rebreathing mask.

Low flow nasal cannula delivers dry oxygen at 1 to 6 litres per minute (L/min). Simple facemask is capable of delivering oxygen concentrations between 40% and 60%, depending on oxygen flow setting from 5 to 10 L/min. Venturi masks give an accurate oxygen concentration, regardless of flow rate. They are available in the concentrations of 24%, 28%, 31%, 35%, 40% and 60% and its use is indicated in patients needing a specific oxygen concentration. Non-rebreathing mask delivers oxygen at concentrations between 60% and 90%, when used at a flow rate of 15 L/min.

According to the British Thoracic Society guidelines for oxygen use [3], every patient with an AE-ILD should be given supplemental oxygen. The target pulse oximetry arterial oxygen saturation (SpO_2) is between 94% to 98% or the highest possible if the target cannot be achieved. Non-rebreathing mask at 15 L/min should be used if SpO_2 at room air is <85%. Otherwise, simple facemask or LFNC would be appropriate.

The use of conventional oxygen therapy has some limitations. The deliver of high flows trough LFNC (>6 L/min) is not tolerated by patients due to drying and irritation of nasal mucosa by the cold dry gas. On the other hand, the use of a facial mask is associated with treatment intolerance due to claustrophobic sensation, discomfort and difficulty in eating and communicating. Moreover, in patients with severe respiratory distress with high respiratory rates, the maximal oxygen flow provided might be lower than patient peak inspiratory flow, resulting in dilution of ambient air and reduction of oxygen concentrations in inspired air.

High-Flow Nasal Cannula Oxygen Therapy (HFNC)

High-flow nasal cannula (HFNC) is a non-invasive respiratory support that allows delivery of a heated, humidified mixture of air and oxygen at flow rates from 15 to 70 L/min and at a defined fraction of inspired oxygen (FiO_2) that ranges from 0.21 to nearly 1.0. For HFNC administration, 4 basic components are necessary: a flow generator capable of providing flow rates up to 60 L/min; an air-oxygen blender that achieves escalation of FiO_2 from 0.21 to 1.0 irrespective of flow rate; a humidifier that saturates the gas mixture at temperatures of 31°C to 37°C; and specifically designed wide bore nasal prongs. To minimize condensation, the heated humidified gas is delivered via heated tubing.

HFNC was initially used in preterm infants and pediatric population. However, recent clinical trials have evaluated its use in adults with ARF. These trials have show that HFNC, compared with either conventional oxygen therapy or non-invasive ventilation (NIV), was associated with better comfort, better rate of dyspnoea improvement, reduced mortality risk, higher ventilator free-days and reduce risk of intubation in patients with moderate to severe hypoxemia [4]. Additionally it was effective in preventing post-extubation respiratory failure [5] and was superior to NIV in managing ARF in immunocompromised patients [5].

Due to its apparent clinical benefit, attention has been devoted to understanding the physiological mechanism of action of HFNC. Currently, it is believed to have 5 mechanisms [5]: heating and humidification of inhaled gas, increasing airway humidification and leading to improved treatment tolerance; washout of anatomic dead space waste gasses including CO_2; reduction of nasopharyngeal resistance to inspiration due to high nasal inspiratory flow; generation of a positive airway pressure with a positive end-expiratory pressure (PEEP) effect; and reduction in ambient air entrainment during inspiration.

Humidification and warming of inspired air are crucial in creating an effective oxygenation system. It allows delivering of high-flow rates of gas at a temperature that is non-irritating to the mucosa making it comfortable for the patient. Moreover, the administration of warmed and humidified gas mixture reduces secretions viscosity and helps to maintain an adequate mucosal function, maximising mucociliary clearance [6].

The high flow rates deliver volumes of air superior to patient ventilation, which increases ventilation and allows washout of CO_2 from the anatomical dead space and its replacement with O_2 excess. This will reduce the minute ventilation requirement and work of breathing. Additionally, it will create an increase in alveolar oxygen partial pressure and a greater oxygen diffusion gradient, potentially improving oxygenation [5].

Through the application of a positive pressure, HFNC accomplishes a reduction of nasopharyngeal airway resistance by dilation of the radius of the nasopharyngeal airways. It increases ventilation and oxygenation potential [6].

Besides providing positive pressure support to the nasopharynx, HFNC creates a PEEP effect to the lower airways. This will lead to recruitment of atelectatic alveoli and impede them from collapsing during exhalation. Consequently, there will be an increase in the surface area available for gas exchange and improvement in V/Q mismatch, oxygenation and respiratory workload; in addition, there is also a consequent reduction in alveolar stress and strain that also contributes to better clinical outcomes. Ritchie et al. [7] reported a PEEP of 7 cmH2O in normal individuals at flow rates of 50 L/min and Parke et al. [8] relates a liner relation between the positive airway pressure and the administered flow-rate with an increase of 0.69 cmH_2O for each increase of 10 L/min; this effect is diluted when breathing with mouth open.

Patients with respiratory distress usually have high inspiratory flow rates that exceed the flow rates of conventional oxygen delivery systems. Incorporated room air dilutes the supplemental oxygen reducing FiO_2. HFNC delivers higher flow rates (up to 70 L/min), which in most cases exceeds patient's peak inspiratory flow, reducing the mixture of room air. In consequence the delivered FiO_2 is more accurate and oxygenation is improved. Breathing with open mouth during HFNC reduces this effect, once enables room air mixing.

Consistent with those HFNC effects, patients improve oxygenation and reduce respiratory rate and inspiratory effort during treatment for ARF [4]. An additional advantage of HFNC is a good tolerance for a long period of treatment, since it enables food intake and communication.

High-Flow Nasal Cannula Oxygen Therapy (HFNC) in AE-ILD

Respiratory support in patients with ARF after an AE-ILD remains a great challenge. Evidence of the usefulness of HFNC in improving oxygenation and reducing respiratory rate and inspiratory effort during treatment for ARF in AE-ILD is still very scarce [9]; however, its use is becoming more common.

Yukihiro et al. [2] describe the successful use of HFNC in 3 patients admitted to the intensive care unit due to AE-ILD. All patients were successfully treated and discharged from the unit. He showed that HFNC immediately improved oxygenation in all patients, whose respiratory failure was not controlled with conventional oxygen therapy. In addition, he suggests that HFNC can be well tolerated for more than 3 weeks.

Another study evaluated the efficacy and tolerability of HFNC for hypoxemic respiratory failure in patients with interstitial lung disease with do-not-intubate orders [10]. It was concluded that, when compared to NIV, HFNC was associated with a significantly lower rate of temporary interruption and discontinuation of treatment as well as significantly lower adverse effects and significantly better in terms of eating and ability to communicate. Although HFNC had a significant impact in respiratory rate reduction, no impact on patients' subjective dyspnoea was observed.

So far, no established guidelines exist for the use of HFNC in patients with AE-ILD. However, it is proposed that it should be initiated when conventional oxygen therapy fails to correct hypoxemia. One study used as initial levels of FiO_2 1.0 at flow rates of 70 L/min [11]; posteriorly adjusted to provide minimum FiO_2 to maintain $SpO_2 \geq 92\%$. In addition, one report suggests treatment weaning to conventional oxygen therapy when FiO_2 has been safely tapered to 0.35-0.4 at flow rates of 35-40 L/min [2].

As any other treatment, the use of HFNC has some issues of concern. These include great expense of care relative to conventional therapy, increased complexity and training to initiate treatment, potential to delay other potential treatments and loss of PEEP effect when breathing with mouth open. In addition, its use is contraindicated in unconscious patients, facial injury, presence of secretion with increased risk of aspiration and haemodynamic instability; all cases where invasive mechanical ventilation should be considered.

References

[1] Kolb M, Bondue B, Pesci A, Miyazaki Y, Song JW, Bhatt NY, et al. Acute exacerbations of progressive - fibrosing interstitial lung diseases. *Eur. Respir Rev.* 2018;27:180071.

[2] Horio Y, Takihara T, Niimi K, Komatsu M, Tomomatsu K, Hayama N, et al. High-flow nasal cannula oxygen therapy for acute exacerbation of interstitial pneumonia: A case series. *Respir. Investig.* [Internet]. Elsevier; 2016;54:125-9. Available from: http://dx.doi.org/10.1016/j.resinv.2015.09.005.

[3] B Ronan O'Driscoll, Luke Howard, John Earis VM, Sabrina Bajwah, Richard Beasley, Katrina Curtis AD, Alistair Dorward, Chris Dyer, Angela Evans LF, Clare Fitzpatrick, Simon Gibbs, Kim Hinshaw RH, Binita Kane, Jeff Keep, Carol Kelly HK, Muhammed Asad Iqbal Khan, Roop Kishen LM eld, et al. Bts guideline for oxygen use in adults in healthcare and emergency settings. *Thorax.* 2017;72:i1-90.

[4] Jean-Pierre Frat, MD, Arnaud W. Thille, MD, PhD, Alain Mercat, MD, PD, Christophe Girault, MD, PhD, Stéphanie Ragot, Pharm. D PD, Sébastien Perbet, MD, Gwénael Prat, MD, Thierry Boulain MD, Elise Morawiec, MD, Alice Cottereau, MD, Jérôme Devaquet MD, Saad Nseir, MD, PhD, Keyvan Razazi, MD, Jean-Paul Mira, MD, PD, Laurent Argaud, MD, PhD, Jean-Charles Chakarian MD, et al. High-Flow Oxygen through Nasal Cannula in Acute Hypoxemic Respiratory Failure. *N. Engl. J. Med.* 2015;472:2185-96.

[5] Fraisse F, At D, Carli P, Spaulding C. Not Just Oxygen? Mechanisms of Benefit from High-Flow Nasal Cannula in Hypoxemic Respiratory Failure Supplemental inhaled oxygen has been used as a therapeutic agent. *Am. J. Respir. Crit. Care Med.* 2017;195:9-12.

[6] Spoletini G, Alotaibi M, Blasi F, Fershill NS. Heated Humidified High-flow nasal oxygen in adults: mechanism of action and clinical complications. *Chest.* 2015;148:253-61.

[7] Ritchie JE, Williams AB, Gerard C, Hockey H. Evaluation of a humidified nasal high-flow oxygen system, using oxygraphy, capnography and measurement of upper airway pressures. *Anaesth. Intensive Care*. 2011;39:1103-10.

[8] Parke RL, Mhsc RN, Rn MLE, Mcguinness SP, Chb MB. The Effects of Flow on Airway Pressure During Nasal High-Flow Oxygen Therapy. *Respir. Care*. 2011;56:1151-5.

[9] Bräunlich J, Beyer D, Mai D, Hammerschmidt S, Wirtz HSH. Effects of Nasal High Flow on Ventilation in Volunteers, COPD and Idiopathic Pulmonary Fibrosis Patients. *Respiration*. 2013;85:319-25.

[10] Koyauchi T, Hasegawa H, Kanata K, Kakutani T, Amano Y, Ozawa Y, et al. Efficacy and Tolerability of High-Flow Nasal Cannula Oxygen Therapy for Hypoxemic Respiratory Failure in Patients with Interstitial Lung Disease with Do-Not-Intubate Orders: *A Retrospective Single-Center Study*. 2018;6:323-9.

[11] Vianello A, Arcaro G, Molena B, Turato C, Braccioni F, Paladini L, et al. High-flow nasal cannula oxygen therapy to treat acute respiratory failure in patients with acute exacerbation of idiopathic pulmonary fibrosis. *Ther. Adv. Respir. Dis*. 2019;13:1-13.

In: Respiratory Ventilatory Strategies …
Editor: Antonio M. Esquinas

ISBN: 978-1-53617-847-0
© 2020 Nova Science Publishers, Inc.

Chapter 20

NON-INVASIVE VENTILATION: CONTINUOUS POSITIVE AIR PRESSURE VENTILATION (CPAP) AND PRESSURE SUPPORT VENTILATION (PSV)

Corrado Mollica[1]*, MD, Angelo Petroianni[2], MD and Edoardo Piervincenzi[3], MD
[1]Department of Cardiovascular & Respiratory Sciences, "Sapienza" University, Rome, Italy
[2]Respiratory Diseases Unit, Policlinico Umberto I, "Sapienza" University, Rome, Italy
[3]Anesthesia and Intensive care Medicine, "Sapienza" University, Rome, Italy

ABSTRACT

Background and objectives: Acute respiratory failure (ARF) in patients (pts) with idiopathic pulmonary fibrosis (IPF) is associated with poor prognosis, therefore a non-invasive approach, such as noninvasive ventilation (NIV) may represent a good option to turn to. NIV modes: continuous positive airway pressure (CPAP) in spontaneous breathing (SB) (range 8-10 cmH_2O level) is applied in the absence of respiratory acidosis in order to treat hypoxemia with tachypnea. Inspired oxygen fraction (FiO_2) is set at the lowest value to keep PaO_2 at more than 60mmHg. Hypercapnia, hypoventilation and respiratory fatigue are treated in assisted/controlled ventilation by face-mask (FM) in pressure support ventilation (PSV). Pressure support (PS) and positive end-expiratory pressure (PEEP) level are set respectively at 12-18 and 4-9 cmH_2O, titrated to provide a moderate tidal volume (TV) (6-8 ml/Kg of predicted body weight). When NIV-Helmet is applied, PS and PEEP baseline levels are respectively set at 10 and 5 cmH_2O, both raising in increments of 2–3 cmH_2O. FM advantages: higher efficacy in improving CO_2

* Corresponding Author's E-mail: c.mollica@libero.it.

elimination and reducing work of breathing while applying PSV in pts with high respiratory muscle load. Disadvantages: not tolerated in pts with prolonged MV necessity. Helmet advantages over FM: improved tolerability and lesser air leaks as with a new helmet that can be performed for prolonged periods of time. Disadvantages: because of its larger inner volume, standard helmet is characterized by less efficient rates of pressurization and triggering function, worsening patient–ventilator synchrony. In pts with high respiratory drive and intense inspiratory effort, the risk of patient self-inflicted lung injury (P-SILI) is highly considerable. Conclusions: NIV with helmet in CPAP mode and face-mask in PSV provides relief from dyspnoea and avoids endo-tracheal intubation (ETI).

Keywords: acute respiratory failure, idiopathic pulmonary fibrosis, non-invasive mechanical ventilation, helmet, face-mask

ABBREVIATIONS

AE-IPF	Acute exacerbation of IPF;
ARDS	Acute respiratory distress syndrome;
ARF	Acute respiratory failure;
CPAP	Continuous positive airway pressure;
DAD	Diffuse alveolar damage;
DNR	Do not resuscitate;
DP	Driving pressure;
ETI	Endotracheal intubation;
ECCO2R	Extracorporeal CO_2 removal;
FEV1	Forced expiratory volume in the 1st second;
FEV1/ FVC ratio	Forced expiratory volume in the 1st second/ Forced vital capacity;
FiO_2	Inspired oxygen fraction;
FMV	Face-mask ventilation;
FVC	Forced vital capacity;
GCS	Glasgow coma scale score;
HFOT	High flow oxygen therapy;
HRCT	High resolution computed tomography;
ICU	Intensive care unit;
ILD	Interstitial lung disease;
IMV	Invasive mechanical ventilation;
IPF	Idiopathic pulmonary fibrosis;
MOF	Multiple organ failure;
MV	Mechanical ventilation;
NMBAs	Neuromuscular blocking agents;

NIV	Non-invasive mechanical ventilation;
PaO_2	Oxygen arterial pressure;
$PaCO_2$	Carbon dioxide arterial pressure;
PBW	Predicted body weight;
PEEP	Positive end-expiratory pressure;
PSV	Pressure support ventilation;
P/F	oxygen arterial pressure(PaO_2)/inspired oxygen (FiO_2) ratio;
p/pts	Patient/s;
P-SILI	Patient self-inflicted lung injury;
%	percentage
RR	Respiratory rate;
RICU	Respiratory intensive care unit;
SaO_2	Arterial oxygen saturation;
SAPS	Simplified acute physiology score;
SB	Spontaneous breathing;
TLC	Total lung capacity;
UIP	Usual interstitial pneumonia;
VAP	Ventilator-associated pneumonia;
VILI	Ventilator-induced lung injury;
TV	Tidal volume;
WOB	Work of breathing
% pred	Percent of predicted value.

INTRODUCTION

Idiopathic pulmonary fibrosis (IPF) is defined as a chronic progressive-fibrosing interstitial pneumonia of unknown cause, with high morbidity and mortality in older adults [1]. While most IPF patients (pts) show a gradually progressive course, others follow a relatively rapid decline. Whether this represents a distinct phenotype remains unexplored [2]. IPF acute exacerbation (AE-IPF) is characterized by a diffuse alveolar damage (DAD), with evidence of new bilateral ground-glass opacity and/or consolidation on an usual interstitial pneumonia (UIP) pattern. It results in the development or severe worsening of dyspnoea, typically < 1 month in duration, without an identifiable cause, and is characterized by evidence of low PaO_2/FiO_2 ratio (P/F) that may lead to severe hypoxemia [1]. In this subset of subjects (5-10%) mechanical ventilation (MV) may be required in order to improve oxygenation when high flow oxygen-therapy is not sufficient, and can represent a palliative therapeutic option, which reduces patient's discomfort and helps avoiding more invasive approaches [3]. AE-IPF has a poor outcome, with a median survival after diagnosis ranging from 3 to 5 years and invasive mechanical ventilation (IMV) seems to be useless to ameliorate prognosis [4].

Mechanical Ventilation in IPF: Basic Topics

Current IPF guidelines recommend that the majority of patients with respiratory failure should not receive IMV [4]. The rationale is that both the structural lung disease and the precipitating condition causing ARF are irreversible and progressive [4]. Poor prognosis data about IMV in IPF are based on previous studies conducted before the lung protective strategies were performed [5]. An agreement was based on the consideration that a more severe baseline hypoxemia, higher mechanical ventilation pressures, and the presence of diffuse ILD are associated with a poorer outcome [6, 7, 8]. Despite numerous aetiologies, interstitial lung disease (ILD) shows a progressive impairment in respiratory mechanics and in physiological lung function. The IPF alterations are of the restrictive kind, with a decreased lung capacity and an increased FEV1/FVC ratio. Reductions in lung compliance occur early, and may be tightly correlated with the degree of lung fibrosis [9]. This leads to a poor recruitment of the lungs, in spite of the use of high pressures needed in mechanical ventilation to obtain adequate tidal volume (TV). AE-IPF presents several patho-physiological features linked to acute respiratory disease syndrome (ARDS) [10]. As reported in Marchioni et al. (2018) in the presence of DAD there is a partial overlap between AE-IPF pts and a fair percentage of ARDS pts [11]. Both ARDS and AE-IPF show an over-expression of pro-inflammatory cytokines produced by alveolar macrophages with chemotaxis of neutrophils [12]. The use of higher positive end-expiratory pressure (PEEP) value in AE-IPF pts may be harmful, just as in ARDS pts who have a low percentage of recruitable lung, since it simply overinflates lung regions that are already open [13]. Performing IMV in IPF pts is not useful, because of both low percentage of recruitable lung areas and the lungs themselves not being edematous. As a result, in this kind of patients an "open lung strategy" with high levels of PEEP (> 10 cm H_2O) may determine ventilator-induced lung injury (VILI) by provoking over-distension injury and bio-trauma. Moreover "the use of high PEEP to keep alveolar units opened during expiration exposes the lung at risk of injury by forming 'squishy ball' lung areas that aggravate the end-inspiratory transpulmonary pressure effects" [14]. Thus, Marchioni et al. (2020) suggest using a "lung resting strategy", as opposed to "open lung approach" in IPF pts (with UIP pattern) under MV, "regardless of the underlying etiology" [14]. When IMV has to be used in IPF pts, low TV and low PEEP should be employed (note that this topic is still under discussion in ARDS) regardless of the mode of ventilation ("volume/pressure controlled") [5]. The use of IMV in AE-IPF pts is associated with high in-hospital mortality rate (86-100%) when it is performed at high TV [(> 8 ml/Kg of PBW)] [7]. However, mortality is reduced when low TV values (< 8 ml/Kg of PBW) at 64% [15] and 67% [16] are used. The same also occurred in a large cohort study, where in-hospital mortality of IPF pts mechanically ventilated (IMV = 51,6% vs NIV = 30,8%) was approximately 50% [17], due to a more frequent use of lung protective strategies that may have improved the outcomes. In conclusion, "these are encouraging results that may help physicians when it comes to making a decision on invasive mechanical ventilation and safer alternatives for patients with IPF" [18]. Despite this, poor prognosis associated with a higher risk of infections occurring during IMV may suggest the use of non-invasive ventilation (NIV).

NON-INVASIVE VENTILATION (NIV)

Indication to start NIV in IPF pts is generally based on the occurrence of moderate-to-severe dyspnoea, respiratory rate above 30 breaths/min, signs of increased work of breathing (WOB), and /or P/F < 200 not responding to the oxygen and pharmacological therapy. In pts with hypoxaemic respiratory failure[1] the use of NIV aims at improving oxygenation, facilitating ventilation, decreasing WOB and dyspnoea, avoiding intubation, and reducing the complications associated with IMV [19]. A recent guideline statement issued by the American Thoracic Society (ATS) / European Respiratory Society (ERS) points to the use of NIV as a life-sustaining measure in some IPF pts who have survived an episode of acute pulmonary fibrosis as a treatment, not least as a bridge to transplant [4].

It is also particularly noteworthy that, in end-stage pts – when palliation is more appropriate for IPF pts – NIV can be taken into account as a major palliative option. Together with appropriate supportive care, it may help reducing patient's discomfort by decreasing breathing work and permits management in a respiratory intensive care unit (RICU) [11]. In a nationwide analysis performed in the USA, IPF patients who received MV were younger with fewer chronic medical conditions; the number of IPF pts treated by NIV was increasing [7.9% (583) in 2009, 8.3% (550) in 2010, and 10.3% (862) in 2011 ($p = 0.112$)] [20]. Retrospective studies show a moderate success of NIV compared to IMV with a lower mortality in responder pts; a percentage between 85 and 100% died within 3 months, regardless of endo-tracheal intubation (ETI) being imposed [21, 22]. The use of NIV instead of IMV in the management of life-threatening AE-IPF, showed a better 60-day survival rate, a shorter high-care unit stay, and preserved oral communication, all the while providing for better quality of life and more rational usage of medical resources [23]. Moreover, NIV may be applied in selected pts, such as those with less severe ARF, to identify early NIV-responder pts and to treat the causes of ARF,

---

1 Hypoxaemic respiratory failure is usually defined as significant hypoxaemia (P/F ≤ 200), tachypnoea (respiratory rate > 30–35 breaths·min–1) or use of accessory respiratory muscles or paradoxical abdominal motion, and a non-COPD diagnosis (e.g. pneumonia and/or acute respiratory distress syndrome (ARDS) [19].

minimizing complications and the poor outcome linked to ETI and IMV [24]. Early NIV application in pts with less severe respiratory failure may improve patients' management and short-term outcomes (better 30-day survival) and can help avoiding complications related to intubation, such as ventilator-associated pneumonias (VAPs) [21, 24]. Stratifying the results on the basis of the causes of ARF and the radiological pattern of ILD, Aliberti et al. (2014) evaluated NIV responsiveness in pts with ILD and ARF [6]. The results show that NIV improved oxygenation in pts with pneumonia, yet not in those with AE-IPF, without differences in terms of radiological pattern [6]. Nevertheless, in mechanically ventilated pts with ILD with autoimmune features, the prognosis was related to the extension of the lung fibrosis and the presence of a UIP pattern on CT scan rather than to the ILD etiology [25].

However, NIV responsiveness did not have a relevant impact on the poor prognosis related to the disease: one-year mortality rate in NIV-responders was $\geq 70\%$ in all the evaluated studies [21].

NIV Mode: PSV vs CPAP

NIV is generally performed in PSV ("*Pressure Support Ventilation*") mode (range: 5-15 cmH_2O), or in CPAP ("*Continuous Positive Air Pressure*") mode (range: 8 - 10 cmH_2O). In the absence of respiratory acidosis, the early NIV mode is often a CPAP. CPAP level is gradually increased with a range 8-10 cmH_2O. Inspired oxygen fraction (FiO_2) is set at the lowest value to keep PaO_2 at more than 60mmHg [6]. During CPAP, which involves exclusively the application of a PEEP in a tight-fitting pressurized system (helmet or mask), all the respiratory work is performed by the patient and the only positive result consists in balancing the effects of the auto-PEEP and the recruitment of hypo-ventilated lung areas. CPAP is thus effective for treating hypoxemia with tachypnea, but does not improve hypercapnia (and acidosis), insofar as it does not correct hypoventilation. Conversely, alveolar hypoventilation and hypercapnia do not occur frequently in the early stage of AE-IPF. This is probably due to the adaptation of the respiratory muscle to the increased respiratory workload which is associated with lung stiffness [9]. In the end stages of the disease, this causes ARF in about 40% of pts. The onset of respiratory fatigue may lead to CO_2 retention and respiratory acidosis (pH< 7.35, $PaCO_2 \geq 45$ mmHg) that forces to perform CPAP mode (mean 10.1+/-2.5 cmH_2O) up to 12 cmH_2O to keep the lung open, and Spontaneous/Timed mode (mean inspiratory positive airway pressure/expiratory positive airway pressure; 15.0+/-3.3 / 10.2+/-2.9 cmH_2O) [21]. Treating a hypoxemic / hypercapnic patient with AE-IPF in NIV support can be extremely challenging for the clinician. PSV in NIV, the most frequent mode used in intensive care unit (ICU), exploits a flow trigger, a pressure supply with a pre-set PEEP level and a loop cycling with a percentage (%) drop in flow. The developed TV depends on the patient's thoraco-pulmonary system compliance. L'Her et al.(2005) showed that in ARDS pts NIV support pressure of 10-15 cmH_2O above a PEEP of 5-10 cmH_2O was the best combination in order to reduce inspiratory effort, dyspnea, and improve oxygenation [26]. Unfortunately, in ILDs, the need for a support pressure level to assure fitted tidal volumes limits the safety margins of the method. In a retrospective study on ILD pts treated with PSV through full face mask with homecare ventilators, Vianello et al. (2014) reported P-support and PEEP level respectively imposed equal to 15.4 ± 2.7 and 6.4 ± 2.5 cmH_2O, titrated to moderate TV (6-8 ml/Kg of PBW) [22]. The days under NIV therapy were 6.8 ± 7.0. The 45% of patients had a successful NIV treatment and did not require IMV, while they all survived during NIV therapy. All the pts in the 55% of NIV failure group died in few days (average 20 days) from multiple organ failure (MOF) / sepsis or cardiac failure [22]. The authors underline that protecting the lung in fragile patients could play a key role in terms of survival rate, especially when an immunosuppressive / corticosteroid therapy is used [21, 22].

According to Marchioni et al. (2020) a "lung resting strategy" should establish a PEEP setting = 4 cmH_2O, TV = 6 ml/kg of PBW, transpulmonary pressure at end-inspiration below 10–12 cmH_2O in inhomogeneous lung parenchyma, "tolerating hypercapnia if the arterial pH remains above 7.25, with a PaO2 above 50–60 mmHg or a SpO2 above 88–90%. In patients in whom a DAD or ground-glass opacities at the CT predominate over the UIP pattern, higher PEEP levels might be considered, similarly to ARDS [14]. Criteria to interrupt the NIV therapy were defined by P/F > 200, respiratory rate (RR) < 20 and clinical improvement of radiological findings [19]. In the presence of acute alteration of consciousness [Glasgow coma scale (GCS < 8)], cardiac arrest, poor mask compliance, inability to clear secretions, or haemodynamic instability, IMV must be performed, unless the patient has previously declared a do not resuscitate (DNR) will [19].

NIV Interface: Helmet vs Face – Mask

A brief trial with face-mask ventilation (FMV) is usually performed during the first 4 hours (range: 2 - 6) in pts with higher $PaCO_2$ values, due to the higher performance of face-mask (*vs* helmet) to determine an improving in CO_2 elimination [27]. In hypoxemic patients, who required prolonged MV, face-mask treatment is not well tolerated and helmet is usually used as an interface. The helmet is a transparent hood that covers the entire head of the patient, with a collar that adheres to the neck and ensures a sealed connection once the helmet is inflated. The ventilator delivers pressure to the patient through the helmet inlet; the patient exhales into the helmet, which is connected to the ventilator expiratory line. *Advantages versus face mask*: no skin lesions due to the helmet's lack of contact with the face; effective application of higher PEEP (i.e., 8-12

cmH_2O) with minimal air leaks during prolonged treatments without interruptions [28]. *Disadvantages*: standard helmet's large inner volume (12–15 L) results in a compressible volume, which interferes with circuit pressurization, trigger sensitivity, and WOB [29], thus facilitating rebreathing [30]. Additionally, the helmet can cause pain and discomfort as a result of the pressure exerted on the skin of the axillary area due to armpit brace, and an upward displacement of helmet during ventilator insufflation, owing to the highly compliant soft collar [31]. Helmet requires high PS values in the early phase of inspiration to pressurize his inner volume. This actually cause a longer time to reach the required level of PS, and can result in patients' less assistance and in a higher risk of asynchrony for a significantly longer inspiratory trigger delay [30,32]. Chiumello et al. (2003) evaluated the breathing pattern and WOB with helmet and face-mask during CPAP and PSV. During CPAP, there was no difference in breathing pattern and WOB; on the contrary, the face-mask significantly reduced the WOB compared to the helmet during PSV [33]. Racca et al., (2005) also compared the helmet and face-mask during PSV with normal and high respiratory muscle load to simulate dyspnoeic pts. Both breathing pattern and respiratory effort were the same in presence of normal muscle load. However, it was also noted that, when a helmet was applied instead of face-mask, to a higher respiratory muscle load corresponded a significantly higher inspiratory effort [30]. These evidences suggest to use helmet in CPAP mode and face-mask in PSV [30]. An increasing in $PaCO_2$ is described while using single-limb-circuit bi-level ventilators which do not have efficient exhalation systems [27]. A new helmet recently introduced into clinical practice features an annular openable ring which, placed underneath an inflatable cushion, secures the helmet without the need of armpit braces, as opposed to the standard helmet. The new design improves comfort, rate of pressurization, and triggering performance, while the procedure can be used in clinical practice in order to determine an improvement in clinical outcome, especially in the most severe pts requiring NIV for prolonged periods of time [31].

Other Side Effects of NIV

There is a significant hyper-activation of the respiratory drive that causes an increase in respiratory rate (RR) and significantly higher effort in patients with AE-IPF (as in ARDS pts) when applying the helmet than with the face-mask, due to the presence of air leaks [30,32,33]. This may be reduced by increasing the PS values [34]. Moreover, if the use of NIV-Helmet in ARDS pts is prolonged over time, the need for high PS values leads to an increase in trans-pulmonary pressures, reaching −30 to −40 cmH_2O, that may exacerbate the danger of developing patient self-inflicted lung injury (P-SILI) [34]. Only ARDS pts with a P/F ratio below 200 mmHg after one hour of PSV-NIV and expired TV exceeding 9-9.5 ml/Kg of PBW are exposed to the development of P-SILI [35]. In these pts the use of neuromuscular blocking agents (NMBAs) may counterbalance the potentially injurious effects of assisted breathing, thus resulting in improved survival [36]. We cannot rule out a P-SILI developing even in AE-IPF, because lung protective ventilator strategies (such as maintaining a low TV of 6 ml/kg of PBW) are more difficult to apply with NIV than with IMV, as the maneuvers (end - inspiratory/expiratory pauses) required for the measurements of trans-pulmonary pressure are difficult to perform in spontaneously breathing pts. This raises a note of caution when using NIV that combines spontaneous effort with ventilator support [35]. Recently, the ventilator-related causes of lung injury have been unified in a single variable, i.e., the mechanical power, that is the mathematical description of the mechanical energy (in joule/min) produced by MV and delivered to the respiratory system over time. The mechanical power is assessed by measuring the pressure-volume loops that can be computed from its components: TV / driving pressure (DP), flow, PEEP and respiratory rate (RR) [37]. It may help to estimate the contribution of the different ventilator-related causes of lung injury and of their variations, although it is still under discussion, in fact "...lung heterogeneity is not readily quantified, and clinicians at the bedside are left with what we can measure about the elements of the equation of motion"[38]. Furthermore, we cannot exclude that even in IPF (as in ARDS) a significant correlation between mechanical power and serum fibrosis biomarkers (TGF-β1 and CTGF) could be found [39].

Predictors of MV Failure in IPF

In subjects who receive NIV, APACHE II scores < 20 and non-continuous demand for NIV show a higher survival compared to older subjects receiving IMV [16]. The presence of diffuse ILD ("widespread opacification") [8], simplified acute physiology score (SAPS II) >34 [7, 40], and the inability to improve P/F after 1hr of NIV, later requiring to switch to IMV, have shown to correlate with a higher mortality [21, 22]. An early start of NIV during AE-IPF is associated as well with a better 30-day survival, improving patients management and short-term outcomes [24]. With regards to the MV setting in ILDs pts, since high PEEP has effect neither on fibrotic, nor on recruitable areas, thus promoting VILI, a high in-hospital mortality rate is referred when high levels of PEEP (> 10 cm H2O) and high VT (> 8 ml/Kg) values are applied [10]. Recently, a comprehensive scale including acidosis, consciousness, oxygenation, heart and respiratory rate (the HACOR Scale) predicts NIV failure after 1 hour-treatment in a large prospective cohort study with high specificity (90%) and good sensitivity (72%) [41].

Conclusion

All strategies used to prevent a worsening in the AE-IPF clinical outcome, not only in terms of mortality but also in terms of quality of life after the acute event, seem to be ineffective. Routine ventilatory modes fitting to safeguard the residual healthy lung parenchyma are difficult to implement in most serious IPF onset, in which plateau and driving pressures "higher than the considered threshold accepted for safety", are often to be applied. If NIV fails, and unless patients have previously declared a DNR will, a protective ventilation strategy in IMV with low TV and low driving pressure could be recommended, similarly to ARDS. However, the least harmful mechanical ventilation strategy is not yet fully elucidated in AE-IPF patients [14]. Additionally, in IPF pts the greater susceptibility of the lung to develop VILI, the impaired ability to repair the acute alveolar damage, and the patients older age may play a role to explain the worse mortality rate. Nevertheless early use of NIV in selected pts might avoid IMV and improve clinical conditions at ICU admission. In this way we can meet the new technologies of extracorporeal CO_2 removal (ECCO2R) and high flow oxygen therapy (HFOT) that are beyond the aim of this chapter [42].

Key Messages

- The abnormalities of the respiratory mechanics are common in patients with idiopathic pulmonary fibrosis. Most alterations are likely to result from the progressive inflammatory process that leads to interstitial fibrosis and re-organization of the lung architecture.
- Several non-invasive ventilation (NIV) modes can be used in IPF patients at different stages of the diseases and with various purposes: treating respiratory fatigue and tachypnea, hypoxemia with or without hypercapnia, palliation. CPAP is generally indicated for treating hypo-normocapnic hypoxemia with tachypnea, while PSV can be considered in late stages in the presence of respiratory fatigue, CO2 retention, respiratory acidosis, and DNR will.
- Invasive Mechanical ventilation (IMV) was more frequent in IPF patients. Its use was associated with an increase in mortality rate. Overall mortality was approximately 50% for IMV and 30% for NIV.
- NIV may be useful for compassionate use, providing relief from dyspnoea while permitting to avoid aggressive approaches. Further advances in IPF treatment and development of IPF-specific decision aids are needed to improve the outcomes and use of MV in IPF.

Acknowledgments

Fabrizio Bigotti, PhD, and Francesca Niutta for revising the final draft of this paper.

References

[1] Raghu G., Collard H. R., Egan J. J., Martinez F. J., Behr J., Brown K. K., et al. (2011). An official ATS/ERS/JRS/ALAT statement: idiopathic pulmonary fibrosis: evidence-based guidelines for diagnosis and management. *Am. J. Respir. Crit. Care Med.*,183:788–824. DOI: 10.1164/rccm.2009-040GL.

[2] Olson A. L., Gifford A.H., Inase N., Fernández Pérez E. R. and Suda T. (2018). The epidemiology of idiopathic pulmonary fibrosis and interstitial lung diseases at risk of a progressive-fibrosing phenotype. *Eur. Respir. Rev.*, 27(150):180077. DOI.org/10.1183/ 16000617.0077-2011.

[3] Collard H.R., Moore B. B., Flaherty K.R, Brown K.K, Kaner R.J, King T.E. Jr, et al. (2007). Idiopathic Pulmonary Fibrosis Clinical Research Network Investigators. Acute exacerbations of idiopathic pulmonary fibrosis. *Am. J. Respir. Crit. Care Med.*,176:636–643.DOI:10.1164/rccm.200703-463PP.

[4] Raghu G., Rochwerg B., Zhang Y., Garcia C.A.C., Azuma A., Behr J., et al. (2015). An official ATS /ERS /JRS /ALAT clinical practice guideline: treatment of idiopathic pulmonary fibrosis. An update of the 2011 clinical practice guideline. *Am. J. Respir. Crit. Care Med.*, 192: e3–19. DOI:10.1164/rccm.201506-1063 ST.

[5] Mallick S. (2008). Outcome of patients with idiopathic pulmonary fibrosis (IPF) ventilated in intensive care unit. *Respir Med*,102:1355–9. DOI: 10.1016/j.rmed. 2008.06.003.

[6] Aliberti S., Messinesi G., Gamberini S., Maggiolin S., Visca D., Galavotti V. et al, (2014). Non-invasive mechanical ventilation in patients with diffuse interstitial lung diseases. *BMC Pulm. Med.*,14:194. DOI.org/10.1186/1471-2466-14-194.

[7] Fernández-Pérez E.R., Yilmaz M., Jenad H., Daniels C.E., Ryu J.H., Hubmayr R.D. and Gajic O. (2008). Ventilator settings and outcome of respiratory failure in chronic interstitial lung disease. *Chest.*,13:1113-9. DOI.org/10.1378/chest.07-1481.

[8] Gacouin A., Jouneau S., Letheulle J., Kerjouan M., Bouju P., Fillatre P., et al. (2015). Trends in prevalence and prognosis in subjects with acute chronic respiratory failure treated with noninvasive and/or invasive ventilation. *Respir. Care*, 60:210 –218. DOI:10.4187/respcare.03467.

[9] Nava S. and Rubini F. (1999). Lung and chest wall mechanics in ventilated patients with end stage idiopathic pulmonary fibrosis. *Thorax,* 54(5):390–5. DOI:10.1136/ thx.54.5.390.

[10] Papiris S.A., Manali E.D., Kolilekas L., Kagouridis K., Triantafillidou C., Tsangaris I., et al. (2010). Clinical review: Idiopathic pulmonary fibrosis acute exacerbations - unravelling Ariadne's thread. *Crit. Care,* 14: 246. DOI: 10.1186/cc9241

[11] Marchioni A., Tonelli R., Ball L., Fantini R., Castaniere I., Cerri S., et al. (2018). Acute exacerbation of idiopathic pulmonary fibrosis: lessons learned from acute respiratory distress syndrome? *Crit. Care*, 22:80. DOI: 10.1186/s13054-018-2002-4.

[12] Dreyfuss D., Ricard J-D. and Saumon G. (2003). On the physiologic and clinical relevance of lung-borne cytokines during ventilator-induced lung injury. *Am. J. Respir. Crit. Care Med.,* 167:1467–147. DOI.org/10.1164/rccm.200206-611CP.

[13] Gattinoni L., Caironi P., Cressoni M., Chiumello D., Ranieri V.M., Quintel M., et al. (2006). Lung recruitment in patients with the acute respiratory distress syndrome. *N. Engl. J. Med.,* 354:1775–1786. DOI:10.1056/NEJMoa052052.

[14] Marchioni A., Tonelli R., Rossi G., Spagnolo P., Luppi F., Cerri S., et al. (2020). Ventilatory support and mechanical properties of the fibrotic lung acting as a "squishy ball". *Ann. Intensive Care.,*10:13-22. DOI.org/10.1186/s13613-020-0632-6.

[15] Gungor G., Tatar D., Salturk C., Cimen P., Saltürk C., Çimen P., et al. (2013). Why Do Patients with Interstitial Lung Diseases Fail in the ICU? A 2-Center Cohort Study. *Respir. Care.* 2013;58: 525–531. DOI: 10.4187/respcare.01734.

[16] Gaudry S., Vincent F., Rabbat A., Nunes H., Crestani B., Naccache J., et al. (2014). Invasive mechanical ventilation in patients with fibrosing interstitial pneumonia. *J. Thorac. Cardiovasc. Surg.*147:47–53. DOI: 10.1016/j.jtcvs.2013.06.039.

[17] Rush B., Wiskar K., Berger L. and Griesdale D. (2016) The use of mechanical ventilation in patients with idiopathic pulmonary fibrosis in the United States: a nationwide retrospective cohort analysis. *Respir. Med.*,111:72–6.DOI: 10.1016/*j.rmed.* 2015.12.005.

[18] Silva Santos P., Cruz C. and Esquinas A.M. (2016). Mechanical ventilation in idiopathic pulmonary fibrosis: Unresolved dilemma. *Respir.Med.*,117:283. DOI:10.1016/ *j. rmed.*2016.04.003.

[19] Rochwerg B., Brochard L., Elliott M.W., Hess D., Hill N.S., Nava S., et al. (members of the task force). (2017). Official ERS/ATS clinical practice guidelines: noninvasive ventilation for acute respiratory failure. *Eur. Respir. J.*, 50: 1602426. DOI: 10.1183/13993003.02426-2016.

[20] Mooney J.J., Raimundo K., Chang E. and Broder M.S. (2017). Mechanical ventilation in idiopathic pulmonary fibrosis: a nationwide analysis of ventilator use, outcomes, and resource burden. *BMC Pulm. Med.*, 17:84. DOI: 10.1186/s12890-017-0426-2.

[21] Yokoyama T., Kondoh Y., Taniguchi H., Kataoka K., Kato K., Nishiyama O., et al. (2010). Noninvasive ventilation in acute exacerbation of idiopathic pulmonary fibrosis. *Intern Med.,* 49:1509–14. DOI:10.2169/internalmedicine.49.3222

[22] Vianello A., Arcaro G., Battistella L., Pipitone E., Vio S., Concas A. et al. (2014). Noninvasive ventilation in the event of acute respiratory failure in patients with idiopathic pulmonary fibrosis. *J. Crit. Care.,* 29:562–7. DOI:10.1016/ j. jcrc.2014.03.019.

[23] Tomii K., Tachikawa R., Chin K., Murase K., Handa T., Mishima M., et al. (2010). Role of non-invasive ventilation in managing life-threatening acute exacerbation of interstitial pneumonia. *Intern. Med. Tokyo Jpn.,* 49:1341–7. DOI:10.2169/ internalmedicine.49.3491.

[24] Faverio P., De Giacomi F., Sardella L., Fiorentino G., Carone M., Salerno F., et al. (2018). Management of acute respiratory failure in interstitial lung diseases: overview and clinical insights. *BMC Pulm. Med.,* 18:70. DOI: 10.1186/s12890-018-0643-3.

[25] Grasselli G., Vergnano B., Pozzi M.R., Sala V., D'Andrea G., Scaravilli V., et al. (2017). Interstitial pneumonia with autoimmune features: an additional risk factor for ARDS? *Ann. Intensive Care.,* 7:98. DOI: 10.1186/s13613-017-0320-3.

[26] L'Her E., Deye N., Lellouche F., Taille S., Demoule A., Fraticelli A., et al. (2005), Physiologic effects of noninvasive ventilation during acute lung injury. *Am. J. Respir. Crit. Care Med.,* 172:1112–8 DOI:10.1164/rccm.200402-226OC.

[27] Navalesi P., Costa R., Ceriana P., Carlucci A., Prinianakis G., Antonelli M., et al. (2007). Non-invasive ventilation in chronic obstructive pulmonary disease patients: Helmet versus facial mask. *Intensive Care Med.,* 33:74-81. DOI 10.1007/s00134-006-0391-3.

[28] Antonelli M., Conti G., Pelosi P., Gregoretti C., Pennisi M.A., Costa R., et al. (2002). New treatment of acute hypoxemic respiratory failure: non invasive pressure support ventilation delivered by helmet--a pilot controlled trial. *Crit. Care Med.*, 30:602-8. DOI:10.1097/00003246-200203000-00019.

[29] Kallet R.H. and Diaz J.V. (2009). The physiologic effects of noninvasive ventilation. *Respir Care* 2009; 54: 102–115. PubMed 19111110.

[30] Racca F., Appendini L., Gregoretti C., Stra E., Patessio A., Donner C.F., et al. (2005). Effectiveness of mask and helmet interfaces to deliver noninvasive ventilation in a human model of resistive breathing. *J. Appl. Physiol.,* 99:1262-71. DOI:10.1152/japplphysiol.01363.2004.

[31] Olivieri C., Longhini F., Cena T., Cammarota G., Vaschetto R., Messina A., et al. (2016). New versus conventional helmet for delivering noninvasive ventilation a physiologic, crossover randomized study in critically ill patients. *Anesthesiology,* 124:101-08. DOI: 10.1097/ALN.0000000000000910.

[32] Esquinas Rodriguez A.M., Papadakos P. J., Carron M., Cosentini R., Chiumello D. (2013). Clinical review: helmet and non-invasive mechanical ventilation in critically ill patients. *Crit. Care,* 17: 223. DOI:10.1097/ ALN.0000000000000910.

[33] Chiumello D., Pelosi P., Carlesso E., Severgnini P., Aspesi M., Gamberoni C., et al. (2003). Noninvasive positive pressure ventilation delivered by helmet vs. standard face mask. *Intensive Care Med.*, 29:1671-9. DOI:10.1007/s00134-003-1825-9.

[34] Yoshida T., Uchiyama A., Matsuura N., Mashimo T. and Fujino Y. (2012). Spontaneous breathing during lung-protective ventilation in an experimental acute lung injury model: high transpulmonary pressure associated with strong spontaneous breathing effort may worsen lung injury. *Crit. Care Med.*,40:1578–85. DOI: 10.1097/CCM.0b013e3182451c40.

[35] Grieco D.L., Menga L.S., Eleuteri D. and Antonelli M. (2019). Patient self-inflicted lung injury: implications for acute hypoxemic respiratory failure and ARDS patients on non-invasive support. *Minerva Anestesiol.,* 5:1014-1023. DOI: 10.23736/S0375-9393.19.13418-9.

[36] Chiumello D. and Brioni M. (2016). Severe hypoxemia: which strategy to choose. *Crit. Care.,* 20: 132. DOI: 10.1186/s13054-016-1304-7.

[37] Gattinoni L., Tonetti T., Cressoni M., Cadringher P., Herrmann P., Moerer O., et al. (2016). Ventilator-related causes of lung injury: the mechanical power. *Intensive Care Med.,* 42:1567–1575. DOI: 10.1007/s00134-016-4505-2.

[38] Marini J.J. and Jaber S. (2016). Dynamic predictors of VILI risk: beyond the driving pressure. *Intensive Care Med.*, 42:1597–1600. DOI: 10.1007/s00134-016-4534-x.

[39] Xie Y., Wang Y., Liu K., Li X. (2019). Correlation analysis between mechanical power, transforming growth factor-β1, and connective tissue growth factor levels in acute respiratory distress syndrome patients and their clinical significance in pulmonary structural remodeling. *Medicine (Baltimore)*, 98(29):e16531. DOI: 10.1097/MD.0000000000016531.

[40] Le Gall J.R., Lemeshow S. and Saulnier F. (1993). A new Simplified Acute Physiology Score (SAPS II) based on a European/North American multicenter study. *JAMA,* 270:2957-63 DOI:10.1001/jama.270.24.2957.

[41] Duan J., Han X., Bai L., Zhou L. and Huang S. (2017). Assessment of heart rate, acidosis, consciousness, oxygenation, and respiratory rate to predict noninvasive ventilation failure in hypoxemic patients. *Intensive Care Med.*, 43:192-199. DOI: 10.1007/s00134-016-4601-3.

[42] Esquinas A.M. (2014). Fibrosing interstitial pneumonia: Is mechanical ventilation always the final alternative for the intensivist? *The Journal of Thoracic and Cardiovascular Surgery*,147: 1113. DOI: 10.1016/j.jtcvs.2013.09.077.

In: Respiratory Ventilatory Strategies …
Editor: Antonio M. Esquinas
ISBN: 978-1-53617-847-0
© 2020 Nova Science Publishers, Inc.

Chapter 21

IDIOPATHIC PULMONARY FIBROSIS DURING INVASIVE MECHANICAL VENTILATION

Berrin Er**, MD
and Ebru Ortac Ersoy, MD
Medical Intensive Care Unit, Hacettepe University Faculty of Medicine,
Ankara, Turkey

ABSTRACT

Idiopathic pulmonary fibrosis (IPF) is a progressive interstitial lung disease. Patients may present with acute respiratory failure, named as acute exacerbation during follow-up, and they often require intensive care and mechanical ventilation support. While mechanical ventilation has been considered as futile treatment due to high mortality rates, recent studies have shown that prognosis is better in patients. However, there are no IPF-specific treatment strategies in mechanical ventilation. Because of the pathophysiological and clinical similarities with acute respiratory distress syndrome, it is considered that lung protective ventilation strategies with low-tidal volume can be applied in IPF. However, high positive end expiratory pressure is not recommended because of the low probability of recrutability due to lung damage.

Keywords: Invasive mechanical ventilation, idiopathic pulmonary fibrosis, acute exacerbation

* Corresponding Author's E-mail: berrinerkus@gmail.com.

INTRODUCTION

Idiopathic pulmonary fibrosis (IPF) is a chronic, progressive fibrosing lung disease of unknown cause, occurring primarily in older adults. Although most patients demonstrate a gradual worsening of lung function over years, a minority group of patients develop an exacerbation clinic leading to acute respiratory failure [1]. Criteria for the definition of exacerbation; previous or concurrent diagnosis of IPF, acute worsening or development of dyspnea typically < 1 month in duration, computed tomography with new bilateral ground-glass opacity and/or consolidation superimposed on a background pattern consistent with usual interstitial pneumonia pattern, deterioration not fully explained by cardiac failure or fluid overload [2]. Acute exacerbations are associated with increased mortality in IPF. Patients with IPF presenting with acute respiratory failure are often referred to intensive care units for respiratory support. Mortality was 90% in patients with IPF requiring ventilation support in a study which was conducted in 2008. Since the prognosis of these patients in the intensive care unit was poor, mechanical ventilation was found to be futile [3]. Due to the high mortality, the mechanical ventilation is a poor recommendation in these patients in 2011 guideline, and a study conducted in a transplant center intensive care unit, recommends that patients without a chance of rapid transplantation not be intubated [1, 4]. However, recent studies show different results. In a US cohort study, mortality was 51% in patients who underwent invasive mechanical ventilation [5]. In the Japanese patient cohort of 209 patients who underwent invasive mechanical ventilation, 30-day mortality was found as 44%. Prognosis has improved significantly in the last decade, so the use of mechanical ventilation should be considered in rapidly progressive patients. It has been reported that mechanical ventilation may not be performed in patients over 80 years of age because of poor prognosis [6]. Mechanical ventilation can be used as a bridge therapy to lung transplantation or in the treatment of reversible non-IPF causes of respiratory failure, other than acute exacerbation therapy in IPF [7].

RESPIRATORY MECHANICS IN MECHANICALLY VENTILATED PATIENTS

In IPF, the alveolar structure was destroyed with chronic inflammation and fibrosis. This leads to changes in dynamic and static lung volumes. There is one study evaluating respiratory mechanics in end-stage IPF patients. In this study, with normal chest wall elastance and elevated lung elastance, total respiratory system elastance was measured elevated. Alveolar fibrosis decreases lung volume, static and dynamic compliance decrease in contracting lung [8]. Reduction of surfactant production in IPF patients may also contribute to decreased compliance [9]. While 30cmH_20 plateau pressure applied, transpulmonary pressure of 27cmH_20 was found to be above the acceptable values. Therefore, the lowest plateau and driving pressure that can provide gas exchange is recommended in patients [8].

VENTILATOR SETTINGS

Data on mechanical ventilation in acute exacerbations of IPF are limited. The fact that the studies were retrospective, differences in the definition of the patient groups, being performed with a small number patients in single centers, not specifying ventilator settings, and differences in the treatments lead to insufficient data. In a recent study in the United States involving a large series of patients, mortality was 51% in patients who underwent invasive mechanical ventilation [5]. Although mortality data is better over time, rates are still higher than acute respiratory distress syndrome (ARDS) [10]. The selection of the patients newly diagnosed, younger, less comorbid with higher chances for transplantation who will be admitted to intensive care unit and applied invasive mechanical ventilation, provided better mortality data [11].

ARDS and IPF acute exacerbation definitions have similar features such as the presence of newly developed opacities in the lungs, acute onset, and absence of fluid overload or cardiac failure leading to respiratory failure. In addition, pathophysiologically overexpression of proinflammatory cytokines and diffuse alveolar damage occurs in acute exacerbation as similar to ARDS [12].

Since ventilator induced lung injury (VILI) is associated with increased mortality, the mechanical ventilation strategy in ARDS has been changed to application of lower tidal volume and higher positive end expiratory pressure (PEEP) to protect the lung from mechanical ventilation damage [13]. Stress and strain over physiological limits are known to be responsible for VILI development [14]. Mechanical ventilation damage was also seen in patient groups other than ARDS [15]. Therefore, applying lung protective mechanical ventilation strategies in ARDS in cases of IPF exacerbation due to having similar pathophysiological and clinical features. In fact, the decrease in mortality over time in IPF patients who require mechanical ventilation may be attirubuted to the application mechanical ventilation strategies in IPF.

On the other hand, alveolar collapse caused by septal wall thickening and alveolar epithelial hyperplasia with excessive proliferation of type 2 pneumocytes prevents the recruitment of lungs with high peep in IPF patients. The high pressure in the airways causes open alveoli to overstretch rather than opening the closed alveoli [16]. In the light of these data, high peep application in mechanical ventilation in interstitial lung disease was associated with increased mortality [17]. In an observational study investigating mechanical ventilation in IPF, high PEEP application in the first 24 hours was associated with increased mortality. High PEEP did not improve oxygenation, and was associated with alveolar overdistension and poor outcome [18]. Considering the possibility of low recruitability, low-medium PEEP application (4 - 6cmH_20) can be performed.

As the main goal is to reduce lung injury due to ventilator, it is recommended to provide <6ml/kg tidal volume based on ideal body weight and <30cmH20 plateau pressure in controlled modes, similar to ARDS [19, 20]. As the dead space is increased in these patients, minute ventilation can be increased by higher respiratory rate [21]. Despite the insufficient data, early neuromuscular blockers use may be recommended for reducing stress and strain in lungs and reducing patient-ventilator asynchrony in severe patients [22].

Transpulmonary pressure can be measured with an esophageal catheter to predict the pressure to which the lungs are exposed. Pressures below 20cmH_20 in homogeneous lungs and under 12cmH_20 in nonhomogeneous lungs are accepted [23].

Spontaneous assisted breathing may contribute to shunt reduction, oxygenation improvement, and maintenance of diaphragm tone in mild/moderate respiratory failure. During assisted spontaneous breaths, inspiratory muscles produce negative pressure in the pleura.

In case of acute exacerbation of IPF, this effort may cause respiratory drive to reach -30 to -40cmH_20. This may increase lung damage by increasing transpulmonary pressure [24]. A high respiratory drive may result in heterogeneous pressure drops in the airways at the end of the expiration, increasing the transmural pressure in the venous bed, leading to pulmonary edema and progression of VILI [25]. In addition, changes in transpulmonary pressure during respiratory effort can lead to heterogeneous distantion without affecting the tidal volume in the lung. This increases lung damage by local stretching [26].

Respiratory drive is not only affected by pressure support, but is also affected by the patient's sedation level, so sedation should be considered as part of preventive ventilation in patients with high respiratory drive.

Prone position is recommended at least 16 hours per day in the early period in patients with moderate to severe ARDS [27]. In pulmonary fibrosis, prone position does not improve oxygenation and increases plateau pressure, therefore it is not recommended in these patients [28].

CONCLUSION

Mechanical ventilation strategies for acute respiratory failure in IPF patients have not yet been fully defined, but lung protective ventilation strategies may have a positive impact on mortality data due to pathophysiological and clinical features similar to ARDS.

REFERENCES

[1] Raghu, G., Collard, H. R., Egan, J. J., Martinez, F. J., Behr, J., Brown, K. K. et al. An official ATS/ERS/JRS/ALAT statement: idiopathic pulmonary fibrosis: evidence-based guidelines for diagnosis and management. *Am. J. Respir. Crit. Care Med.,* 2011; 183(6):788 - 824.

[2] Collard, H. R., Ryerson, C. J., Corte, T. J., Jenkins, G., Kondoh, Y., Lederer, D. J. et al. Acute Exacerbation of Idiopathic Pulmonary Fibrosis. An International Working Group Report. *Am. J. Respir. Crit. Care Med.,* 2016; 194(3):265 - 75.

[3] Mallick, S. Outcome of patients with idiopathic pulmonary fibrosis (IPF) ventilated in intensive care unit. *Respir. Med.,* 2008; 102(10):1355 - 9.

[4] Magro, C. M., Allen, J., Pope-Harman, A., Waldman, W. J., Moh, P., Rothrauff, S. et al. The role of microvascular injury in the evolution of idiopathic pulmonary fibrosis. *Am. J. Clin. Pathol.,* 2003; 119(4):556 - 67.

[5] Rush, B., Wiskar, K., Berger, L., Griesdale, D. The use of mechanical ventilation in patients with idiopathic pulmonary fibrosis in the United States: A nationwide retrospective cohort analysis. *Respir. Med.,* 2016; 111:72 - 6.

[6] Oda, K., Yatera, K., Fujino, Y., Ishimoto, H., Nakao, H., Hanaka, T. et al. Efficacy of concurrent treatments in idiopathic pulmonary fibrosis patients with a rapid progression of respiratory failure: an analysis of a national administrative database in Japan. *BMC Pulm. Med.,* 2016; 16(1):91.

[7] Weill, D., Benden, C., Corris, P. A., Dark, J. H., Davis, R. D., Keshavjee, S. et al. A consensus document for the selection of lung transplant candidates: 2014--an update from the Pulmonary Transplantation Council of the International Society for Heart and Lung Transplantation. *J. Heart Lung Transplant.,* 2015; 34(1):1 - 15.

[8] Nava, S., Rubini, F. Lung and chest wall mechanics in ventilated patients with end stage idiopathic pulmonary fibrosis. *Thorax,* 1999; 54(5):390 - 5.

[9] Robinson, P. C., Watters, L. C., King, T. E., Mason, R. J. Idiopathic pulmonary fibrosis. Abnormalities in bronchoalveolar lavage fluid phospholipids. *Am. Rev. Respir. Dis.,* 1988; 137(3):585 - 91.

[10] Bellani, G., Laffey, J. G., Pham, T., Fan, E., Brochard, L., Esteban, A. et al. Epidemiology, Patterns of Care, and Mortality for Patients with Acute Respiratory Distress Syndrome in Intensive Care Units in 50 Countries. *JAMA,* 2016; 315(8):788 - 800.

[11] Mooney, J. J., Raimundo, K., Chang, E., Broder, M. S. Mechanical ventilation in idiopathic pulmonary fibrosis: a nationwide analysis of ventilator use, outcomes, and resource burden. *BMC Pulm. Med.,* 2017; 17(1):84.

[12] Marchioni, A., Tonelli, R., Ball, L., Fantini, R., Castaniere, I., Cerri, S. et al. Acute exacerbation of idiopathic pulmonary fibrosis: lessons learned from acute respiratory distress syndrome? *Crit. Care,* 2018; 22(1):80.

[13] Petrucci, N., De Feo, C. Lung protective ventilation strategy for the acute respiratory distress syndrome. *Cochrane Database Syst. Rev.,* 2013(2):CD003844.

[14] Protti, A., Cressoni, M., Santini, A., Langer, T., Mietto, C., Febres, D. et al. Lung stress and strain during mechanical ventilation: any safe threshold? *Am. J. Respir. Crit. Care Med.,* 2011; 183(10):1354 - 62.

[15] Neto, A. S., Simonis, F. D., Barbas, C. S., Biehl, M., Determann, R. M., Elmer, J. et al. Lung-Protective Ventilation with Low Tidal Volumes and the Occurrence of Pulmonary Complications in Patients without Acute Respiratory Distress Syndrome: A Systematic Review and Individual Patient Data Analysis. *Crit. Care Med.,* 2015; 43(10):2155 - 63.

[16] Lutz, D., Gazdhar, A., Lopez-Rodriguez, E., Ruppert, C., Mahavadi, P., Gunther, A. et al. Alveolar derecruitment and collapse induration as crucial mechanisms in lung injury and fibrosis. *Am. J. Respir. Cell Mol. Biol.,* 2015; 52(2):232 - 43.

[17] Papiris, S. A., Manali, E. D., Kolilekas, L., Kagouridis, K., Triantafillidou, C., Tsangaris, I. et al. Clinical review: idiopathic pulmonary fibrosis acute exacerbations--unravelling Ariadne's thread. *Crit. Care,* 2010; 14(6):246.

[18] Fernandez-Perez, E. R., Yilmaz, M., Jenad, H., Daniels, C. E., Ryu, J. H., Hubmayr, R. D. et al. Ventilator settings and outcome of respiratory failure in chronic interstitial lung disease. *Chest,* 2008; 133(5):1113 - 9.

[19] Terragni, P. P., Rosboch, G., Tealdi, A., Corno, E., Menaldo, E., Davini, O. et al. Tidal hyperinflation during low tidal volume ventilation in acute respiratory distress syndrome. *Am. J. Respir. Crit. Care Med.,* 2007; 175(2):160 - 6.

[20] Gaudry, S., Vincent, F., Rabbat, A., Nunes, H., Crestani, B., Naccache, J. M. et al. Invasive mechanical ventilation in patients with fibrosing interstitial pneumonia. *J. Thorac Cardiovasc. Surg.,* 2014; 147(1):47 - 53.

[21] Bhatti, H., Girdhar, A., Usman, F., Cury, J., Bajwa, A. Approach to acute exacerbation of idiopathic pulmonary fibrosis. *Ann. Thorac Med.,* 2013; 8(2):71 - 7.

[22] Papazian, L., Forel, J. M., Gacouin, A., Penot-Ragon, C., Perrin, G., Loundou, A. et al. Neuromuscular blockers in early acute respiratory distress syndrome. *N Engl. J. Med.,* 2010; 363(12):1107 - 16.

[23] Mauri, T., Yoshida, T., Bellani, G., Goligher, E. C., Carteaux, G., Rittayamai, N. et al. Esophageal and transpulmonary pressure in the clinical setting: meaning, usefulness and perspectives. *Intensive Care Med.,* 2016; 42(9):1360 - 73.

[24] Brochard, L., Slutsky, A., Pesenti, A. Mechanical Ventilation to Minimize Progression of Lung Injury in Acute Respiratory Failure. *Am. J. Respir. Crit. Care Med.,* 2017; 195(4):438 - 42.

[25] Bellani, G., Grasselli, G., Teggia-Droghi, M., Mauri, T., Coppadoro, A., Brochard, L. et al. Do spontaneous and mechanical breathing have similar effects on average transpulmonary and alveolar pressure? A clinical crossover study. *Crit. Care,* 2016; 20(1):142.

[26] Yoshida, T., Torsani, V., Gomes, S., De Santis, R. R., Beraldo, M. A., Costa, E. L. et al. Spontaneous effort causes occult pendelluft during mechanical ventilation. *Am. J. Respir. Crit. Care Med.,* 2013; 188(12):1420 - 7.

[27] Kallet, R. H. A Comprehensive Review of Prone Position in ARDS. *Respir. Care,* 2015; 60(11):1660 - 87.

[28] Nakos, G., Tsangaris, I., Kostanti, E., Nathanail, C., Lachana, A., Koulouras, V. et al. Effect of the prone position on patients with hydrostatic pulmonary edema compared with patients with acute respiratory distress syndrome and pulmonary fibrosis. *Am. J. Respir. Crit. Care Med.,* 2000; 161(2 Pt 1):360 - 8.

In: Respiratory Ventilatory Strategies … ISBN: 978-1-53617-847-0
Editor: Antonio M. Esquinas © 2020 Nova Science Publishers, Inc.

Chapter 22

IDIOPATIC PULMONARY FIBROSIS AND MECHANICAL VENTILATION INTERACTION – PATIENT VENTILATOR ASYNCHRONY

Martin Scharffenberg[1,*], MD and Esme O'Loughlin[2], MD
[1]Dept. of Anaesthesiology and Intensive Care Medicine, University Hospital Carl Gustav Carus at Technische Universität Dresden, Dresden, Germany
[2]Department of Trauma and Orthopaedics, Univeristy Hospitals Birmingham NHS Trust, Birmingham, United Kingdom

ABSTRACT

Non-invasive ventilation may represent a valuable option in certain patients with idiopathic pulmonary fibrosis and respiratory worsening. Despite technical improvements, subject-ventilator asynchrony may occur, which is shown to be a major factor promoting failure of non-invasive ventilation and is associated with decreased survival. This chapter summarizes different asynchrony entities and their treatment during non-invasive ventilation in patients with idiopathic pulmonary fibrosis.

Keywords: patient ventilator asynchrony, patient ventilator interaction, subject ventilator asynchrony, mechanical ventilation, non-invasive ventilation

---

* Corresponding Author's E-mail: martin.scharffenberg@ukdd.de.

Abbreviations

CPAP	Continuous positive airway pressure
EADi	Electrical activity of the diaphragm
F_iO_2	Inspiratory fraction of oxygen
HFNO	High-flow nasal oxygen
IPF	Idiopathic pulmonary fibrosis
MV	Mechanical ventilation
NAVA	Neurally Adjusted Ventilatory Assist
NIV	Non-invasive ventilation
PAV	Proportional assist ventilation
PEEP	Positive end-expiratory pressure
PEEPi	Intrinsic positive end-expiratory pressure
SVA	Subject-ventilator asynchrony

Introduction

Idiopathic pulmonary fibrosis (IPF) is associated with a progressive decrease of lung function and low survival rates (Marchioni et al. 2018). Acute deterioration of lung function, so-called acute exacerbations, have prognostic significance and frequently induce acute hypoxemic respiratory failure often requiring mechanical ventilation (MV). Although the majority of patients should be managed without invasive MV (Raghu et al. 2011), non-invasive ventilation (NIV) may be a reasonable intervention (Yokoyama et al. 2010; Vianello et al. 2019; Mollica et al. 2010; Güngör et al. 2013). Recently, the use of NIV for patients with IPF increased. Cautiously interpreting clinical trials regarding a possible selection bias in terms of less severe clinical presentations, NIV was associated with reduced complication and mortality rates in IPF patients (Yokoyama et al. 2010; Vianello et al. 2014). In general, a good patient-ventilator interaction is essential for the success of the therapy, but subject-ventilator asynchrony (SVA) may occur frequently during NIV. SVA was identified as a major factor of NIV tolerance and was associated with increased mortality (Blanch et al. 2015). However, it remains unclear if SVA is a cause of mortality or a symptom of more severe illness. While incidences and effects of SVA in the special cohort of patients with IPF have not been investigated in detail yet, and recently published studies on NIV in IPF patients did not report results regarding SVA, this chapter will assess the framework of subject-ventilator interaction in non-invasively ventilated patients with IPF.

SUBJECT-VENTILATOR ASYNCHRONY: GENERAL ASPECTS

Subject-ventilator asynchrony is defined as the mismatch between the inspiratory times of the patient and the ventilator, or in other words, a mismatch between the patient´s need and the mechanical respiratory support. The nomenclature is not uniform in the literature, but SVA can be classified into different entities. In brief, an inspiratory effort, which is not answered by the ventilator, is usually called ineffective or missed effort. In contrast, an unintendedly applied breath by the ventilator represents and auto-triggered breath. Both types can be summarized as rate asynchronies. Besides these two extremes, different intra-cycle asynchronies result from inadequately applied respiratory support, e.g., when the respiratory support is successfully triggered but undercuts or exceeds the patient´s respiratory effort.

A respiratory support with a significant delay between the onset of the patient´s inspiratory effort and the breath is called delayed trigger. If a respiratory support is stopped before or after the end of the patient´s inspiratory effort, premature cycling off, or delayed cycling off, is present respectively. Two consecutive breaths without complete expiration in between, or with less than 30% of the usual expiratory time in between, are called double trigger or double cycling. Ineffective trigger, auto-trigger, and trigger delay are sometimes summarized as triggering asynchronies, while an inadequate inspiratory flow, double trigger, and premature cycling off, as well as delayed cycling off are sometimes referred to as asynchronies within the respiratory cycle. Furthermore, SVA was classified by some authors as major (ineffective trigger, auto-trigger, double trigger) and minor (delayed trigger, premature or delayed cycling off) asynchrony events (Longhini et al. 2017).

Moreover, there is another special SVA type: Reverse triggering describes the activation of the patient´s respiratory center with consecutive muscle contraction due to a passive insufflation of the lung (Akoumianaki et al. 2013). Because this leads to a second inspiration directly after the mechanical inspiration, it may be confused with double trigger and thus this asynchrony type is usually rarely recognized. However, if the inflation-induced muscle contraction during a reverse trigger does not induce the second breath, it will in turn represent an ineffective effort.

POTENTIAL CAUSES OF SUBJECT-VENTILATOR ASYNCHRONY

Different problems may cause SVA: They can be classified as patient-related causes vs. non-patient-related causes. One of the main factors promoting SVA during NIV are air leaks. Table 1 summarizes potential causes.

Besides this general causes of SVA, pathological lung mechanics in advanced stages of IPF, e.g., increased lung elastance (Nava and Rubini 1999), may further promote SVA. However, there is no specific evidence regarding SVA in IPF patients.

Table 1. Potential causes of asynchrony events

Type of Subject-Ventilator Asynchrony	Potential causes
Ineffective effort/Missed effort	Severe air leaks, inadequately high trigger threshold or low trigger sensitivity, very low inspiratory flow, excessive ventilator over-assistance, high intrinsic positive end-expiratory pressure, decreased respiratory effort, deep sedation
Auto-trigger	Air leaks, artefacts in airway pressure due to manipulation, high trigger sensitivity, water in the ventilator circuit, cardiac oscillations
Delayed trigger	Inadequately high trigger threshold or low trigger sensitivity
Double trigger	Severe air leaks, low inspiratory flow, very low trigger sensitivity, short inspiratory time, very high or other pathological respiratory drive
Premature cycling off	Inadequate cycling-off threshold, high inspiratory flow
Delayed cycling off	Inadequate cycling-off threshold, severe air leaks (not reaching cycling off-threshold), low inspiratory flow
Reverse trigger	Mechanical inflation of the lung, deep sedation, intrinsic positive end-expiratory pressure

Potential Consequences of Subject-Ventilator Asynchrony

SVA is a major factor of NIV intolerance and for NIV failure. Depending on the incidence and type, SVA can significantly increase the work of breathing and induce an excessive load to respiratory muscles in the case of under-assistance. This is usually associated with impaired breathing comfort and sleep quality as well as with an increased oxygen consumption. Furthermore, SVA may impair gas exchange and result in air hunger and hypoxia and/or hypercapnia. This can further increase the respiratory drive of patients with acute exacerbations of IPF and lead to even more pronounced SVA, promoting a vicious circle. Accordingly, SVA may induce an activation of the sympathic vegetative system with all its related feedback and reflex loops (Evans et al. 2002). SVA can induce or aggravate anxiety, and different ventilation-related worries, e.g., anxiety of choking, which have been frequently reported by survivors of a critical illness who have been on MV (Tate et al. 2012). While this anxiety again activates the sympathic nervous system and increases oxygen consumption, whichi leads to the already described vicious circle, SVA may increase the need of deeper sedation of patients undergoing NIV.

Apart from subjective impairments, SVA may contribute to ventilator-induced lung injury. Double triggering increases the applied tidal volume to values exceeding the limits of lung-protective ventilation. More negative pleural pressures, due to increased respiratory drive to compensate an ineffective ventilation, which may be induced by SVA, may promote development of pulmonary edema. In presence of inhomogeneous aeration of the lungs, lung injury may result from regionally different effects of heavy inspiration on dependent and non-dependent lung areas. To date, it remains unclear if the reverse trigger can induce lung and diaphragmatic injury. In general, IPF patients are more susceptible to the development of a ventilator-induced lung injury, due to fibrosis-related reduced lung compliance and impaired pulmonary repair mechanisms (Marchioni et al. 2018). Furthermore, in invasively ventilated patients, SVA was associated with longer time on ventilation and increased mortality. However, it remains unclear if this also applies to SVA during NIV.

Despite this evidence, pathomechanisms directly linking SVA to lung injury and survival rates, remain unclear, especially during NIV. Currently it remains elusive if SVA is a symptom or a cause. Mortality rates of patients with IPF and respiratory deterioration are very high and are mostly affected by the severity of the underlying disease and the exacerbation of IPF itself. Thus it remains unclear and questionable if the incidence of SVA has a major influence on the survival rates in this population. However, improving comfort, and reducing work of breathing is an important aim and should be achieved in all patients undergoing mechanical ventilation.

Detection of Subject-Ventilator Asynchrony

The correct and reliable detection of SVA is challenging and not standardized. Theoretically, SVA entities can be detected by observing and interpreting the flow and pressure wave forms provided on the ventilator screen. However, different studies showed that even experienced clinicians failed to recognize all episodes and to classify asynchrony events correctly. Thus, errors may occur frequently as some SVA entities are hard to recognize by only watching airway and flow profiles for a certain time. In addition to this, the correct identification requires deep understanding of respiratory physiology and the continuous attendance of skilled personnel. Especially observing limited periods may lead to an underestimation of the SVA incidence, because asynchrony events were shown to occur in episodes, e.g., clusters, where more than 30 events occur in three minutes within phases without any SVA (Vaporidi et al. 2017). Even more importantly than solely checking ventilation waveforms, is the direct observation of the patient to recognize signs of distress and fighting against the ventilator, and to diagnose technical problems, e.g., significant air leaks or water in the ventilator circuit.

Additional measurements may allow better understanding and more easy detection of SVA events, e.g., measuring esophageal pressure or the electrical activity of the diaphragm (EADi). Negative deflections in the esophageal pressure as well as amplitudes of the EADi signal represent inspiratory efforts of the patient and can be compared with corresponding airway pressure and flow wave forms regarding occurrence and timing. Without these additional measurements, SVA rates are usually underestimated. However, measuring the esophageal pressure reguires the placement of a special esophageal balloon catheter and measuring the EADi signal requires a special naso-/orogastric feeding tube equipped with electrodes attached to a special ventilator. Those do not belong to the clinical routine in most intensive care units. Furthermore, these catheters may represent a source of additional discomfort and/or air leaks. The current evidence does not support routine use of these two additional measurements.

Interestingly, computer-based software programs have been developed recently, which incorporate different input signals from the ventilator while being able to automatically detect different SVA entities. Also automatic detection using big data is emerging and corresponding systems have already been developed. However, these are not yet commercially available and the clinical relevance remains unclear.

Knowing its limitations and pitfalls, observation of the ventilator screen still represents the currently most frequently used method of detecting SVA.

PREVENTION AND TREATMENT OF SUBJECT-VENTILATOR ASYNCHRONY: ADJUST THE VENTILATOR, NOT THE PATIENT

In general, prevention is usually better than therapy. Thus, measures should be taken to avoid SVA. Studies showed that asynchrony rates were lower when dedicated NIV ventilators were used instead of regular intensive care ventilators. Furthermore, air leaks should be minimized, or well compensated for, while other disruptive factors should be excluded. Therefore, choosing the optimal NIV interface, e.g., a well-fitting NIV mask of proper size, as well as its correct placement and fixation, are essential.

According to the predominantly detected type of SVA, ventilator settings should be titrated (trigger sensitivity, pressure support level, and cycling-off thresholds, if applicable) until subjective signs of distress and fighting, as well as occurrence of SVA in ventilator wave forms diminish. A possible intrinsic positive end-expiratory pressure should be detected and treated. If double triggers appear frequently, measures may be taken to distinguish between a double trigger due to insufficient respiratory support and a reverse trigger, which may appear similar in airway pressure and flow waveforms but require different treatments (see Table 2). Therefore, measurement of esophageal pressure or EADi may be helpful. Patients should be monitored closely and treatment effects should be re-evaluated regularly.

Table 2 summarizes treatment options according to the different types of asynchrony.

Table 2. Treatment options according to the different types of asynchrony

Type of Subject-Ventilator Asynchrony	Treatment option
Ineffective effort/Missed effort	Compensate or eliminate air leaks, increase trigger sensitivity, increase inspiratory flow, detect and treat intrinsic positive end-expiratory pressure, check for and treat causes of decreased respiratory drive, consider reduction of sedation, consider inspiratory muscle training with physical therapy (if possible)
Auto-trigger	Compensate or eliminate air leaks, reduce trigger sensitivity, remove water from ventilator circuit
Delayed trigger	Adjust trigger sensitivity
Double trigger	Compensate or eliminate air leaks, ensure adequate minute ventilation by adequate inspiratory flow and time, consider increasing trigger sensitivity
Premature cycling off	Adjust cycling-off threshold, compensate or eliminate air leaks, decrease inspiratory flow
Delayed cycling off	Adjust cycling-off threshold, compensate or eliminate air leaks, increase inspiratory flow
Reverse trigger	Detect and treat intrinsic positive end-expiratory pressure, consider reduction of sedation

The current evidence on the effects of sedation on SVA are conflicting. Clinical trials showed that increasing the sedation for patients submitted to the intensive care unit with frequent double trigger, did not reduce SVA, and, the incidence of ineffective triggers increased with deepened sedation. However, in another trial, deep sedation improved asynchrony but did not completely eliminate it. In an observational trial, administration of opioids without other sedation reduced SVA without impairment of consciousness. Thus, sedation management should be titrated cautiously using opioids in order to improve patient ventilator interaction.

Finally, changing the mode of ventilation can be considered.

High-flow nasal oxygen (HFNO) is a relatively new method of non-invasive respiratory support. In contrast to conventional oxygen insufflation, which is usually applied with an oxygen flow up to 15 L/min, HFNO allows a continuous inspiratory flow of up to 70 L/min with an adjustable inspiratory fraction of oxygen (F_iO_2). The benefits of HFNO include application of humidified and warmed gas with precise F_iO_2 adjustment, a wash-out effect of carbon dioxide from the anatomical deadspace, and a small PEEP-like effect depending on the applied flow. HFNO is usually well tolerated by patients and clinical trials reported only a few complaints about tolerance. Its value has been primarily established in patients with acute respiratory failure caused by other diseases than IPF. However, a small clinical trial revealed some positive effects of HFNO on respiratory variables in IPF patients with global respiratory insufficiency and hypercapnia (Bräunlich et al. 2013). Also in ambulatory IPF patients without acute respiratory distress, HFNO showed positive effects. Furthermore, case reports and retrospective trials reported application of HFNO in IPF and other interstitial lung diseases. As there is no support pressure during HFNO, SVA is not possible per definition in this kind of respiratory support. Thus, if high-flow nasal oxygen was successful during respiratory worsening of IPF, respiratory support without asynchrony could be achieved. In conclusion, HFNO may offer respiratory support to IPF patients who do not need urgent intubation and may be tried in absence of contraindications. But it remains unclear, if there is a significant reduction of intubation or mortality rates.

In one very small clinical trial on IPF patients with acute exacerbation, continuous positive airway pressure (CPAP) of up to 12 cmH_2O was used alone or as spontaneous/timed mode, which was successfully applied in half of the patients (Yokoyama et al. 2010). In analogy to HFNO, CPAP without pressure support excludes any asynchrony. However, data on SVA were not reported in this trial.

In one retrospective clinical trial, patients were non-invasively ventilated using flow-triggered pressure support with positive end-expiratory pressure (Mollica et al. 2010). NIV temporarily improved oxygenation and reduced the respiratory rate, however, in some patients NIV was withdrawn due to poor compliance. Unfortunately, data on SVA were not reported. Interestingly, the patients who had NIV and died, did not decease due to respiratory problems.

If SVA is not manageable during common pressure support modes, it may be helpful to switch to other ventilation modes, which were shown to improve the patient-ventilator interaction. In Neurally Adjusted Ventilatory Assist (NAVA), breaths are primarily triggered by the EADi signal. NAVA was shown to decrease asynchrony compared with conventional pressure support ventilation. Furthermore, proportional assist ventilation (PAV and PAV+) was shown to increase patient comfort. However, it remains unclear if there is a benefit of one of these modes for patients with IPF.

Conclusion

The survival rate of patients with IPF and acute respiratory failure is low, and probably mostly affected by the underlying disease itself. Thus, it remains unclear and questionable if the incidence of asynchrony events has a major influence on the mortality and other clinically relevant outcomes in this certain population. Reliable evidence is needed. However, achieving favourable short-term effects, e.g., improving comfort and work of breathing, reducing dyspnea, allowing communication, and bridging to other treatments, is a valuable goal and should be achieved in all patients undergoing NIV. This justifies cautious monitoring and treatment of SVA in order to let the IPF patient benefit from NIV.

REFERENCES

Akoumianaki, Evangelia, Aissam Lyazidi, Nathalie Rey, Dimitrios Matamis, Nelly Perez-Martinez, Raphael Giraud, Jordi Mancebo, Laurent Brochard, and Jean-Christophe Marie Richard. 2013. "Mechanical Ventilation-Induced Reverse-Triggered Breaths: A Frequently Unrecognized Form of Neuromechanical Coupling." *Chest* 143 (4): 927-38. https://doi.org/10.1378/chest.12-1817.

Blanch, Lluís, Ana Villagra, Bernat Sales, Jaume Montanya, Umberto Lucangelo, Manel Luján, Oscar García-Esquirol, et al. 2015. "Asynchronies during Mechanical Ventilation Are Associated with Mortality." *Intensive Care Medicine* 41 (4): 633-41. https://doi.org/10.1007/s00134-015-3692-6.

Bräunlich, Jens, Denise Beyer, David Mai, Stefan Hammerschmidt, Hans-Jürgen Seyfarth, and Hubert Wirtz. 2013. "Effects of Nasal High Flow on Ventilation in Volunteers, COPD and Idiopathic Pulmonary Fibrosis Patients." R*espiration; International Review of Thoracic Diseases* 85 (4): 319-25. https://doi.org/10.1159/000342027.

Evans, Karleyton C., Robert B. Banzett, Lewis Adams, Leanne McKay, Richard S. J. Frackowiak, and Douglas R. Corfield. 2002. "BOLD FMRI Identifies Limbic, Paralimbic, and Cerebellar Activation during Air Hunger." *Journal of Neurophysiology* 88 (3): 1500-1511. https://doi.org/10.1152/jn.2002.88.3.1500.

Güngör, Gökay, Dursun Tatar, Cüneyt Saltürk, Pinar Çimen, Zuhal Karakurt, Cenk Kirakli, Nalan Adıgüzel, et al. 2013. "Why Do Patients with Interstitial Lung Diseases Fail in the ICU? A 2-Center Cohort Study." *Respiratory Care* 58 (3): 525-31. https://doi.org/10.4187/respcare.01734.

Longhini, Federico, Davide Colombo, Lara Pisani, Francesco Idone, Pan Chun, Jonne Doorduin, Liu Ling, et al. 2017. "Efficacy of Ventilator Waveform Observation for Detection of Patient-Ventilator Asynchrony during NIV: A Multicentre Study." *ERJ Open Research* 3 (4). https://doi.org/10.1183/23120541.00075-2017.

Marchioni, Alessandro, Roberto Tonelli, Lorenzo Ball, Riccardo Fantini, Ivana Castaniere, Stefania Cerri, Fabrizio Luppi, Mario Malerba, Paolo Pelosi, and Enrico Clini. 2018. "Acute Exacerbation of Idiopathic Pulmonary Fibrosis: Lessons Learned from Acute Respiratory Distress Syndrome?" *Critical Care* (London, England) 22 (1): 80. https://doi.org/10.1186/s13054-018-2002-4.

Mollica, Corrado, Gregorino Paone, Vittoria Conti, Daniela Ceccarelli, Giovanni Schmid, Paolo Mattia, Nicola Perrone, et al. 2010. "Mechanical Ventilation in Patients with End-Stage Idiopathic Pulmonary Fibrosis." *Respiration; International Review of Thoracic Diseases* 79 (3): 209-15. https://doi.org/10.1159/000225932.

Nava, S., and F. Rubini. 1999. "Lung and Chest Wall Mechanics in Ventilated Patients with End Stage Idiopathic Pulmonary Fibrosis." *Thorax* 54 (5): 390-95. https://doi.org/10.1136/thx.54.5.390.

Raghu, Ganesh, Harold R. Collard, Jim J. Egan, Fernando J. Martinez, Juergen Behr, Kevin K. Brown, Thomas V. Colby, et al. 2011. "An Official ATS/ERS/JRS/ALAT Statement: Idiopathic Pulmonary Fibrosis: Evidence-Based Guidelines for Diagnosis and Management." *American Journal of Respiratory and Critical Care Medicine* 183 (6): 788-824. https://doi.org/10.1164/rccm.2009-040GL.

Tate, Judith Ann, Annette Devito Dabbs, Leslie A. Hoffman, Eric Milbrandt, and Mary Beth Happ. 2012. "Anxiety and Agitation in Mechanically Ventilated Patients." *Qualitative Health Research* 22 (2): 157-73. https://doi.org/10.1177/1049732311421616.

Vaporidi, Katerina, Dimitris Babalis, Achilleas Chytas, Emmanuel Lilitsis, Eumorfia Kondili, Vasilis Amargianitakis, Ioanna Chouvarda, Nicos Maglaveras, and Dimitris Georgopoulos. 2017. "Clusters of Ineffective Efforts during Mechanical Ventilation: Impact on Outcome." *Intensive Care Medicine* 43 (2): 184-91. https://doi.org/10.1007/s00134-016-4593-z.

Vianello, Andrea, Giovanna Arcaro, Laura Battistella, Emanuela Pipitone, Stefania Vio, Alessandra Concas, Luciana Paladini, et al. 2014. "Noninvasive Ventilation in the Event of Acute Respiratory Failure in Patients with Idiopathic Pulmonary Fibrosis." *Journal of Critical Care* 29 (4): 562-67. https://doi.org/10.1016/j.jcrc.2014.03.019.

Vianello, Andrea, Giovanna Arcaro, Beatrice Molena, Cristian Turato, Fausto Braccioni, Luciana Paladini, Stefania Vio, et al. 2019. "High-Flow Nasal Cannula Oxygen Therapy to Treat Acute Respiratory Failure in Patients with Acute Exacerbation of Idiopathic Pulmonary Fibrosis." *Therapeutic Advances in Respiratory Disease* 13 (December): 1753466619847130. https://doi.org/10.1177/1753466619847130.

Yokoyama, Toshiki, Yasuhiro Kondoh, Hiroyuki Taniguchi, Kensuke Kataoka, Keisuke Kato, Osamu Nishiyama, Tomoki Kimura, Ryuichi Hasegawa, and Keishi Kubo. 2010. "Noninvasive Ventilation in Acute Exacerbation of Idiopathic Pulmonary Fibrosis." *Internal Medicine* (Tokyo, Japan) 49 (15): 1509-14. https://doi.org/10.2169/internalmedicine.49.3222.

In: Respiratory Ventilatory Strategies …
Editor: Antonio M. Esquinas
ISBN: 978-1-53617-847-0
© 2020 Nova Science Publishers, Inc.

Chapter 23

WEANING FROM MECHANICAL VENTILATION: HOW TO APPROACH

***Lokesh Tiwari*[1,*] *and Shashank Shekhar*[2]**
[1]Associate Professor and Head of Pediatrics,
Incharge Pediatric Intensive Care Unit,
All India Institute of Medical Sciences Patna, Patna, India
[2]Senior Resident, Pediatric Intensive Care Unit,
All India Institute of Medical Sciences Patna, Patna, India

ABSTRACT

Indications for putting patient on NIV are well-defined but there are no established guidelines for weaning patients from NIV though it is very important to reduce the complications related to prolonged ventilation and hospital stay. There are several weaning criteria that need to be considered while withdrawing NIV. Current data on weaning strategies from NIV is limited. NIV withdrawal strategies include progressive weaning or immediate withdrawal. In progressive weaning strategies step wise reduction of NIV duration or ventilator pressure support is attempted while in immediate withdrawal strategy, NIV is discontinued abruptly as soon as patient meets weaning criteria. Stepwise reduction of NIV use seems reasonable and may be adopted in day to day practice. Well-designed randomized studies with adequate sample size are needed to find the best strategy for weaning from NIV that would shorten the length of hospital/ICU stay and improve outcome parameters.

* Corresponding Author's E-mail: lokeshdoc@yahoo.com.

Introduction

Mechanical ventilation (MV) is known to cause several complications including ventilator associated pneumonia. Weaning is the process of withdrawing mechanical ventilatory support and transferring the work of breathing from the ventilator to the patient. Weaning may be done abruptly with patient being directly transitioned from full ventilatory support to unassisted spontaneous breathing simply by discontinuing the ventilator in certain conditions where ventilatory support is needed for very short period of time and there are no associated morbidities. For other patients where ventilatory support is prolonged, weaning process is more gradual. The process is individualized for each patient and it may take from days to weeks depending upon underlying disease and various patient related conditions. Daily assessment of readiness for extubation with a spontaneous breathing trial (SBT), regular breaks in sedation, early mobilisation and protocolised rehabilitation is recommended to help with weaning. Pressure support ventilation (PSV) and spontaneous breathing trial (SBT) are established weaning modes from invasive mechanical ventilation [1, 2].

Noninvasive ventilation (NIV) is defined as the use of a mask or nasal prongs to provide ventilator support through a patient's nose and/or mouth bypassing the use of invasive artificial airway (endotracheal tube or tracheostomy tube). Utility of non-invasive positive pressure ventilation (NIV) in many acute and chronic conditions leading to respiratory failure is well established to reduce the requirement of endotracheal intubation, Intensive Care Unit (ICU) stay, cost of care and mortality [3]. NIV has become an integral maneuver in ICU for adult and pediatric patients with both chronic and acute respiratory failure of various etiologies. Extubation to non-invasive ventilation (NIV) following a failed SBT is also used as a weaning strategy from invasive mechanical ventilator, commonly in hypercapnic respiratory failure patients.

Indications for putting patient on NIV are well-defined but there are no established guidelines for weaning patients from NIV. Complications of NIV include gastric distension, skin breakdown and interface discomfort. All efforts should be made to minimize the duration of ventilator support to reduce NIV associated complications as well as complications due to prolonged hospital stay. There are several parameters that need to be considered while withdrawing NIV though there are very few studies which have compared specific weaning protocols with treating team guided weaning from NIV. Most of these studies have a small sample size hence, are largely inconclusive.

Weaning Success and Failure

After the weaning process, if patient is able to maintain spontaneous breathing for a prescribed period of time, it is considered as weaning success. Weaning failure generally means that patient is returned to mechanical ventilation after any length of weaning trial or a period of un-sustained spontaneous breathing.

NIV as a Weaning Strategy from Mechanical Ventilation

A systematic review and meta-analysis comparing non-invasive ventilation (NIV) with invasive ventilation weaning protocols concludes that use of NIV in weaning from mechanical ventilation decreases hospital mortality, the incidence of VAP and ICU length of stay. NIV as a weaning strategy appears to be most beneficial in patients with COPD. This conclusion is derived from twenty-five relevant studies involving 1609 patients. Mortality at hospital discharge was lower in the NIV weaning group compared to the invasive weaning group [pooled odds ratio (OR) 0.58, 95% highest density interval (HDI) 0.29-0.89]. NIV weaning reduced the duration of invasive ventilation in patients and ICU length of stay. Reported rates of ventilator associated pneumonia (VAP) were lower in the NIV group. NIV weaning did not reduce overall hospital length of stay or long-term mortality [4].

Recent RCT comparing protocol directed versus physician directed weaning in patients using NIV for any cause of respiratory failure found that the protocol directed weaning decreased the duration of NIV and ICU stay in the patients with exacerbation of COPD [5].

Weaning from NIV

In absence of evidence based NIV weaning protocols, physicians often use their clinical judgment to wean the patient from NIV using various parameters similar to weaning from invasive ventilation such as cardiovascular stability/hemodynamic stability, good gas-exchange, control of pulmonary edema, atelectases, secretions, and bronchospasm, GCS, >10, stable blood gas and electrolytes etc.

Weaning Strategies

Successful weaning from NIV is defined as no deterioration of arterial blood gases or clinical condition resulting in restarting of NIV from time of initiation of weaning to 48 h after complete withdrawal of NIV. In the absence of universal guidelines, rapid withdrawal may lead to failed weaning warranting hiking of NIV support or endotracheal intubation in some patients while on other hand a significant number of patients would stay on NIV for a longer time than necessary with risk of hospital acquired infections [6]. This necessitates the need for uniform NIV weaning protocols. The Royal College of Physicians (RCP) and the British Thoracic Society (BTS) in 2008 suggested a weaning protocol for NIV following progressive reduction in duration of NIV use [7]. Other studies have used similar progressive protocols (gradual increasing off NIV periods or decreasing pressure support) and compared it with immediate weaning [8, 9].

NIV Weaning Initiation Criteria

Before attempting weaning, it is important to assess patient's readiness for weaning. Clinical improvement and stability of the patient's condition are the most important factors in determining when NIV may be safely withdrawn. A patient who has recovered from the underlying condition and has acceptable clinical and physiological parameters (weaning criteria), is ready for weaning from NIV. The clinical and physiological parameters used in this setting include –

1. Arterial pH $\geq$ 7.35, PaO2 > 60mmHg, PaO2/FiO2 > 150,
2. Oxygen haemoglobin saturation (SpO_2) >90% on $FiO_2 \leq 50\%$,
3. Systolic blood pressure $\geq$90 mmHg or age appropriate SBP for children (without vasopressor)
4. No signs of respiratory distress like agitation, diaphoresis or anxiety.
5. Glasgow Coma Scale $\geq$13
6. Heart Rate between <110 beats/minute (age appropriate for children)
7. Respiratory Rate <24 breaths/minute (age appropriate for children) without use of respiratory accessory muscles.

Patient satisfying these criteria can be weaned from NIV by 3 ways –

1. Stepwise reduction of duration of NIV use,
2. Stepwise reduction in pressure support and
3. Immediate withdrawal of NIV.

Stepwise Reduction of Duration of NIV Use

This strategy involves gradually increasing the NIV free interval over few days (usually 2-3 days) and then complete removal of NIV. The Royal College of Physicians (RCP) and the British Thoracic Society (BTS) in 2008 suggested a weaning protocol as below [7].

- Initially weaning should be during the day with extended periods off the ventilator for meals, physiotherapy, nebulised therapy etc.
- After successfully weaning during the day, many patients require an additional night on NIV.
  - Continue NIV for 16 hours on day 2
  - 12 hours on day 3 including 6-8 hours overnight use
  - NIV may be discontinued on day 4 unless continuation is clinically indicated
  - Some patients improve rapidly and a clinical decision to wean early can be made, some may self-wean.
  - Long-term nocturnal support may be indicated in selected patients following assessment by the respiratory team.

For safety reason, NIV would be immediately restored if pH fell below 7.35, or there was a clinical deterioration. If patients deteriorated, NIV use would be restarted at 20 h per day.

In the study by Lun et al., stepwise reduction in the duration of NIV use was followed. The NIV use duration was reduced as below under regular monitoring of vital signs and pulse oximetry (SpO2).

- 16 hours on the day 0
- 12 hours on day 1
- 8 hours on day 2 and
- 0 h on days 3, respectively.

This was compared with immediate weaning protocol and there was no statistically significant difference in weaning success rate (74.3% versus 56%, $p = 0.139$). Significantly lower NIV duration in immediate weaning group (median of 0, IQ: 0-3) vs median of 3, IQ: 3-3) ($p < 0.001$) was observed. There was no significant difference between G1 for duration of hospital stay (median of 5, IQ, 5-7 vs median of 5; IQ 3-6.5; $p = 0.14$) [10].

According to Damas and colleagues, the weaning protocol was based on gradually increasing NIV free duration during a three days period [11].

- On day 1, during the day, for every 3 hours one hour was without NIV and two hours with NIV. During the night, patients were under continuous NIV.
- On day 2, during the day, for each 3 hours two hours were without NIV and one hour with NIV, keeping NIV continuously during the night.
- On day 3, patients were without NIV during the day (only with supplementary oxygen delivered by mask) and with continuous NIV during the night.

This protocol was found safe and Success rate of 83.7%.

Stepwise Reduction of Pressure Support

In the study by Momii et al., progressive reduction in FiO2 and pressure was followed. The SpO2 values served as the initial basis for the reduction of the inspired fraction of oxygen (FiO2) and as soon as the patients maintained SpO2 ≥ 95% with FiO2 of 40%, the authors progressively reduced the NIV pressure values until its withdrawal [9].

- Once SpO2 remained ≥99% for 30 min, in the first step, FiO2 was decreased by 20% every 30 minutes, if SpO2 ≥ 95%, until it reached 40%.
- If the patient's condition remained stable for 30 minutes, IPAP and EPAP were decreased by 3cm of H_2O every 30 minutes while SpO2 was maintained above 95%.
- If SpO2 remained above this value for another 30 minutes, the NIV was removed and 3l/min of oxygen was administered through nasal cannula.
- If worsening of SPO2 or other symptoms were noted at any step of the weaning protocol, FiO2 and pressures were returned to the previous values.

Following this protocol, Mean duration of NIV requirement was 19.5 (±28) hours.

In most of the studies progressive weaning has been found to be effective in NIV though all the studies have small sample size and most of the patients studied are COPD adults. It is reasonably safe to progressively wean duration of ventilation or pressure (IPAP and EPAP) as patient is able to maintain SpO2 above 94% and other vital signs. Gradual reduction (2 cm – 4 cm of H_2O) of inspiratory positive airway pressure (IPAP) and expiratory positive airway pressure (EPAP) should be attempted every 4 h – 6 h. The NIV can be removed once patient is able to tolerate the IPAP of 6 cm – 8 cm of H_2O and EPAP of 4 cm – 6 cm of H_2O [12].

Immediate Withdrawal of NIV

In immediate withdrawal strategy, NIV is removed and O2 is administered with a nasal cannula up to 5 L/min once patient is fulfilling weaning criteria such as hemodynamic stability, good gas-exchange, control of pulmonary edema, atelectases, secretions, and bronchospasm, GCS, >10, stable blood gas and electrolytes. If the patient fails weaning attempt, they should be reconnected to NIV with the previous parameters.

Repeat weaning attempt should be considered 24 hours later only if the patients satisfy the weaning criteria.

Immediate weaning was compared by Lun et al., with progressive weaning protocol and there was no statistically significant difference in weaning success rate (74.3% versus 56%, $p = 0.139$). Significantly lower NIV duration in immediate weaning group (median of 0, IQ: 0-3) vs median of 3, IQ: 3-3) ($p < 0.001$) was observed. There was no significant difference between two groups for duration of hospital stay (median of 5 days, IQ, 5-7 vs median of 5 days; IQ 3-6.5; $p = 0.14$) [10].

There is need of prospective randomized studies with adequate sample size to compare different NIV weaning strategies. Some studies are going on to compare the success rate and the duration of NIV after randomization between 3 NIV weaning methods: gradual decrease in duration of NIV vs level of pressure.

Conclusion

Current data on weaning strategies from NIV is limited. Protocol-directed weaning reduces the duration of NIV and the duration of the ICU stay. However, of all the three weaning strategies, immediate withdrawal from NIV has the highest failure rate leading to re-institution of NIV. Stepwise reduction of NIV use seems reasonable and may be adopted in day-to-day practice. Well-designed randomized studies with adequate sample size are needed to find the best strategy for weaning from NIV that would shorten the length of hospital/ICU stay and improve outcome parameters.

References

[1] Esteban A., Frutos F., Tobin M. J., Alía I., Solsona J. F., Valverdú I., et al., A comparison of four methods of weaning patients from mechanical ventilation. Spanish Lung Failure Collaborative Group. *N Engl J Med.* 1995; 332:345-50.

[2] Brochard L., Rauss A., Benito S., Conti G., Mancebo J., Rekik N., et al., Comparison of three methods of gradual withdrawal from ventilatory support during weaning from mechanical ventilation. *Am J Respir Crit Care Med.* 1994; 150:896-903.

[3] Girou E., Schortgen F., Delclaux C., Brun-Buisson C., Blot F., Lefort Y., et al., Association of noninvasive ventilation with nosocomial infections and survival in critically ill patients. *JAMA.* 2000; 284:2361-7.

[4] Yeung J., Couper K., Ryan E. G., Gates S., Hart N., Perkins G. D. Non-invasive ventilation as a strategy for weaning from invasive mechanical ventilation: a

systematic review and Bayesian meta-analysis. *Intensive Care Med.* 2018; 44(12):2192-2204.

[5] Duan J., Tang X., Huang S., Jia J., Guo S. Protocol-directed versus physician-directed weaning from noninvasive ventilation: The impact in chronic obstructive pulmonary disease patients. *J Trauma Acute Care Surg.* 2012; 72:1271-5.

[6] Khilnani G. C., Jain N. Do we need a protocol for weaning patients from noninvasive ventilation? *Indian J Crit Care Med.* 2014; 18(12):775-777.

[7] Royal College of Physicians, British Thoracic Society, Intensive Care Society. Chronic obstructive pulmonary disease: non-invasive ventilation with bi-phasic positive airways pressure in the management of patients with acute type 2 respiratory failure. *Concise Guidance to Good Practice series,* No 11. London: RCP, 2008.

[8] Duan J., Tang X., Huang S., Jia J., Guo S. Protocol-directed versus physician-directed weaning from noninvasive ventilation: The impact in chronic obstructive pulmonary disease patients. *J Trauma Acute Care Surg.* 2012; 72(5):1271-75.

[9] Momii H., Tashima Y., Kadokami T., Narita S., Yoshida M., Ando S. Experience of step-wise protocol using noninvasive positive pressure ventilation for treating cardiogenic pulmonary edema. *Eur J Emerg Med.* 2012; 19(4):267-70.

[10] Lun C. T., Chan V. L., Leung W. S., Cheung A. P. S., Cheng S. L., Tsui M. S. N., et al., A pilot randomized study comparing two methods of non-invasive ventilation withdrawal after acute respiratory failure in chronic obstructive pulmonary disease. *Respirology.* 2013; 18(5):814-9.

[11] Damas C., Andrade C., Araújo J. P., Almeida J., Bettencourt P. Weaning from non-invasive positive pressure ventilation: experience with progressive periods of withdraw. *Rev Port Pneumol.* 2008; 14(1):49-53.

[12] Hadda V., Kumari R. Protocols for Weaning From NIV: Appraisal of Evidence. *Insights Chest Dis.* 2016, 1:14.

In: Respiratory Ventilatory Strategies … ISBN: 978-1-53617-847-0
Editor: Antonio M. Esquinas © 2020 Nova Science Publishers, Inc.

Chapter 24

How Pulmonary Hypertension Influences Weaning from Mechanical Ventilation

Miguel Guia[1,*], MD, Andrea Machado[2], MD, Cátia Pereira[2], MD, João Carvalho[2], MD and Paula Pinto[2,3], MD

[1]Serviço de Pneumologia do Hospital Professor Doutor Fernando Fonseca EPE, Lisbon, Portugal

[2]Departamento de Tórax do Centro Hospitalar Universitário Lisboa Norte, Lisbon, Portugal

[3]ISAMB Faculdade de Medicina de Lisboa; Lisbon, Portugal

Abstract

Pulmonary hypertension (PH) is defined as an increase in mean pulmonary arterial pressure to values ≥ 25 mmHg at rest as assessed by right heart catheterization. Right ventricle (RV) failure is the most frequent cause of death in PH patients.

Cardiovascular performance can be independently influenced by positive intrathoracic pressure due to a decrease in RV preload. Also both lung hyperinflation and lung volumes under functional residual capacity lead to increased pulmonary vascular resistance.

PH is associated with an increased afterload on the RV, conditioning mechanical ventilation strategy and its weaning. Special attention is required to avoid hypoxia, hypercapnia and high PEEP (levels should be (<10 cmH_2O). Low tidal volume ventilation strategies are a good option, however $PaCO_2$ levels should be closely monitored. PH also hinders weaning from mechanical ventilation, since it worsens some of the weaning potential negative effects on cardiovascular function.

* Corresponding Author's E-mail: miguelguia7@gmail.com.

Pulmonary Hypertension

Pulmonary hypertension (PH) is defined as an increase in mean pulmonary arterial pressure (PAPm) $\geq$ 25 mmHg at rest as assessed by right heart catheterization (RHC). Normal PAPm at rest is 14 +/- 3mmHg with an upper limit of normal of approximately 20 mmHg. PH is subdivided into 5 groups: group I includes pulmonary arterial hypertension of idiopathic, heritable origin or induced by drugs and toxins and other associated causes; group II PH is associated with left heart diseases; group III PH is associated with chronic lung diseases and/or hypoxia; group IV is chronic thromboembolic PH and PH associated with other pulmonary artery obstructions; group V PH includes PH from unclear and multifactorial mechanisms. The mechanisms involved in group III include hypoxic vasoconstriction, mechanical stress of hyperinflated lungs, lost of capillaries, inflammation and toxic effects of cigarette smoke.

Right Heart Failure

The right ventricle (RV) is characterized for having a thin-wall and a crescent-shaped structure with the function of ejecting blood into the pulmonary circulation, whose vascular circuit has low resistance, high compliance and low impedance [1]. RV failure is the most frequent cause of death in PH patients, mainly in the patients with pulmonary arterial hypertension or chronic thromboembolic pulmonary hypertension. RV adapts poorly to sudden increases in afterload, which may overwhelm its contractile capability leading to hemodynamic collapse [1].

RV failure is a manifestation of disease progression in PH patients despite targeting therapy [1].

The left ventricle (LV) is interrelated to the RV through the interventricular septum and the surrounding pericardium, meaning the effect of filling of one ventricle directly influences the other [1, 2]. In PH, RV enlargement leads to septal wall motion towards the left side by pressure and volume overload of the RV, reducing LV filling [1, 2].

Right Heart Effects of Mechanical Ventilation

Cardiovascular performance, in the form of preload, afterload, heart rate and myocardial contractility, can be furthermore independently influenced by intrathoracic pressure and lung volume. Alterations in intrathoracic pressure affect thoracic structures (specifically the heart) and lung volume changes influence pulmonary vascular resistance [2].

In spontaneous inspiration there is a reduction in intrapleural pressure producing a reduction in intrathoracic pressure that is transmitted to the right atrium. There is also an increase in intrabdominal pressure due to the diaphragmatic descent [2].

During spontaneous inspiration there is an increase in the gradient between the extrathoracic veins and the pressure of the right atrium, leading to an increase of systemic venous return. Therefore in spontaneous inspiration the RV preload and stroke volume increase [2]. Conversely, during positive pressure ventilation (PPV) there is an increase in intrathoracic pressure during inspiration and consequently an increase in right atrium pressure. This causes deceleration of systemic venous return and therefore a decrease in RV preload and cardiac output [2].

Changes in lung volume directly affect the pulmonary vascular resistance (PVR), which is the main determinant of RV afterload, since there is an increase in the PVR at both extremes of lung volume [2]. This happens because when the lung is over the functional residual capacity (FRC), and therefore hyperinflated, there is compression of the alveolar vessels due to alveolar distention, leading to increase in PVR [2].

On the other hand, when the lung volume is under FRC it results in hypoxic pulmonary vasoconstriction due to the collapse of terminal airways at low lung volumes resulting in alveolar hypoxia. Also the parenchymal vessels become more tortuous and consequently predisposed to collapse, elevating the PVR [2].

Invasive Mechanical Ventilation Strategies

PH is associated with an increased afterload on the RV which increases the risk of developing right heart failure in the critically ill patient, conditioning mechanical ventilation strategy and its weaning. Special attention is required to avoid hypoxia, hypercapnia and high PEEP.

Hypoxia and Hypercapnia

In contrast to systemic circulation, the pulmonary circulation vasoconstricts in the presence of hypoxia. Hypoxic pulmonary vasoconstriction is a protective reflex contraction of vascular smooth muscle in the pulmonary circulation in response to a low regional oxygen partial pressure, which is a mechanism for matching regional perfusion and ventilation. However these areas of high resistance in the pulmonary circulation promote the development of PH [3].

The effect of carbon dioxide (CO_2) on pulmonary vascular tone is controversial, as there is evidence of both vasoconstriction and vasodilation effects. However, high partial pressure of CO_2 ($PaCO_2$) levels seems to increase the extracellular ionized calcium influx, which promotes vasoconstriction in the pulmonary circulation [4]. Hypoxic pulmonary vasoconstriction is also potentiated by acidaemia independently of $PaCO_2$ levels [3].

PEEP

Many studies have demonstrated that increasing PEEP improves alveolar recruitment and oxygenation, and also may shorten the duration of mechanical ventilation. However, elevated airway pressure levels has a negative effect on right ventricle function and hemodynamic.

A study on 16 acute respiratory distress syndrome (ARDS) patients compared groups after PEEP titration. The group with titrated PEEP of 13 +/- 4 cmH_2O showed increased right ventricle outflow impedance (by Doppler analysis of pulmonary artery flow velocity) during tidal ventilation versus the group with titrated PEEP of 6 +/- 3 cmH_2O. Zero end-expiratory pressure (ZEEP) strategy was also associated to a greater impact than 6 cmH_2O PEEP (but less than 13 cmH_2O PEEP) on right ventricular outflow impedance. This effect of PEEP on cardiac output may be explained by the curvilinear shape of the relationship between lung volume and pulmonary vascular resistance [5]. Another study showed that high PEEP levels (10-12 cmH_2O) were associated with higher end-diastolic right ventricle/left ventricle area ratio, evaluated by echocardiography [6]. These findings strength the importance of avoiding high PEEP levels on patients with pulmonary hypertension.

Tidal Volume

Besides its protective effect on the lung, low tidal volume ventilation may also have a positive hemodynamic effect on PH patients. As mentioned before, the pulmonary vascular resistance is high both at low and high lung volumes, since, on one hand, at low volumes lung parenchyma elastic recoil leads to extra-alveolar vessel collapse and terminal airway collapse, favoring hypoxia and hypoxic pulmonary vasoconstriction. On the other hand, at high volumes, stretching of alveolar walls leads to alveolar vessels collapse. However CO_2 levels must be closely monitored, since, as previously mentioned, hypercapnia promotes pulmonary vasoconstriction.

Ventilatory strategies that result in augmented $PaCO_2$ levels may be deleterious, especially if it occurs abruptly. Acidosis and hypercapnia induced by tidal volume reduction were found to be associated with impaired right ventricular function and hemodynamics on a study with ARDS patients. RV stroke index was significantly correlated to arterial pH and end-systolic eccentricity index. Multivariate analysis of the results showed that RV stroke index and end-systolic eccentricity were associated with respiratory acidosis, but not with PEEP levels [6].

RV protective strategy, for example in ARDS patients, implies optimizing lung recruitment without producing pulmonary over-distension phenomena, which can lead to greater deterioration of RV function [7].

In conclusion, the strategy of low tidal volume ventilation proposed for PH is similar to the one used to ventilate patients with ARDS, but permissive hypercapnia should be avoided [8].

Weaning from Mechanical Ventilation

PH and RV failure may predispose the patient to failure on weaning from mechanical ventilation. In fact, weaning may increase right ventricle afterload, due to increased work of breathing, hypoxemia and high intrinsic PEEP. This adverse effect over the right ventricle promotes its enlargement and shifting of intra-ventricular septum towards the left ventricle, affecting its filling and output, which can lead to pulmonary edema, that also contributes to the difficulties experienced while weaning patients with PH from mechanical ventilation. The increased RV afterload may also induce RV enlargement, impending diastolic filling of the left ventricle (due to biventricular interdependence mechanisms) [9].

In a study in which spontaneous breathing trials were monitored, it was found that weaning-induced pulmonary edema was present in 59% of failed trials [10].

Weaning-induced pulmonary edema should be suspected in cases of intolerance to a spontaneous breathing trial. Combined increase in arterial pressure and heart rate during unsuccessful weaning are suggestive of pulmonary edema.

Right heart catheterization during unsuccessful spontaneous breathing trial allows pulmonary wedge pressure evaluation (increased values are suggestive of cardiogenic pulmonary edema). During weaning, lung protective ventilation strategies should be gradually adopted, but not forgetting to monitor CO2 levels. Progressive decrements of pressure support levels and keeping a low PEEP level may reduce weaning-induced cardiogenic pulmonary edema [9].

The strategies referred in the previous section are fundamental during weaning, since it is essential to minimize pulmonary artery pressure and its deleterious effects on RV function.

Pulmonary vasodilators may also play an important role in weaning form mechanical ventilation.

Noninvasive Ventilation and Pulmonary Hypertension

As in invasive mechanical ventilation, noninvasive ventilation may lead to a reduction in RV preload and an increase RV afterload, whereas left ventricular preload and afterload diminishes. Application of NIV in PH is thus controversial. Most existing studies show that PH is an unfavorable prognostic factor to NIV response, namely in the acute setting. More studies have to be designed and implemented, and efficacy of NIV in PH has to be demonstrated in future studies.

Conclusion

There is a lack of studies on mechanical ventilation in PH patients. Most of the data comes from the evaluation of mechanical ventilation effects on right ventricle function and hemodynamic in ARDS patients.

Key Messages

- During mechanical ventilation of patients with PH, hypoxia and hypercapnia should be avoided due to their pulmonary vasoconstriction effects.
- PEEP levels should remain relatively low (<10 cmH_2O)
- Low tidal volume ventilation strategies are a good option, however $PaCO_2$ levels should be closely monitored
- PH hinders weaning from mechanical ventilation, since it worsen some of the weaning potential negative effects on cardiovascular function

References

[1] Hoeper MM, Granton J. Intensive care unit management of patients with severe pulmonary hypertension and right heart failure. *Am J Respir Crit Care Med.* 2011;184:1114–1124.

[2] Shekerdemian L, Bohn D. Cardiovascular effects of mechanical ventilation. *Arch Dis Child.* 1999;80:575-480.

[3] Tarry D, Powell M. Hypoxic pulmonary vasoconstriction; *BJA Education.* 2017;17(6):208-213.

[4] Chuang I, Dong H, Yang R, Wang T, Tsai J, Yang P, Huang M. Effect of carbon dioxide on pulmonary vascular tone at various pulmonary arterial pressure levels induced by endothelin-1; *Lung.* 2010;188(3):199-207.

[5] Schmitt J, Vieillard-Baron A, Augarde R, Prin S, Page B, Jardin F. Positive end-expiratory pressure titration in acute respiratory distress syndrome patients: impact on right ventricular outflow impedance evaluated by pulmonary artery Doppler flow velocity measurements. *Crit Care Med.* 2001;29(6):1154-1158.

[6] Dessap A, Charron C, Devaquet J, Aboab J, Jardin F, Brochard L, Vieillard-Baron A. Impact of acute hypercapnia and augmented positive end-expiratory pressure on right ventricle function in severe acute respiratory distress syndrome. *Intensive Care Med.* 2009;35:1850-1858.

[7] Gordo-Vidal F, Enciso-Calderón Acute respiratory distress syndrome, mechanical ventilation and right ventricular function. *Med Intensiva*. 2011;36(2):138-142.

[8] Zamanian R, Haddad F, Doyle R, WeinackerA. Management strategies for patients with pulmonary hypertension in the intensive care unit; *Crit Care Med.* 2007;35(9):2037-2050.

[9] Teboul J, Monnet X, Richard C. Weaning failure of cardiac origin: recent advances. *Critical Care.* 2010;14:211.

[10] Liu J, Shen F, Teboul K, Anquel N, Beurton A, Bezaz N, Richard C, Monnet X. Cardiac dysfunction induced by weaning from mechanical ventilation: incidence, risk factors, and effects of fluid removal; *Crit Care*. 2016;(20)1:369.

In: Respiratory Ventilatory Strategies …
Editor: Antonio M. Esquinas
ISBN: 978-1-53617-847-0
© 2020 Nova Science Publishers, Inc.

Chapter 25

PREOPERATIVE EVALUATION OF PATIENTS WITH IDIOPATHIC PULMONARY FIBROSIS

Habib Md Reazaul Karim**, Chinmaya Kumar Panda and Subrata Kumar Singha
All India Institute of Medical Sciences, Raipur, India

ABSTRACT

Preoperative evaluation is the indispensable component for caring for a surgical patient planned to undergo surgery. Although the practice is nearly universal now, a robust pathway is still lacking. The objective of preoperative evaluation is to assess the patient's disease and comorbid conditions, their impact on the different vital organ systems and functional reserve of the patient. The evaluation also aims to find out the different risk factors that can have an impact on the perioperative morbidity and mortality of the patients. The respiratory system is very critical for perioperative physicians, intensivists, and health care providers caring for surgical patients. Idiopathic pulmonary fibrosis is a progressive lung disease with hampered oxygen transport. As it can affect the morbidity and mortality of the patient during the perioperative period, it is essential to assess the patient, risk-stratify accurately, and optimize the patient before proceeding for elective surgery. This chapter briefly describes the preoperative evaluation and management approach to a patient with idiopathic pulmonary fibrosis planned for both thoracic and non-cardiac surgeries. A flow algorithm is also proposed to help the perioperative health care provider.

Keywords: idiopathic pulmonary fibrosis, anesthesia, preanesthetic assessment, risk stratification, postoperative pulmonary complication

* Corresponding Author's E-mail: drhabibkarim@gmail.com.

ABBREVIATIONS

ASA	American Society of Anesthesiologists
COPD	Chronic obstructive pulmonary disease
CPET	cardiopulmonary exercise testing
CXR	chest X-ray
ECG	electrocardiogram
HRCT	high resolution computerized tomography
IPF	idiopathic pulmonary fibrosis
METs	Metabolic equivalent of tasks
NICE	National Institute for Health and Care Excellence
OSA	obstructive sleep apnoea
PPCs	Postoperative pulmonary complications

INTRODUCTION

Preoperative evaluation is an integral and critical component of perioperative patient care. It aims in reducing the perioperative morbidity and mortality and is achieved by preoperative assessment, risk stratification, and optimization of the patients. Although the preoperative evaluation is primarily the job of Anaesthesiologists, a multidisciplinary approach is often required for the optimization of the comorbid conditions. A Pulmonary or Respiratory physician often needs to get involved in the optimization process of the patients who are having respiratory diseases and planned for surgery. The present chapter is intended to outline the framework for the preoperative evaluation of patients with known or suspected idiopathic pulmonary fibrosis.

PREOPERATIVE ASSESSMENT

Preoperative assessment of the patient includes a thorough history taking of the patients, clinical examination, reviewing the investigations done, and if required ordering further relevant laboratory tests. If the patient is already a known case, clinical history and examination are required to correlate the findings with the diagnosis, assess the disease progression, reviewing the drugs and their effects and complications. If the case is a suspected case of idiopathic pulmonary fibrosis, history, clinical examination, and laboratory tests should be done to diagnose or rule out idiopathic pulmonary fibrosis. IPF is usually a disease of the elderly and rarely presents before the fifth decade of life. The patient mostly presents with insidious onset and progressively worsening dyspnoea but rarely can present with acute exacerbation. A family history of interstitial lung disease may be present, and a good number of patients have other respiratory comorbidities like emphysema, pulmonary artery hypertension, sleep apnoea, and lung cancer. A detailed history of cigarette smoking and other environmental exposure at home, workplace, or other frequently visited places, exposure to drugs are essential and recommended. While serum biomarker testing for the diagnosis of IPF is not recommended, serological testing for excluding other connective tissue disorder is required to diagnose IPF. High-resolution computed tomography (HRCT) is recommended in suspected cases, and IPF shows features of usual interstitial pneumonia in the subpleural and basal areas, but often the distribution is heterogeneous. Bronchoalveolar lavage and lung biopsy may be done. A pulmonologist or a respiratory physician has well conversed with these skills and tests, and the present chapter is not intended to discuss further details in this aspect. Auscultatory findings of the respiratory system like wheezing, crepitations, altered breath sounds can indicate active pathology. If the anaesthesiologist suspects a case to have IPF or encounters a known case of IPF, the case can be referred to a specialist for further evaluation, diagnosis and optimization as required based on other clinical circumstances [1].

PREOPERATIVE LABORATORY TESTING

A preoperative laboratory testing or investigation should be patient and surgery specific and currently routine preoperative investigations are not recommended by the ASA as well as the NICE [2, 3]. Perioperative impact of routine laboratory tests even with abnormal test results are minimal even in elderly patients [4]. Moreover, a diagnostic test (tests required for diagnostic evaluation) and preoperative tests should not be mixed. Reviewing the tests or investigations that are already done can give the perioperative team/anaesthesiologists good information and always essential. It is the patients clinical finding history of illness that should dictate the requirement of the preoperative tests.

Coronary artery disease is associated with co-morbidity in such patients. Moreover, dyspnoea may be because of either or both respiratory and cardiovascular origin. Therefore, the systemic examination of the cardiorespiratory system plays a crucial role. Furthermore, information about the patients' cardiopulmonary reserve is indispensable. This can be measured in terms of METs, and an idea of METs can be obtained from the history itself; CPET is mostly not required. A 6-minute walk test and fall in peripheral oxyhemoglobin saturation can give valuable information. Although resting 12-lead ECG has minimal value, as these patients are often elderly and comorbid, a baseline ECG may be helpful if the patient is planned to undergo NICE grade 2 and above surgeries. Routine chest X-ray in patients has limited information and impact in the perioperative management of patients [5]. Preoperative CXR is likely to be helpful in patients with symptoms and signs of acute or unstable cardiopulmonary disease [6]. Moreover, IPF often has the HRCT done, and unless there is a new onset or acute worsening of the pulmonary condition, preoperative CXR will not be useful. The need for echocardiography should also be based on the patient's condition. If the patients have unexplained shortness of breathing with an abnormal electrocardiogram or chest X-ray findings, a known case of ischemic or structural heart disease, or not a known case but having a new onset murmur, the feature of heart failure with metabolic equivalents of task ≤ 4 are the candidates for preoperative echocardiography [7]. However, in patients with IPF, cardiac origin dyspnoea may be masked. Moreover, cardiac function may also be affected because of the pulmonary condition, and these aspects should also be considered.

Pulmonary function tests are often done during the diagnostic evaluation and if there is no change in the symptoms and signs. A routine or repeat PFT will not be required if planned for non-thoracic surgeries [8]. As such, preoperative spirometry has failed to show evidence as a tool to stratify the risk of postoperative pulmonary complications in non-cardiothoracic surgery [9]. However, if the patient is in acute exacerbation or worsening, planned for thoracic surgery, and a recent PFT is not available after starting any treatment, it can be done to access the current condition and response to the treatment. Therefore, preoperative spirometry should not done as a risk stratifying tool, rather as a management tool to optimize the preoperative lung function.

On the other hand, if the patient is planned for a lung resection surgery, then the "three-legged stool" of respiratory assessment is required which includes assessment for lung mechanical function, pulmonary parenchymal function, and cardiopulmonary reserve [10]. This requires spirometry, lung diffusing capacity for carbon monoxide, exercise tolerance, arterial blood gases, and imaging of regional lung function.

Treatment of IPF vary, and the patient may be on either on no medication or taking steroids, N-acetyl cysteine, antifibrotic drugs like pirfenidone, immunosuppressant like azathioprine, cyclophosphamide, etc. [11]. The medication dose, route, and possible complications should be assessed and noted. As the patients are elderly, polypharmacy for other comorbidities is common and the other drugs like anticoagulants, hypoglycemics, antihypertensives, etc., if taking needs to be noted for appropriate perioperative management. Antifibrotic therapy like pirfenidone has been associated with gastrointestinal disorders like anorexia, dyspepsia, nausea and may indicate towards electrolyte imbalance and malnutrition and hepatic dysfunction. Investigations in this aspect may be required if the physical examination and history indicates.

RISK ASSESSMENT

The ASA physical status (ASA-PS) classification is a good and reliable indicator of overall morbidity and mortality. However, additional organ-specific risk assessment is also required when for better risk assessment, planning management, and explanation and consent. Patients with IPF, whether undergoes thoracic or non-thoracic surgery, are prone to postoperative respiratory failure and other postoperative pulmonary complications. Although there is a lack of specific risk assessment tool for IPF, several risk assessment tools are used and found to be useful in predicting PPCs. Assessment of Respiratory Risk in Surgical patients in Catalonia (ARISCAT) and Prospective Evaluation of a RIsk Score for postoperative pulmonary COmPlications in Europe (PERISCOPE) are two well-known studies in this aspect [12, 13]. The ARISCAT was also externally validated with the European cohort of the PERISCOPE group [14].

ARISCAT takes patients age, preoperative peripheral oxyhemoglobin saturation, respiratory infection, surgical incision site, duration, and nature of surgery in calculating the risk. The scoring system assigns the parameters with different scores based on their severity for calculating a composite value for predicting the risk of postoperative pulmonary complications [12]. The cumulative score of the ARISCAT gives three risk groups, i.e., low, intermediate and high-risk group with ARISCAT score of <v26, 26-44 and >45 having a risk of in-hospital postoperative pulmonary complications of 1.6%, 13.3%, and 42.1% respectively.

Additionally, regression modeling of the PERISCOPE data also identified preoperative chronic liver disease, history of congestive heart failure as independent risks [13]. Another systematic review indicated good evidence to support ASA class 2 or higher, functional dependence, COPD, and serum albumin level less than 30 g/L as a predictor of postoperative pulmonary complications [9]. Current smoking has been implicated as a risk for postoperative pulmonary morbidity in patients undergoing curative-intent lung cancer surgery [15]. Furthermore, a nationwide inpatient sample from the United Kingdom comprising about 12000 patients with interstitial lung disease who underwent lung biopsy showed that increasing comorbidity was also a predictor of postoperative pulmonary morbidity and mortality [16]. Obstructive sleep apnea has been linked with a seven-fold increase in need of postoperative tracheal intubation and mechanical ventilation [17]. The National Veterans Administration Surgical Quality Improvement Program also developed a multifactorial risk factor for predicting postoperative respiratory failure and found a preoperative blood urea nitrogen >30 mg/dl as another risk [18]. These additional risk factors, excluding the common risk factors as of ARISCAT study, are enumerated in Table 1. A flow diagrammatic algorithmic approach is suggested in Figure 1. However, as the increasing comorbidity also indicates and correlates with increasing ASA physical class (ASA-PS II and above), the ASA-PS II and above, and increasing comorbidity is taken as one risk factor.

Table 1. Different Risk factors of postoperative pulmonary morbidities and additional risk factors over and above ARISCAT scoring for the algorithmic approach of preoperative evaluation of patients with IPF

Author (year)	Study name/brief	Risk Factors for PPCs
Canet J et al. (2010)	ARISCAT	Age, Preoperative peripheral oxyhemoglobin saturation, Respiratory infection, Surgical incision site, Surgical duration, Nature of surgery (elective/emergency)
Canet J et al. (2015)	PERISCOPE	Low preoperative SpO_2, At least one preoperative respiratory symptom, Preoperative chronic liver disease, History of congestive heart failure, Open intrathoracic or upper abdominal surgery, Surgical procedure lasting at least 2 h, Emergency surgery.
Smetana GW et al. (2006)	Systematic Review	Patient-related (Advanced age, American Society of Anesthesiologists class 2 or higher, Functional dependence, Chronic obstructive pulmonary disease, Congestive heart failure). Procedure-related (Aortic aneurysm repair, Nonresective thoracic surgery, Abdominal surgery, Neurosurgery, Emergency surgery, General anesthesia, Head and neck surgery, Vascular surgery, and Prolonged surgery). Laboratory predictor - serum albumin level less than 30 g/L
Hutchinson JP et al. (2016)	Epidemiological study (Nationwide survey)	Non-elective surgery, Male sex, Increasing age, Increasing comorbidity, Open surgery, A provisional diagnosis of idiopathic pulmonary fibrosis or connective tissue disease-related interstitial lung
Lugg ST et al. (2017)	A prospective study with consecutive patients as a cohort	Current smoker
Arozullah AM et al. (20000	Multifactorial risk index from the National Veterans Administration Surgical Quality Improvement Program	Type of the operation (i.e., abdominal aortic aneurysm repair, neurosurgery, and thoracic, upper abdominal, peripheral vascular, neck) Nature of the operation- Emergency surgical procedures) Laboratory abnormalities (albumin, <3.0 g/dl; blood urea nitrogen, >30 mg/dl), Patients' clinical characteristics (older age, low functional status, and COPD)
Memtsoudis S, et al.	Retrospective analysis	OSA
Additional risk factors over and above ARISCAT Male Sex, ASA-PS II and above or increasing comorbidity, Preoperative chronic liver disease, History of congestive heart failure, other respiratory comorbidity (COPD, OSA), General anesthesia, serum albumin <3.0 g/dl, blood urea nitrogen >30 mg/dl.		

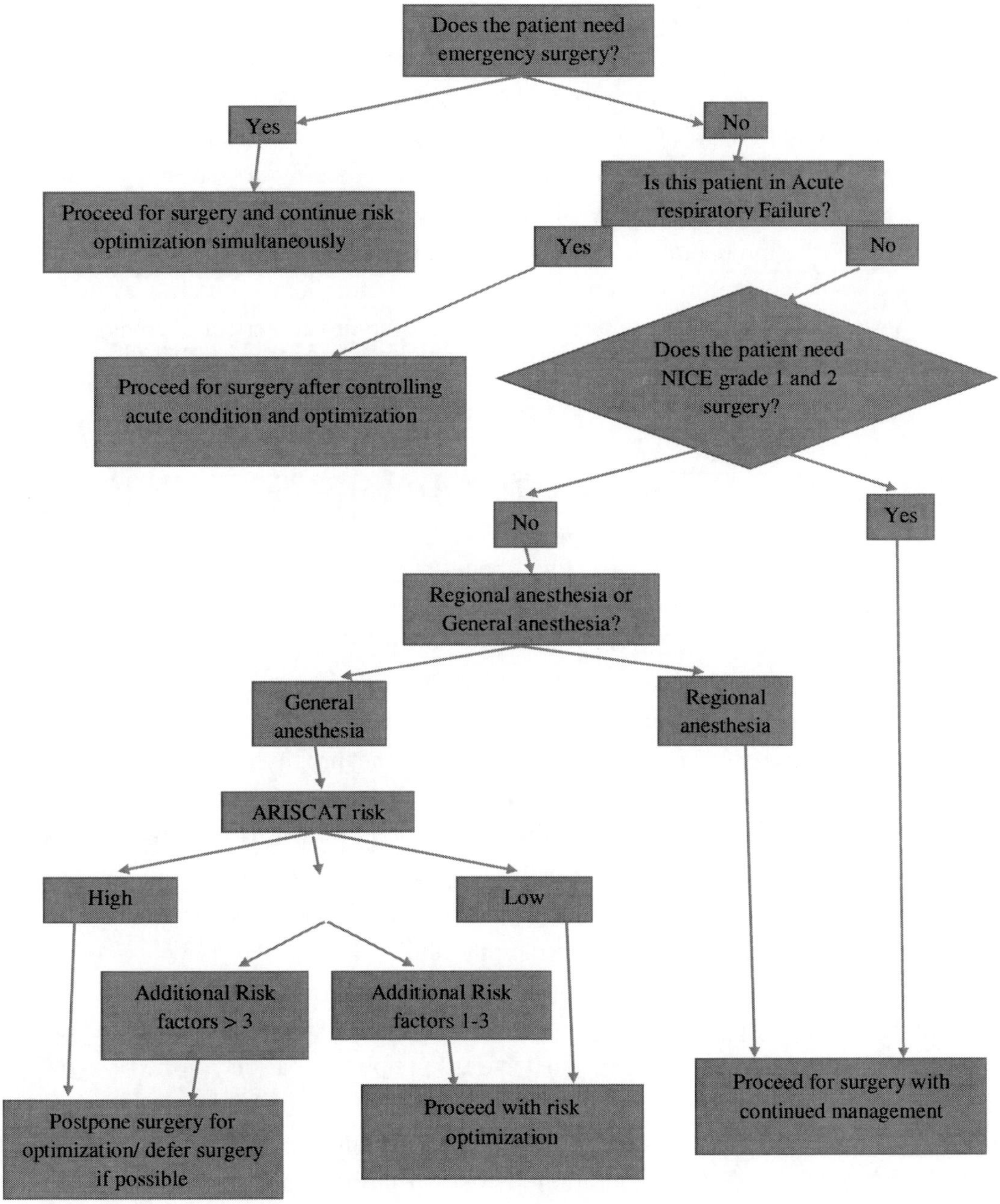

Figure 1. Algorithmic approach of preoperative evaluation and optimization of patients with IPF.

RISK OPTIMIZATION

Postoperative complications were significantly higher in patients with the presence of pulmonary symptoms and physical examination signs [19]. Therefore, it is prudent to control the signs and symptoms of the patients before taking up for an elective procedure as far as possible; infections need to be treated, COPD, and OSA optimized. As the IPF is a progressively worsening disease with no specific treatment for a cure yet, a complete clinical resolution of the symptoms and signs for IPF may not be possible. Similarly, other comorbid conditions, if any also needs to be optimized as far as possible depending on the planned nature of surgery. Preoperative physiotherapy in patients undergoing upper abdominal surgery has been shown to reduce postoperative pneumonia [20]. Evidence shows that preoperative exercise program in patients undergoing lung cancer resection is also helpful in preventing PPCs [21]. Although there is no clear evidence for a 6-week abstinence from smoking as a demarcation line in smokers, it is advised to stop the smoking.

PREOPERATIVE ADVISES

Usual pulmonary medications like beta-2 agonists, anticholinergics, steroid inhalation, etc., are usually continued. Presently good evidence is lacking to advise for or against of continuation of fibrotic therapy. Whether pirfenidone prevents acute exacerbation or not is not yet very clear [22]. A recent study in patients with IPF who underwent lung resection for cancer found a reduced incidence of acute exacerbation in the postoperative period when treated with pirfenidone prophylactically [23]. Similar results for the prevention of acute exacerbation and the good safety profile was also shown by a phase II trial by West Japan Oncology Group 6711 L (PEOPLE Study) [24]. Expert opinion indicates that unless there is unbearable side-effects and/or lack of efficacy, these drugs should not be discontinued [25]. Therefore, it appears to be a good clinical practice to continue antifibrotic therapy until we get better evidence against it. Preoperative physiotherapy and incentive spirometry may be advisable. The other medications for comorbid conditions need to be managed as per current evidence. Gastroesophageal reflux is often associated and also implicated as one of the risks of IPF. Therefore prophylaxis appears to be reasonable. Nil per oral can be followed as per the recommendation of the ASA. Preoperative anxiolysis should not be routine and based on the patients' cardiorespiratory condition. Broad-spectrum antibiotic effective against respiratory flora should be administered [26].

POSTOPERATIVE CARE PLAN

IPF patients undergoing general anesthesia may deteriorate and should be managed under intensive monitoring with a frequent assessment of the condition. A multidisciplinary approach for early mobilization, chest physiotherapy, patient education, incentive spirometry, mouth care, head-end elevation, sputum clearance is likely to help in preventing postoperative pulmonary complications, and morbidity [27]. Mucolytic medications, 3% NS nebulization, can be effectively used to decrease PPC [26].

Conclusion

At present specific and good quality evidence is lacking to recommend a framework for perioperative evaluation and management of patients with IPF. Most of the data are preliminary and extrapolated from broader disease class, i.e., interstitial lung disease and restrictive lung disease. As IPF is a disease of elderly, is progressively worsening fatal condition with 2-5 years of survival after the diagnosis, the decision to carry out an elective surgery needs to be weighted with multiple factors and risk-benefit. Patients with higher risks of postoperative pulmonary complications, with other comorbidities, and who require major surgery for a chronic non-fatal disease condition, may not be a candidate for surgery. If at all surgery is required, preoperative risk optimization and preventive measures with a multidisciplinary approach is probably the better strategy.

Key Message

- IPF itself is a risk for postoperative pulmonary morbidity and mortality
- A thorough history, clinical examination, medical record review is essential for preoperative evaluation. Preoperative investigations should be patient and surgery specific and target risk assessment and optimization too.
- A multidisciplinary approach for preoperative risk optimization and postoperative management plan is required for elective and non-emergent surgeries.

References

[1] Raghu G, Remy-Jardin M, Myers JL, et al.; American Thoracic Society, European Respiratory Society, Hapanese Respiratory Society, and Latin American Thoracic Society. Diagnosis of Idiopathic Pulmonary Fibrosis. An Official ATS/ERS/JRS/ALAT Clinical Practice Guideline. *Am. J. Respir. Crit. Care Med.* 2018 Sep 1;198(5):e44-e68. doi: 10.1164/rccm.201807-1255ST.

[2] Committee on Standards and Practice Parameters. Apfelbaum JL, Connis RT, Nickinovich DG; American Society of Anesthesiologists Task Force on

Preanesthesia Evaluation. Practice advisory for preanesthesia evaluation: an updated report by the American Society of Anesthesiologists Task Force on Preanesthesia Evaluation. *Anesthesiology*. 2012;116:522-538.

[3] National Guideline Centre (UK). *Preoperative Tests (Update): Routine Preoperative Tests for Elective Surgery.* 2016 Apr. Available from: https://www.ncbi.nlm.nih. gov/pubmed/27077168.

[4] Reazaul Karim HM, Sahoo SK, Prakash A, Rajaram N, Kumar S, Narayan A. Abnormal routine preoperative test results and their perioperative anesthetic impact in patients aged 60 years and more: An observational study. *Indian Anaesth Forum* 2018;19:6-10. doi: 10.4103/TheIAForum.TheIAForum_41_17.

[5] Archer C, Levy AR, McGregor M. Value of routine preoperative chest x-rays: a meta-analysis. *Can. J. Anaesth.* 1993 Nov;40(11):1022-7.

[6] Young EM, Farmer JD. Preoperative Chest Radiography in Elective Surgery: Review and Update. *S. D. Med.* 2017 Feb;70(2):81-87.

[7] Shim CY. Preoperative cardiac evaluation with transthoracic echocardiography before non-cardiac surgery. *Korean J. Anesthesiol.* 2017;70(4):390-397. doi: 10. 4097/kjae.2017.70.4.390.

[8] Carter JB. Pulmonary Function Testing. In: Raj T. (eds) *Data Interpretation in Anesthesia*. Springer, Cham. 2017. doi: 10.1007/978-3-319-55862-2_68.

[9] Smetana GW, Lawrence VA, Cornell JE; American College of Physicians. Preoperative pulmonary risk stratification for noncardiothoracic surgery: systematic review for the American College of Physicians. *Ann. Intern. Med.* 2006 Apr 18;144(8):581-95.

[10] Slinger P, Darling G. Preanesthetic assessment for thorcic surgery. In: Slinger P, editor. *Principles and Practice of Anesthesia for Thoracic Surgery*. New York: Springer; 2011. p. 19.

[11] Behr J, Kreuter M, Hoeper MM, et al. Management of patients with idiopathic pulmonary fibrosis in clinical practice: the INSIGHTS-IPF registry. *Eur. Respir. J.* 2015 Jul;46(1):186-96. doi: 10.1183/09031936.00217614. Epub 2015 Apr 2.

[12] Canet J, Gallart L, Gomar C, et al. Prediction of postoperative pulmonary complications in a population-based surgical cohort. *Anesthesiology* 2010; 113: 1338-50.

[13] Canet J, Sabaté S, Mazo V, et al.; PERISCOPE group. Development and validation of a score to predict postoperative respiratory failure in a multicentre European cohort: A prospective, observational study. *Eur. J. Anaesthesiol.* 2015 Jul;32(7): 458-70. doi: 10.1097/EJA.0000000000000223.

[14] Mazo V, Sabaté S, Canet J, et al. Prospective external validation of a predictive score for postoperative pulmonary complications. *Anesthesiology.* 2014 Aug;121 (2):219-31. doi: 10.1097/ALN.0000000000000334.

[15] Lugg ST, Tikka T, Agostini PJ, et al. Smoking and timing of cessation on postoperative pulmonary complications after curative-intent lung cancer surgery. *J. Cardiothorac. Surg.* 2017;12(1):52. Published 2017 Jun 19. doi: 10.1186/s13019-017-0614-4.

[16] Hutchinson JP, Fogarty AW, McKeever TM, et al. Inhospital mortality after surgical lung biopsy for interstitial lung disease in the United States: 2000 to 2011. *Am. J. Respir. Crit. Care Med.* 2016;193(10):1161-1167.

[17] Memtsoudis S, Liu SS, Ma Y, et al. Perioperative pulmonary outcomes in patients with sleep apnea after noncardiac surgery. *Anesth. Analg.* 2011;112:113-121.

[18] Arozullah AM, Daley J, Henderson WG, Khuri SF. Multifactorial risk index for predicting postoperative respiratory failure in men after major noncardiac surgery: the National Veterans Administration Surgical Quality Improvement Program. *Ann. Surg.* 2000;232:242-253.

[19] Turan MO, Uluorman F. The Analysis of Pulmonary Risk Factors in Preoperative Evaluation. *Eur. Respir. J.* 2017 50: PA742. doi: 10.1183/1393003.congress-2017.PA742.

[20] Boden I, Skinner EH, Browning L, et al. Preoperative physiotherapy for the prevention of respiratory complications after upper abdominal surgery: pragmatic, double blinded, multicentre randomised controlled trial [published correction appears in BMJ. 2019 Apr 25;365:l1862]. *BMJ.* 2018;360:j5916. Published 2018 Jan 24. doi: 10.1136/bmj.j5916.

[21] Steffens D, Beckenkamp PR, Hancock M, et al. Preoperative exercise halves the postoperative complication rate in patients with lung cancer: a systematic review of the effect of exercise on complications, length of stay and quality of life in patients with cancer. *Br. J. Sports Med.* 2018 Mar;52(5):344. doi: 10.1136/bjsports-2017-098032. Epub 2018 Feb 1.

[22] Noble PW, Albera C, Bradford WZ, et al. Pirfenidone in patients with idiopathic pulmonary fibrosis (CAPACITY):two randomised trials. *Lancet* 2011; 377: 1760-1769.

[23] Iwata T, Yoshida S, Fujiwara T, et al. Effect of Perioperative Pirfenidone Treatment in Lung Cancer Patients with Idiopathic Pulmonary Fibrosis. *Ann. Thorac. Surg.* 2016 Dec;102(6):1905-1910. doi: 10.1016/j.athoracsur.2016.05.094. Epub 2016 Aug 18.

[24] Iwata T, Yoshino I, Yoshida S, et al. A phase II trial evaluating the efficacy and safety of perioperative pirfenidone for prevention of acute exacerbation of idiopathic pulmonary fibrosis in lung cancer patients undergoing pulmonary resection: West Japan Oncology Group 6711 L (PEOPLE Study). *Respir. Res.* 2016;17(1):90. Published 2016 Jul 22. doi: 10.1186/s12931-016-0398-4.

[25] Torrisi SE, Pavone M, Vancheri A, Vancheri C. When to start and when to stop antifibrotic therapies. *Eur. Respir. Rev.* 2017 Oct 3;26(145). pii: 170053. doi: 10. 1183/16000617.0053-2017. Print 2017 Sep 30.

[26] Villeneuve PJ. Interventions to avoid pulmonary complications after lung cancer resection. *J. Thorac. Dis.* 2018;10(Suppl 32):S3781-S3788. doi:10.21037/jtd.2018. 09.26.

[27] Cassidy MR, Rosenkranz P, McCabe K, et al. I COUGH: reducing postoperative pulmonary complications with a multidisciplinary patient care program. *JAMA Surg.* 2013 Aug;148(8):740-5. doi: 10.1001/jamasurg.2013.358.

In: Respiratory Ventilatory Strategies …
Editor: Antonio M. Esquinas

ISBN: 978-1-53617-847-0
© 2020 Nova Science Publishers, Inc.

Chapter 26

Idiopathic Pulmonary Fibrosis in Postoperative Conditions

Güniz Koksal**, MD and Cigdem Akyol Beyoglu*†, MD
Istanbul University- Cerrahpasa, Cerrahpasa School of Medicine,
Department of Anesthesiology and Reanimation, Istanbul, Turkey

Abstract

Idiopathic pulmonary fibrosis (IPF) constitutes progressive inflammation resulting in fibrotic areas in the lung parenchyma and causing chronic respiratory distress. These fibrotic areas disrupt the gas exchange and cause a decrease in compliance of the lungs and lung volumes. It is an invasive disease and progresses with acute worsening periods.

The criteria and results of non-invasive or invasive mechanical ventilation for these patients have not been established yet. However, it is important not to delay mechanical ventilation.

Patients with IPF should have high-resolution computed tomography examinations preoperatively. Early postoperative noninvasive mechanical ventilation may be required in patients with IPF after extubation.

High oxygen concentration used in mechanical ventilation during general anesthesia (any oxygen concentration above 21% counts as high oxygen concentration), single lung ventilation, and ischemia-reperfusion injury may cause acute exacerbations and respiratory insufficiency in the postoperative period.

Patients with IPF should be kept in negative fluid balance in the postoperative period to avoid disrupting gas exchange. Drugs such as "pirfenidone" and anticoagulants should be continued and lung protective measurements should be done in the perioperative period.

* Corresponding Author's E-mail: gunizkoksal@hotmail.com.
† Corresponding Author's E-mail: akyolbeyoglu@gmail.com

Keywords: idiopathic pulmonary fibrosis, mechanical ventilation, acute exacerbation, mortality

ABBREVIATIONS

IPF	Idiopathic Pulmonary Fibrosis.
HRCT	High-resolution Computed Tomography.
Ppeak	Peak Airway Pressure.
CPAP	Continuous Positive Airway Pressure.
PaO_2	Partial Arterial Oxygen Pressure.
$PaCO_2$	Partial Arterial Carbon dioxide Pressure.
FiO_2	Fractional Inspired Oxygen Concentration.

INTRODUCTION AND DEFINITIONS

Idiopathic pulmonary fibrosis (IPF) constitutes progressive inflammation resulting in fibrotic areas in the lung parenchyma and causing chronic respiratory distress. These fibrotic areas disrupt the gas exchange and cause a decrease in compliance of the lungs and lung volumes. It is an invasive disease and progresses with acute worsening periods [1]. Average survival time is 2-3 years after the diagnosis of the disease. Patients with IPF are treated in intensive care units during periods of acute worsening. Even if they are discharged from intensive care units, they have a high mortality rate in the first 6 months of discharge [2]. The criteria and results of non-invasive or invasive mechanical ventilation for these patients have not been established yet. However, it is important to emphasize not to delay mechanical ventilation. Mortality rate is supposed to be 49.2% in patients who are applied invasive mechanical ventilation, while 48.8% in non-invasive mechanical ventilation. The mean ICU mortality of patients with IPF is reported as 50% [1].

METHODOLOGY

Since lung biopsy is necessary for IPF diagnosis, general anesthesia and mechanical ventilation is required for biopsy in addition to respiratory insufficiency during acute exacerbations. Apart from this indication, patients may have to undergo surgery and general anesthesia with different diagnoses (hernia repair, lobectomy or pneumonectomy due to lung cancer, cholelithiasis etc.) [3].

There are some key points to take into consideration in preanesthetic examination before surgery. Firstly, patients use pirfenidone containing growth factor, collagen I and II to reduce lung fibrosis. This medication can impair liver function. The liver dysfunction may start with elevated liver enzymes and progresses to Child 1 and 2. Anesthesiologists should be aware of any sign of liver failure, and essential precautions should be taken. Pirfenidone should be continued in perioperative period [4]. Besides the majority of the surgery may have an impact on an increase in the frequency of attacks in the postoperative period [3].

High-resolution computed tomography (HRCT) examination in the preoperative period is necessary in patients with IPF. It will provide detailed information whether the IPF is active or not. In addition, it will provide information about lung parenchyma and pleural effusion in the preoperative period [5]. It is known that mortality is lower in patients without mechanical ventilation. Studies have shown that mechanical ventilation is an independent risk factor on mortality [1].

The role of invasive or non-invasive mechanical ventilation in patients with IPF is unclear. Observational studies are single-center and have a limited number of patients. Therefore, no definite results can be established [1].

High oxygen concentration used in mechanical ventilation during general anesthesia (any concentration above 21% is counted as high oxygen concentration), single lung ventilation (especially preferred in lung biopsy and lobectomy) and ischemia-reperfusion injury leads to respiratory insufficiency and acute exacerbation of the disease in the postoperative period in patients with IPF [6]. In addition, mechanical ventilation may lead to high airway pressures and high tidal volumes during surgery. Increased lung damage has been shown in patients with IPF who underwent hyperventilation with high airway pressures. These applications accelerate the deterioration in the postoperative period. Tidal volumes should not exceed 7-10 ml/kg during mechanical ventilation and maximum inspiratory pressure (Ppeak) should be kept below 35 cm H_2O. Pathological changes in IPF are heterogeneously distributed. Therefore, the tidal volume applied to the patient will be distributed only to the alveoli within normal lung areas. This means that the stretch on the intact alveoli will be higher [7, 8, 9].

When IPF patients with postoperative acute respiratory failure were examined, it was found that these patients had to use 100% fractional inspired oxygen concentration (FiO2) during 40-170 minutes on average. However, PaCO2 levels remained within normal limits. In addition, during surgery and mechanical ventilation alveoli open and close. Cyclic opening and closing of the alveoli will cause tears and further deteriorate the gas exchange. Ruptured alveoli will heal with the development of new fibrosis. Shear stress caused by hyperinflation should be avoided. In IPF, the amount of surfactant in the alveoli is reduced, and the production of inflammatory cytokines (pro-inflammatory) is increased, thus deteriorating the capillary structure. This will increase the damage occurred by free oxygen radicals released by high FiO2. For this reason, applying oxygen concentration appropriate levels keeping PaO2 value below 100 mmHg and avoiding hypoxia in the perioperative period is vital [6, 9].

Early postoperative noninvasive mechanical ventilation may be recommended in patients with PIF just after extubation in the postoperative period. Cosenti et al., [10] showed that the application of CPAP reduces the risk of intubation in PIF patients with pneumonia. Carillo et al., [11] reported that non-invasive mechanical ventilation increases pulmonary tidal volumes in patients with interstitial fibrosis during acute exacerbations but does not guarantee recovery of oxygenation. They also note that non-invasive mechanical ventilation may lead to pneumothorax and pneumomediastinum in patients with PIF. Aliberti et al., [6] state that each patient should be decided individually rather than routine non-invasive mechanical ventilation therapy.

Kondoh et al., [3] showed that the incidence of acute worsening after biopsy in IPF is 2.1% and this worsening occurs in 2-3 weeks following surgery. Ghotol et al., [15] found a high mortality incidence in patients with IPF undergoing pulmonary or non-pulmonary surgery in their review of the literature involving case reports. Therefore, acute attack criteria should be closely monitored and treated rapidly in the postoperative period. These criteria are listed below [12]:

1. Dyspnea aggravated within the last month,
2. PaO2/FiO2 < 225 or decrease in PaO2 level more than 10 mm Hg,
3. The development of new pulmonary infiltrations on chest radiography,
4. No heart disease or new signs of infiltration,
5. Absence of acute worsening pathologies such as pulmonary embolism, congestive heart failure, pneumothorax.

In the postoperative period, it is important to keep the negative fluid balance of PIF patients in order not to affect the gas exchange. In the perioperative period, it is important to perform lung protective measurements and to continue "pirfenidone" and anticoagulant drugs. Continuing high-dose steroid therapy in the perioperative period is considered to be a risk factor increasing incidence of acute attack [5].

About Our Research

Learning Points

1. Surgery and invasive mechanical ventilation in patients with pulmonary fibrosis increase the acute exacerbations of the disease.
2. High airway pressures should be avoided when performing mechanical ventilation in patients with pulmonary fibrosis.

3. High oxygen concentrations worsen the prognosis of pulmonary fibrosis.
4. We should be careful when performing single lung ventilation.

Critical Points

1. In patients with interstitial pulmonary fibrosis "pirfenidone" should be continued during the perioperative period.
2. Patients should be monitored in the postoperative period.
3. Preoperative lung and pleura should be examined in detail with HRCT. It should be established that the patient is not currently in an acute period.
4. 4-Individual non-invasive mechanical ventilation can be applied to the patients in the postoperative period.

CONCLUSION

It is known that mortality is lower in patients with IPF without mechanical ventilation. Studies have shown that mechanical ventilation is an independent risk factor in mortality. High oxygen concentration used in mechanical ventilation during general anesthesia (any concentration above 21% is counted as high oxygen concentration), single lung ventilation (especially preferred in lung biopsy, lobectomy) and ischemia-reperfusion injury leads to acute exacerbation of respiration in the postoperative period in patients with IPF.

REFERENCES

[1] Barret, R., Wiskar, K., Berger, L., Griesdale, D. (2016). The use of mechanical ventilation in patients with idiopathic pulmonary fibrosis in the United States: A nationwide retrospective cohort analysis. *Respiratory Medicine,* 111:72-76].

[2] Stephane, G., Vincent, F., Rabbat, A., Nunes, H., Crestani, B., Naccache J.M., Wolff, M., Thabut, G., Valeyre, D., Cohen, Y., Mal, H. (2014). Invasive mechanical ventilation in patients with fibrosing interstitial pneumonia. *Thorac Cardiovasc Surg,* 147(I):47-53].

[3] Yasuhiro, K.,Taniguchia, H., Kitaichib, M., Yokoic, T., Johkohd, T., Oishie, T., Kimuraa, T., Nishiyamaa, O., Katoa, K., M. du Bois, R. (2006). Acute exacerbation of interstitial pneumonia following surgical lung biopsy. *Respiratory Medicine,* 100(X), 1753-1759].

[4] Manni, Z., Wu, C., Wu, Z., Ren, G., Ji, N., Zhang, I., Huang, M. (2019). Acute exacerbation of interstitial lung disease after radical surgery for lung cancer: a case report. *Ann Transl Med,* 7(VIII):182].

[5] Xiaojun, M., Chen, Z., Liu, Y., Chu, H.(2016). Acute exacerbation of idiopathic pulmonary fibrosis after total hip replacement. *Journal of Clinical Anesthesia,* 34, 518-519].

[6] Stefano, A., Messinesi, G., Gamberini, S., Maggiolini, S., Visca, D., Galavotti, V., Giuliani, F., Cosentini, R., Maria Brambilla, A., Blasi, F., Scala, R., Carone, M., Luisi, F., Harari, S., Voza, A., Esquinas, A., Pesci, A. (2014). Non-invasive mechanical ventilation in patients with diffuse interstitial lung diseases. *BMC Pulmonary Medicine,* 14:194].

[7] Susumu, S., Homma, S., Mun, M., Fujii, T., Kurosaki, A., Yoshimura, K. (2011). Acute Exacerbation of Idiopathic Interstitial Pneumonia Following Lung Surgery in 3 of 68 Consecutive Patients: A Retrospective Study. *Intern Med,* 50: 77-85].

[8] Atsushi, S., Taniguchi, H., Ando, M., Kondoh, Y., Kimura, T., Kataoka, K., Matsuda, T., Yokoyama, T., Sakamoto, K., Hasegawa, Y. (2018). Prognostic evaluation by oxygenation with positive end-expiratory pressure in acute exacerbation of idiopathic pulmonary fibrosis: A retrospective cohort study. *Clin Respir J,* 12(III):895-903].

[9] Meihua, Q., Chen, Y., Ye, Q. (2018). Risk factors for acute exacerbation of idiopathic pulmonary fibrosis: A systematic review and meta-analysis. *Clin Respir J,* 12(III):1084-1092].

[10] Cosentini, R., Brambilla, A. M., Aliberti, S., Bignamini, A., Nava, S., Maffei, A., Martinotti, R., Tarsia, P., Monzani, V., Pelosi, P. (2010). Helmet continuous positive airway pressure vs oxygen therapy to improve oxygenation in community-acquired pneumonia: a randomized, controlled trial. *Chest*, 138(I):114-120].

[11] Carrillo, A., Gonzalez-Diaz, G., Ferrer, M., Martinez-Quintana, M.E., Lopez-Martinez, A., Llamas, N., Alcazar, M., Torres, A. (2012). Non-invasive ventilation in community acquired pneumonia and severe acute respiratory failure. *Intensive Care Med*, 38(III):458-466].

[12] Atsushi, W., Kawaharada, N., Higami, T. (2011). Postoperative Acute Exacerbation of IPF after Lung Resection for Primary Lung Cancer. *Pulmonary Medicine,* doi:10.1155/2011/960316

In: Respiratory Ventilatory Strategies …
Editor: Antonio M. Esquinas ISBN: 978-1-53617-847-0
© 2020 Nova Science Publishers, Inc.

Chapter 27

Extracorporeal Life Support and Unconventional Mode of Respiratory Management

Federica Lo Presti*[*] *and Luca S. De Santo
Department of Translational Medical Sciences,
Università degli Studi della Campania "L. Vanvitelli", Naples, Italy

Abstract

Acute respiratory failure is very common in interstitial lung diseases and optimal ventilatory management in this setting is still under investigation. The dismal prognosis of patients needing mechanical ventilation urged the search for alternative strategies, such as extracorporeal life support. Since its first use as a bridge to lung transplant, extracorporeal membrane oxygenation (ECMO) improved its technology and results. Despite available data on the topic mostly derive from small non-homogeneous case series or reports, usually with a single center setting and a retrospective design, the literature shows that the use of ECMO bridging transplants has risen. Clinical success is more related to appropriate candidacy and timely deployment rather than to device-specific complications. Anyway, further efforts need to be done to improve outcomes and to increase the bridge to transplant/bridge to no-where ratio.

Keywords: acute respiratory failure, extracorporeal membrane oxygenation, bridge to transplant, carbon dioxide removal

[*] Corresponding Author's E-mail: nicopap@hotmail.it.

INTRODUCTION

The treatment of patients with interstitial lung disease (ILD) and acute respiratory failure (ARF) is challenging. Lung transplantation is, currently, the only effective therapy in pharmacologically refractory ILD that are already on the waiting list [1]. Due to gross imbalance between the limited organ supply and the large numbers of recipients listed, mean waiting time averages 12 up to 24 months [2]. Chances of acute decompensation and development of refractory respiratory failure, with an inherent dismal prognosis, are thus concerning.

For patients not yet listed, on the other hand, prognosis following intensive care unit (ICU) admission is usually very poor. Most patients who develop ARF are unlikely to benefit from extended intensive care treatment. High-flow oxygen through a nasal cannula and noninvasive ventilation (NIV) are potential options to avoid intubation in cases of mild ARF. NIV failure is common in case of moderate and severe ARF but avoiding all the cases of evitable mechanical ventilation is the real target for patients with ILD who would normally require intubation. Pre-damaged pulmonary parenchyma is susceptible to ventilator-induced lung injury (VILI) and oxygen toxicity. These likely trigger further disease progression. Right ventricular dysfunction is also very common. Hypoxemia, in fact, increases pulmonary vasoconstriction and mechanical ventilation increases thoracic pressure, adding to the right ventricular afterload elevation.

Mechanical ventilation carries high mortality (70-90%), worsening the already poor prognosis of the underlying disease.

In this setting, Extracorporeal Membrane Oxygenation (ECMO) may be a viable strategy. In patients on ECMO, oxygen supply and CO_2 removal are mainly independent from mechanical ventilation. This enables lung protective ventilation and might prevent VILI and further right ventricular dysfunction. The possibility to keep patients non-sedated/intubated (so-called "awake ECMO") has further enhanced its clinical impact despite the lack of a consensus.

All in all, ECMO has been proved to be successful as "bridge to transplant", when employed with correct timing in selected cases. Sometimes it allows transplant candidacy in patients who had not evaluated and listed before acute decompensation ("salvage transplant"). On the other side, inappropriate deployment could bring to ECMO removal or death during support, thus transforming a bridge to decision – to another type of extracorporeal life support or to palliative care – into so-called "bridge to no-where".

GENERAL PRINCIPLES OF ECMO AND ECCO$_2$-R

Extracorporeal Membrane Oxygenation (ECMO) represents the most commonly used system of extracorporeal life support (ECLS) warranting a temporary support of heart and/or lung function that can last from days up to a few months, depending on the patient's conditions. It represents the natural evolution of conventional cardiopulmonary bypass (CPB), i.e., the heart lung machine, reshaped for prolonged cardiopulmonary support using intrathoracic or extrathoracic cannulation and new matherials aiming at reducing the biologic impact of the device [3].

The ECMO system consists of a circuit composed of a membrane oxygenator, a centrifugal pump, and, if patient needs temperature modification, a heat exchanger. The membrane oxygenator is based on solid hollow fiber, a thin plasma resistant layer of polymethylpentene, which prevents plasma leak. Membrane surface area and blood flow are the principal determinants of the maximal oxygen delivery. The capacity of oxygen exchange for specific membranes, acknowledged as rated flow, represents the volume of desaturated blood (SO_2 = 75%) that the membrane can return to an SO_2 of 95% per minute (L/min). Oxygenation function depends on: inlet SvO_2, FiO_2, membrane capacity, red cell exposure to gas exchange area (in terms of duration of time), [Hb] and blood flow. Full ECMO is able to ensure complete blood oxygenation and decarboxylation, with the counterpart to request high flows of at least 2-5 L per minute, with low recirculation. To provide total extracorporeal support the circuit requires large diameter cannulas, with relatively wide priming volumes and high doses of anticoagulant.

CO_2 removal is more efficient than oxygenation because of its solubility and diffusion properties. Therefore, CO_2 removal can be done with low flows. Hence membranes with a low rated flow are enough for this purpose, such as relatively smaller diameter cannulas and lower priming volumes. Carbon dioxide removal, in fact, mainly depends on CO_2 gradient and gas flow rate (L/min) called sweep flow, while it is relatively independent of blood flow.

The basic principle of ECMO is to collect the patient's venous blood into a pump connected to the oxygenator and restore the oxygenated and decarboxylated blood to the patient.

ECMO is a highly flexible life support technology since it can be implemented both as pure pulmonary support (veno-venous circuit) as well as concomitant cardiac support (veno-arterial circuit); these two modalities maybe even adopted subsequently as patient's condition worsens.

ECMO deployment and management requires ECMO teams. These are multidisciplinary team involving surgeons, anesthetists, intensive care physicians and nursing staff that merge their competencies to achieve the best clinical outcome.

Indeed, ECMO patients may face a huge number of complications including thrombosis, hemorrhage, nosocomial infection, neurological injury, vessel injury, multiple organ failure and device failure.

History and Results of ECMO as a Bridge to Pulmunary Transplantation

Extracorporeal membrane oxygenation (ECMO) was introduced to manage patients on the lung transplant waiting list dying of acute respiratory failure refractory to mechanical ventilation [4]. First ECMO use dates to 1975: the patient survived transplantation but died shortly after from infectious complications. Later, a randomized trial demonstrated worse outcome associated with ECMO in comparison with mechanical ventilation. Therefore, ECMO bridging to lung transplant was almost abandoned.

During the following 3 decades, thanks to improvements in technology, safety profile, and manageability of extracorporeal life support strategies, ECMO has been reintroduced. The burden of lung transplant recipients deemed as potential ECMO candidates is steeply increasing. United Network of Organ Sharing (UNOS) data support that, despite complex management and potential side effects, the use of ECLS as a bridge to lung transplant has risen by 150% in two years compared to the previous decades (1970 to 2010) [2].

The shortage of transplantable lungs has raised ethical concerns. There is a definite potential for dismal lung transplant outcomes when selecting marginal recipients on ECMO support. Lung allocation score (LAS) system emerged as an effective strategy to allocate the organs to patients with higher transplant benefit.

An increased amount of data has demonstrated the potential of ECMO as an alternative to mechanical ventilation in awake, spontaneously breathing patients. Awake-ECMO patients may preserve muscle tone improving the chance of early mobilization reversing the inability and improving the global clinical status prior to lung transplant and making for a better post-transplant outcome.

Besides, there have been significant improvements in ECMO technology, since its initial development. The most valuable are, indeed, the development of heparin-coated circuits and polymethyl pentene oxygenators, widespread usage of centrifugal pumps, implementation of alternative cannulation strategies and development of dual lumen cannulas. Application of ECMO over mechanical ventilation entails several clinical advantages. The most important perceived benefits are reduction/avoidance of ventilator-induced morbidity, preserved/enhanced hemodynamic stability, preservation of oral feeding and spontaneous coughing, minimization of muscular deconditioning and higher chances for early mobilization and intense rehabilitation. On the other side, rates of bleeding, infection and renal failure and, to a lesser extent, those of gas embolism, stroke, and limb ischemia, are still substantial. Length of extracorporeal support, center expertise, timely reassessment of transplant candidacy, and emergent listing are crucial for successful bridging [5].

Chiumello and colleagues produced a systematic review to assess the current evidence on the use of ECMO in patients with advanced respiratory failure awaiting lung transplant and fill the lack of definitive data on the efficacy of ECMO as bridge to lung transplantation. This review including 14 studies evaluated patients with mixed diseases bridged to transplantation with ECMO as an alternative to invasive mechanical ventilation and showed better 6-months survival compared with mechanical ventilation (62% and 35%, respectively).

Back in 2013, Hoopes and colleagues [6] published a retrospective study of their institutional experience on ECMO bridging. They reviewed 31 patients from 2 institutions placed on ECMO as a bridge to lung transplantation compared with similar patients without ECMO at the same institutions and comparison groups queried from the UNOS Database. Pulmonary fibrosis (42%), cystic fibrosis (20%) and pulmonary hypertension (16%) were the most common diagnostic codes, and acute corpulmonale (48%) and hypoxia (39%) were the most common indications to artificial lung support. Authors demonstrated a satisfactory early and long-term post-transplant survival after ECMO bridging (93%, 80% and 66% at 1-, 3- and 5-years respectively). Intriguingly it was comparable to that achieved by a control group of high acuity transplant recipients that needed conventional mechanical support. The study challenged previously issued management algorithms of patients with end-stage lung disease and suggested that implementation of salvage transplantation is technically feasible, logistically viable and, above all, effective in carefully selected patients. In this respect, Authors critically underscored that clinical failure in ECMO bridging was not related to device-specific complications, but rather to inappropriate candidacy and delayed artificial lung deployment. Routinely precluding the active listing of ECMO-supported patients with UNOS until they reach a "threshold of viability", the ECMO bridge to transplant can provide an effective method of pulmonary allograft resource allocation to the sickest of patients, who are likely to benefit. If ECMO is to become for pulmonary transplantation what ventricular assist devices have become for cardiac transplantation, the parameters of effective device deployment will need to be integrated into the current lung allocation system.

The most cited and relevant study on ILD patients was published by Trudzinski and colleagues in the American Journal of Respiratory and Critical Care Medicine in 2016 [1]. It is a series of 21 consecutive patients in whom the cause of respiratory failure was deemed reversible and/or there was a potential for lung transplant candidacy. ECMO was both implemented as an adjunct to unsuccessful conventional mechanical ventilation or to avoid intubation. ECMO was initiated if the pH was below 7.20 for respiratory causes despite mechanical ventilation with high peak and plateau pressure (generally both higher than 35 cm H_2O). All patients were primarily treated with veno-venous ECMO using the femoral (draining) and the jugular (return) veins as standard cannula entry sites. The most frequent ILD etiology in these patients was idiopathic (33.3%), followed by connective tissue disease (23.8%). Reasons for deterioration were mainly ILD exacerbations and infection/sepsis, accounting for 17 of 21 cases (81%). The other 4 of 21 (19%) had a pneumothorax, deteriorated after open lung biopsy or had pulmonary hemorrhage under acetylic acid and clopidogrel. Thirteen of them (61.9%) received continuous veno-venous hemodialysis. Patients previously mechanically ventilated were placed on ECMO with hypoxemic ventilatory failure and severe respiratory acidosis in high or very high ventilator settings. Patients put on ECMO while awake and nonintubated were at risk for intubation (listed for salvage transplantation). These had severe hypoxemia despite high-flow oxygen. Although all patients were cannulated veno-venous when placed on ECMO, the circuit was changed because of progressive right ventricular failure to veno-veno-arterial and later to total cardiopulmonary bypass (n = 2). Five external patients accepted as transplant candidates were finally not listed. Of all patients with ILD placed on ECMO, eight (50%) were listed for lung transplant. Five of the six (83.3%) patients who received a transplant were discharged from hospital. In contrast, 14 of 15 (93.3%) patients who did not receive a transplant died on ECMO. In five patients, ECMO therapy was withdrawn; the other patients died because of (septic) multiorgan failure.

In this setting, ECMO was initiated regardless of whether they could be candidates for lung transplant. The main finding was that patients with ILD on ECMO that were not lung transplant candidates had a high mortality rate, comparable with the mortality rate of these patients when mechanically ventilated. In this cohort, additionally, ECMO had no value in the sense of transplant-independent outcome improvement in ILD. In contrast, patients with an option for lung transplantation benefited from ECMO therapy. The main reason for this benefit was the time gained on ECMO.

Its retrospective nature limited this study and the low number of patients included in. The main messages of the study were:

1. 33% of ECMO patients had the chance to be successfully transplanted or even bridged to a recovery;
2. awake ECMO allowed transplant candidacy in four patients who had not been evaluated and listed before acute decompensation;
3. deferred ECMO deployment after prolonged initial mechanical ventilation significantly affected the management of acutely decompensated ILD and ultimately jeopardized resource utilization and implied dismal survival;
4. inappropriate deployment was dramatically frequent as the severity of illness prevented transplant listing in six patients who had ECMO removal o died during support (so-called "bridge to no-where").

In conclusion, salvage transplantation opens a window for patients that are deteriorating and are not listed for lung transplant: in this perspective, patients with imminent NIV- or high-flow-failure who are eligible for lung transplantation but not yet listed should immediately be referred to a center with the option for both ECMO and salvage lung transplantation.

The latest study published by Hayanga and colleagues on July 2019 is a comparative outcome analysis of MV and ECMO as a bridge to lung transplantation [7]. It analyzed the UNOS database for recipients in 2005-2017.

There were 21,576 lung transplant recipients, categorized into 3 groups: no bridge (n = 19,783), MV (n = 1,129), and ECMO (n = 664). Use of ECMO increased significantly between early (2005-2011) and late (2012-2017) eras (1% vs. 5%). Compared with no bridge, patients with MV and ECMO had greater odds for peri-operative ventilator support > 48 hours, acute rejection, and dialysis. Patients with MV had reduced odds for ventilator support > 48 hours, dialysis, post-operative ECMO, and greater odds for reintubation compared with ECMO. Patients in both MV and ECMO groups had a greater risk for 5-year mortality, but the two groups did not differ, although the risk for mortality in the ECMO group decreased in the later era.

In conclusion, ECMO as a bridge to lung transplant has increased by 271%, while MV has decreased 38% over the past decade. Survival with ECMO has significantly improved and is now equivalent to survival in recipients bridged on MV, thus suggesting its gains in use, outcomes, and safety.

LONG-TERM ECMO SUPPORT: TWO STRICKING REPORTS FROM JAPAN

The Extracorporeal Life Support Organization claims that the average duration of veno-venous ECMO (VV ECMO) in adults with acute respiratory failure is 10.5-13.5 days, though there have been reports of prolonged VV ECMO.

In countries such as Japan in which lung transplant is not based on medical urgency, patients on ECMO must wait for a really extended period for donor lungs. Indeed, the candidates typically wait 2.5-3 years after being listed on the lung transplant waiting list. This clinical setting generated two notable clinical cases.

Last year (2018) Umeiand colleagues reported their limit experience of an idiopathic pulmonary fibrosis 50-year-old Japanese man supported with ECMO for 403 days while waiting for a lung transplant [8]. The ECMO was deployed for severe hypoxia despite intubation and mechanical ventilation, positioning a drainage cannula in the left femoral vein and a return cannula in the right femoral vein and controlling ECMO blood flow around 4 L/min. The patient underwent tracheostomy and the mechanical ventilation settings were switched to a "lung rest" setting. The condition gradually improved, achieving weaning from mechanical ventilation on day 38. He was fully awake, oriented and frequently communicating with his family. In the eighth month, the configuration was switched to venovenous-arterial (VVA) for the impairment of the right ventricle. Two months later, the ECMO configuration was converted back to VV and he was finally listed on the lung transplant registry. While awaiting transplant, the membrane oxygenator was changed 23 times and the cannula 10 times. After a year of extracorporeal life support, septic shock occurred and any attempt to further change the cannulation site failed because echography showed no flow in any vein. The patient died soon after ECMO discontinuation on day 403.

More recently, Sato and colleagues [9] described their experience with a 29-year-old man who had suffered from acute myeloid leukemia nine years before and achieved a complete remission after an allogeneic unrelated bone marrow transplant. Chronic graft-versus-host disease caused the onset of bronchiolitis obliterans, making it necessary continuous home ventilator management for 3 years, after which he progressed to type 2 respiratory failure. The Autors successfully performed bilateral lung transplantation in 2019 as soon as a matched lung donor was found, after 5 months of intensive care management on ECMO.

EXTRACORPOREAL CO_2 REMOVAL IN LIFE THREATENING HYPERCAPNIA

After the Austrian group led bySchellongowski and colleagues at the Medical University of Vienna showed its efficacy, the reported number of patients with primarily hypercapnic terminal respiratory failure receiving extracorporeal CO_2 removal ($ECCO_2$-R) has increased due to lower complexity and invasivity [10].

Twenty patients with hypercapnic respiratory failure underwent arteriovenous (AV) or venovenous (VV) $ECCO_2$-R utilizing the interventional lung assist (ILA®, Novalung) device as bridge to planned primary lung transplant (n = 13) or re-transplant (n = 7) during ten-years. All patients presented with severe hypercapnia ($PaCO_2$: 109 mmHg) and respiratory acidosis (pH: 7.20). The type of ILA was the pumpless arteriovenous ILA membrane ventilator or the novel pump-driven venovenous system (ILA Activve®, Novalung) in ten patients each.

Authors claimed hypercapnia and acidosis were effectively corrected in all patients within the first 12 h of ILA therapy: $PaCO_2$ levels declined from a median of 109 to 57 mmHg and pH increased from a median of 7.20 to 7.39.

Fifteen of twenty patients were intubated and, within the first 12 h of ILA therapy, their ventilator settings (peak inspiratory pressure and tidal volumes) could be rendered more lung protective. Three patients were extubated and remained on ILA until lung transplant, one patient was weaned from ILA and remained intubated until lung transplant, and one patient was extubated and weaned from ILA prior to lung transplant.

Nine of the initially intubated patients and all the initially nonintubated patients received active physical therapy at least once daily.

A reduction on ventilator support was achieved in all invasively ventilated patients, allowing for spontaneous breathing and early mobilization.

Intubation was prevented in all but one noninvasively ventilated patient, thus suggesting that the "awake ECMO" concept by Fuehner et al. [11] can be successfully translated into an "awake ILA" concept in patients with hypercapnic respiratory failure.

As highlighed by many reports, the upgrade to full ECMO could represent a necessary strategy for patients ongoing to progressive hypoxia and/or additional circulatory failure. In the reported paper, four patients were switched from ILA to full ECMO (VV-ECMO: n = 1, VA-ECMO: n = 3) after 2 days on ILA support.

The high rate of patients that achieved the successful transplant (95%) after a median bridging time of 8 days was one of the most convincing data in support of this new strategy. Regarding the intraoperative management, in 18 patients intra-operative support with VA-ECMO was employed and in eight of them (42%) it was prolonged into the postoperative period and lasted 2-3 days.

The complications of such an approach, experienced in about thirty percent of the patients, were mostly related to bleeding and heparin-induced thrombocytopenia with clotting of the membrane. Many patients required hemofiltration due to acute renal failure but most patients (n = 13) were successfully weaned from mechanical ventilation over a tracheostomy. Time on mechanical ventilation after lung transplant was 10 (6-25) days mostly driven by the cases of reperfusion edema with primary graft dysfunction grade 3. Hospital and 1-year survival were 75 and 72%, respectively.

Authors focused on the differences between full ECMO and $ECCO_2$-R: in support of the latter remains the fact that $ECCO_2$-R can be reached by circuits with relatively smaller diameter cannulas and lower priming volumes, thus requiring lower doses of heparin and easier insertion techniques than the first.

Several case series described the deployment of some VV $ECCO_2$-R devices at blood flows of 0.3-0-5 L/min in patients with acute respiratory distress syndrome [12], even though the amount of CO_2 elimination at these very low blood flow is limited and the data on the efficacy of these systems in bridge to lung transplant are still lacking. The ILA membrane ventilator, conversely, can eliminate up to the half of CO_2 production at intermediate blood flows of 1-2 L/min.

By the way, an observational study by Kalbhenn and colleagues [13] valued the occurrence of hemolysis and coagulation disorders during $ECCO_2$-R. For the first time, it assessed the effects of carbon dioxide removal on blood cells (in terms of hemolysis and thrombocytopenia) and coagulation system (regarding factor XIII deficiency and acquired von Willebrand syndrome - due to shear stress and consequent multimers cleavage by metalloprotease ADAMTS-13 -), in order to evaluate whether low flows are actually less invasive about blood injury. They analyzed eight patients treated with the

Hemolung respiratory assist system, observing relevant clinical bleeding symptoms in half of them and continuous platelet decrease in all of them. Only in one patient transfusion of blood products was not necessary. The study confirmed the appearance of the same coagulation disorders known from ECMO in $ECCO_2$-R, thus demonstrating that the blood flow is not of necessity the main factor for blood injury and that it's still early to consider safe this system.

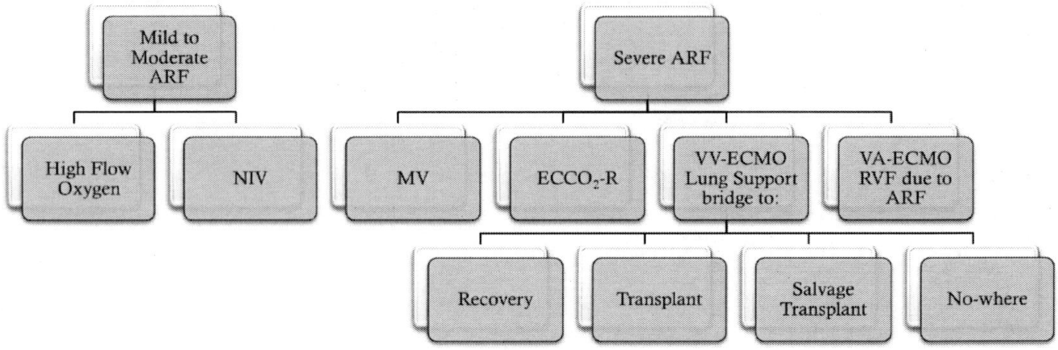

Figure 1. Decisional algorythm in acute respiratory failure.

Despite their retrospective nature and single center setting, these studies claimed that invasively and noninvasively ventilated patients with life threatening hypercapnia can effectively be bridged to lung transplantation by $ECCO_2$-R. The natural history and the progression of the illness may cause severe hypoxia and right ventricular failure: in these cases, a convertion to high-flow VV or VA ECMO - respectively - is available on the shelf (see Figure 1). All in all, the choice of the mode of extracorporeal therapy should be patient-tailored, considering individual features, such as the invasiveness of ventilation and the anticipated course of the respiratory failure.

Conclusion

Despite available data on ECMO bridging in ILD mostly derive from small non-homogeneous case series or reports, usually with a single center setting and a retrospective design, the overall evidence has paved the way for new management algorithms and disclosed both the indication seeking nature of this strategy and the tremendous practical and ethical burden inherent to the treatment of acute respiratory failure in this setting.

The clinical bottom line from published data is that ECMO implementation in the setting of acutely decompensated ILD patients requires judicious clinical evaluation and rapid deployment to avoid the need for mechanical ventilation. Absolute contraindications to ECMO bridging are untreated infections, coexisting organ failure, recent malignancy, active substance abuse, poor social support and history of nonadherence [14].

ECMO allows transplant candidacy both in the term of effective bridging in those already listed or as a rescue pathway for a salvage procedure in carefully selected subjects that had notbeen previously screened. Awake ECMO should be the goal of management algorithms as it allows the most effective environment for post-transplant survival in highly experienced hands. Inappropriate ECMO deployment is futile and entails tremendous implications for institutions, care providers, patients and their relatives.

REFERENCES

[1] Trudzinski, F. C., Kaestner, F., Schäfers, H. J., Fähndrich, S., Seiler, F., Böhmer, P., et al. (2016). "Outcome of patients with interstitial lung disease treated with extracorporeal membrane oxygenation for acute respiratory failure." *Am J Respir Crit Care Med.*, *193*, 527–33. doi: 10.1164/rccm.201508-1701OC.

[2] Diaz-Guzman, E., Hoopes, C. W. & Zwischenberger, J. B. (2013). "The evolution of extracorporeal life support as a bridge to lung transplantation." *ASAIO J.*, *59*(1), 3-10. doi: 10.1097/MAT.0b013e31827461c2.

[3] Chauhan, S. & Subin, S. (2011). "Extracorporeal membrane oxygenation, an anaesthesiologist's perspective: Physiology and principles. Part 1." *Ann Card Anaesth*, *14*, 218-29. doi: 10.4103/0971-9784.84030.

[4] Chiumello, D., Coppola, S., Froio, S., Colombo, A. & Del Sorbo, L. (2015). "Extracorporeal life support as a bridge to lung transplantation: a systematic review." *Crit Care*, *19*, 19. doi: 10.1186/s13054-014-0686-7.

[5] Oto, T., Rosenfeldt, F., Rowland, M., Pick, A., Rabinov, M., Preovolos, A., Snell, G., Williams, T. & Esmore, D. (2004). "Extracorporeal membrane oxygenation after lung transplantation: evolving technique improves outcomes." *Ann Thorac Surg*, *78*(4), 1230-5 doi: 10.1016/j.athoracsur.2004.03.095.

[6] Hoopes, C. W., Kukreja, J., Golden, J., Davenport, D. L., Diaz-Guzman, E. & Zwischenberger, J. B. (2013). "Extracorporeal membrane oxygenation as a bridge to pulmonary transplantation." *J Thorac Cardiovasc Surg*, *145*(3), 862-7, discussion 867-8. doi: 10.1016/j.jtcvs.2012.12.022.

[7] Hayanga, J. W. A., Hayanga, H. K., Holmes, S. D., Ren, Y., Shigemura, N., Badhwar, V. & Abbas, G. (2019). "Mechanical ventilation and extracorporeal membrane oxygenation as a bridge to lung transplantation: Closing the gap." *J Heart Lung Transplant*, pii: S1053-2498(19)31587-6. doi: 10.1016/j.healun.2019.06.026.

[8] Umei, N., Ichiba, S. & Sakamoto, A. (2018). "Idiopathic pulmonary fibrosis patient supported with extracorporeal membrane oxygenation for 403 days while waiting for a lung transplant: A case report." *Respir Med Case Rep.*, *26*, 24, 86-88. doi: 10.1016/j.rmcr.2018.04.015.

[9] Sato, S, Tanaka, E., Tachibana, T., Fukai, R., Kamio, T., Ichiba, S., Sato, M. & Tamai, Y. (2019). "Successfull lung transplantation after long-term ventilator and extracorporeal membrane oxygenation support in a patient with severe bronchiolitis obliterans following allogenic bone marrow transplantation." *Rinsho Ketsueki*, *60*(8), 920-923. doi: 10.11406/rinketsu.60.920.

[10] Schellongowski, P., Riss, K., Staudinger, T., Ullrich, R., Krenn, C. G., Sitzwohl, C., Bojic, A., Wohlfarth, P., Sperr, W. R., Rabitsch, W., Aigner, C., Taghavi, S., Jaksch, P., Klepetko, W. & Lang, G. (2015). "Extracorporeal CO2 removal as bridge to lung transplantation in life-threatening hypercapnia." *Transplant*, *28*(3), 297-304. doi: 10.1111/tri.12486.

[11] Fuehner, T., Kuehn, C., Hadem, J., Wiesner, O., Gottlieb, J., Tudorache, I., Olsson, K. M., Greer, M., Sommer, W., Welte, T., Haverich, A., Hoeper, M. M. & Warnecke, G. (2012). "Extracorporeal membrane oxygenation in awake patients as bridge to lung transplantation." *Am J RespirCrit Care Med*, *185*(7), 763-8. doi: 10.1164/rccm.201109-1599OC.

[12] Terragni, P. P., Del Sorbo, L., Mascia, L., Urbino, R., Martin, E. L., Birocco, A., Faggiano, C., Quintel, M., Gattinoni, L. & Ranieri, V. M. (2009). "Tidal volume lowerthan 6 ml/kg enhanceslungprotection: role of extra- corporeal carbon dioxideremoval." *Anesthesiology*, *111*(4), 826-35. doi: 10.1097/ ALN.0b013e3181b764d2.

[13] Kalbhenn, J., Neuffer, N., Zieger, B. & Schmutz, A. (2017). "Is Extracorporeal CO2 Removal Really "Safe" and "Less" Invasive? Observation of Blood Injury and Coagulation Impairment during ECCO2R." *ASAIO J*, *63*(5), 666-671. doi: 10.1097/MAT.0000000000000544.

[14] Gulack, B. C., Hirji, S. A. & Hartwig, M. G. (2014). "Bridge to lung transplantation and rescue post-transplant: the expanding role of extracorporeal membrane oxygenation." *J Thorac Dis*, *6*(8), 1070-9. doi: 10.3978/j.issn.2072-1439.2014.06.04.

In: Respiratory Ventilatory Strategies …
Editor: Antonio M. Esquinas
ISBN: 978-1-53617-847-0
© 2020 Nova Science Publishers, Inc.

Chapter 28

DO-NOT-INTUBATE (DNI) ORDER IN ACUTE RESPIRATORY MANAGEMENT

A. Úbeda, MD, PhD and I. Fernández, MD
Intensive Care Unit, Hospital Punta de Europa,
Algeciras, Spain

ABSTRACT

Noninvasive ventilation is a treatment option in patients with acute respiratory failure who have declined tracheal intubation. Moreover, NIV may be considered questionable for patients with hypercapnic coma. NIV can relieve dyspnea, improve comfort, and serve as a rescue therapy that can facilitate hospital discharge for some patients who are terminally ill and want to go home. The impact of NIV on the clinical and health-related quality of life is not known. In the case of severe acute respiratory failure in patients with DNI orders, NIV may avoid the need for endotracheal mechanical ventilation.

INTRODUCTION

Despite the cumulative evidence that supports noninvasive ventilation (NIV) for acute hypercapnic respiratory failure, NIV may be considered questionable for vulnerable patients with do-not-intubate (DNI) orders, especially when hypercapnic coma occurs. However, NIV can relieve dyspnea, improve comfort, and serve as a rescue therapy that can facilitate hospital discharge for some patients who are terminally ill and want to go home [1]. Because emergency medical services (EMS) protocol is designed to provide full treatment, including attempted resuscitation and transport to an emergency department, people who prefer otherwise need to plan in advance and make their wishes known. In addition to willingness to make a plan, one needs a mechanism to turn that plan into actions that the health system will respect [2].

A limitation of invasive life support is commonly discussed in frail individuals with end-stage chronic respiratory disease because such patients are considered poor candidates for intubation and prolonged mechanical ventilation. According to good ethical practice and standards of care, the DNI order status of the subjects resulted from a consensual decision-making process by either the patient or the appointed trusted person whenever possible [3].

The prevalence of do-not-resucitate (DNR) and DNI orders has increased in the past several decades (from 9% in 2000 - 2004 to 32% in 2015 - 2019), with studies suggesting most hospitalized and institutionalized patients die with active DNR/DNI orders documented in their medical record. In addition, demographic trends towards increasing numbers of elderly patients who may lack capacity underline the growing importance of clarifying patient preferences and assessing limitations of their documentation [4, 5].

Noninvasive ventilation (NIV) has been shown to be effective in treating acute respiratory failure (ARF) in different conditions, often preventing the need for invasive mechanical ventilation. The goals of treatment and expected outcomes of NIV vary significantly depending on whether patients want to receive all possible life-sustaining treatments, have elected to have preset limits to life support, such as a DNI approach, or prefer to pursue a comfort-measures-only approach. Some experts have called into question the utility of considering NIV for patients with preset limits on life support, arguing that the burdens of NIV may outweigh potential benefits and could merely extend the dying process without providing an acceptable quality of life in survivors or an acceptable quality of death in nonsurvivors [4].

Lemyze et al[1] studied 86 frail subjects in acute respiratory hypercapnic failure (AHRF) who had DNI orders. They found that most of the comatous hypercapnic subjects with DNI orders survived after hospital discharge secondary to the use of NIV as a ceiling of care. They suggested that NIV should be attempted when AHRF occurs even in the case of extreme respiratory acidosis with hypercapnic coma at admission. Those who survived, despite poor quality of life, would choose to be placed on NIV again if a new episode of AHRF occurred.

Wilson et al. [6] performed a meta-analysis on 27 studies evaluating 2.020 patients with DNI orders. Survival was 56%, being 68% for COPD and for pulmonary edema, 41% for pneumonia, and 37% for patients with malignancy. A large proportion of patients who were treated by NIV survived at 1 year, but scant data on quality of life in survivors were available. According to authors, quality of life in survivors, as well as quality of death in nonsurvivors, are crucial issues that warrant to be investigated.

Azoulay et al. [7] performed a large multi-center observational study where they saw that survivors of an episode of acute respiratory failure treated with NIV as a ceiling of care did not exhibit a lower health-related quality of life or higher symptoms of depression, anxiety, and post-ICU burden compared with baseline and with subjects without any treatment limitation decisions. Yet, implementing a ventilatory support for frail patients with an underlying terminal disease, such as end-stage chronic respiratory failure, may be regarded as an excessive, unreasonable escalation that merely prolongs the dying process. The latter seems reasonable when these already frail patients present with reduced consciousness or coma.

Chu et al. [8]. performed a prospective study that examined the long-term outcome of COPD patients with the DNI code who suffered an exacerbation complicated by AHRF requiring NIV. One-year survival of the DNI group was 29.7% compared with 65.1% of the usual care group. One-year event-free survival was 16.2% in the DNI group and 46.5% in the usual care group. Readmission rate to hospital was also high. Survivors in both groups spent a median of 9% to 11% of their time in the hospital in the ensuing year. The DNI patients were generally older and had more severe disease and worse premorbid conditions. This combination of adverse factors was the basis why intubation was felt unjustified in the first place. The DNI group received a higher level of NIV; the inspiratory positive airway pressure level was higher and the duration of NIV was also longer in the DNI group. For the DNI group, the majority of survivors would develop another episode of life-threatening recurrent AHRF requiring NIV or intubation in the ensuing year. Whether if it is appropriate to use NIV to treat AHRF in DNI patients with COPD, their study showed that the 1-year survival was 30% in this group, which was comparable to some patients with advanced malignancies. Also, they we were unable to predict which of these patients would die despite treatment with NIV [8].

Moreover, Wilson et al. [5] conducted a systematic review of observational studies that enrolled 10.755 patients with acute respiratory failure requiring noninvasive ventilation or high-flow nasal cannula oxygen. One in four patients who receive noninvasive ventilation or high flow nasal cannula oxygen had a DNI order. There was a high inter-study variability in published rates of DNI orders, even when accounting for factors such as age, illness severity and decision making processes.

Future considerations may also include evaluating the impact of DNI orders and noninvasive ventilation on short and long-term outcomes as well as the development of interventions to improve DNI decision making.

Key Messages

- A limitation of invasive life support is commonly discussed in frail individuals with end-stage chronic respiratory disease.
- Rates of DNI orders appear to be increasing over time.

- NIV should be attempted in acute respiratory hypercapnic failure when presented with reduced consciousness or coma.
- NIV can increase survival in patients with DNI orders, but scant data on quality of life in survivors is available.

REFFERENCES

[1] Lemyze, M., De Palleja, G., Guiot, A., Bury, Q., Jonard, M., Granier, M. et al. Outcome of Frail Do-Not-Intubate Subjects With End-Stage Chronic Respiratory Failure and Their Opinion of Noninvasive Ventilation to Reverse Hypercapnic Coma. *Resp. Care,* 2019; 64:1023 - 30.

[2] Fromme, E. K., Zive, D., Schmidt, T. A., Cook, J. N., Tolle, S. W. Association between physician orders for life-sustaining treatment for scope of treatment and in-hospital death in Oregon. *J. Am. Geriatr. Soc.,* 2014; 62:1246 - 51.

[3] Brummel, N. E., Bell, S. P., Girard, T. D., Pandharipande, P. P., Jackson, J. C., Morandi, A. et al. Frailty and subsequent disability and mortality among patients with critical illness. *Am. J. Respir. Crit. Care Med.,* 2017; 196:64 - 72.

[4] Jesus, J. E., Allen, M. B., Michael, G. E., Donnino, M. W., Grossman, S. A., Hale, C. P. et al. Preferences for resuscitation and intubation among patients with do-not-resuscitate/Do-not-intubate orders. *Mayo Clin. Proc.,* 2013; 88:658 - 65.

[5] Wilson, M. E., Mittal, A., Karki, B., Dobler, C. C., Wahab, A., Curtis, J. R. et al. Do-not-intubate orders in patients with acute respiratory failure: a systematic review and meta-analysis. *Intensive Care Med.,* 2019; doi:10.1007/s00134-019-05828-2. [Epub ahead of print].

[6] Wilson, M. E., Majzoub, A. M., Dobler, C. C., Curtis, J. R., Nayfeh, T., Thorsteinsdottir, B. et al. Noninvasive Ventilation in Patients With Do-Not-Intubate and Comfort-Measures-Only Orders: A Systematic Review and Meta-Analysis. *Crit. Care Med. Crit. Care Med.,* 2018; 46:1209 - 16.

[7] Azoulay, E., Kouatchet, A., Jaber, S., Lambert, J., Meziani, F., Schmidt, M. et al. Noninvasive mechanical ventilation in patients having declined tracheal intubation. *Intensive Care Med.,* 2013; 39:292 - 301.

[8] Chu, C., Chan, V., Wong, I., Leung, W. S., Lin, A. W., Cheung, K. F. Noninvasive ventilation in patients with acute hypercapnic exacerbation of chronic obstructive pulmonary disease who refused endotracheal intubation. *Crit. Care Med.,* 2004; 32:372 - 7.

In: Respiratory Ventilatory Strategies …
Editor: Antonio M. Esquinas
ISBN: 978-1-53617-847-0
© 2020 Nova Science Publishers, Inc.

Chapter 29

MANAGEMENT OF IDIOPATHIC PULMONARY FIBROSIS IN PNEUMOLOGY DEPARTMENT

Antoine Froidure*[1,2]*, MD, PhD
[1]Pneumology department, Cliniques universitaires Saint-Luc,
Bruxelles, Belgium
[2]Université catholique de Louvain,
Ottignies-Louvain-la-Neuve, Belgium

ABSTRACT

Idiopathic pulmonary fibrosis (IPF) is the most prevalent of interstitial lung diseases (ILD). The disease consists in the replacement of lung alveoli by a fibrotic tissue. Median survival in the absence of treatment is 3 to 5 years. Pirfenidone and nintedanib, two recently approved antifibrotic drugs, are able to slow disease course and prevent IPF-related exacerbations. For all these reasons, proper diagnosis and management are mandatory. The American (ATS), European (ERS), Latin American (ALAT) and Japanese (JRS) respiratory societies published joined updated guidelines for IPF diagnosis end of 2018(1). Those guidelines clearly highlight the role of a multidisciplinary discussion (MDD)-based management. First step consists in ruling out concurrent diagnosis through an appropriate interpretation of clinical, biological and radiological features by the members of the MDD. Optimal and holistic IPF management includes pharmacological and non-pharmacological interventions.

INTRODUCTION

Idiopathic pulmonary fibrosis (IPF) is the most prevalent of interstitial lung diseases (ILD). The disease consists in the progressive replacement of lung alveoli by a fibrotic scar tissue. Although the disease cause is still unknown, several risk factors are identified: IPF usually affects elderly patients (median age of 65) and is more frequent in men (sex ratio F/M 0.7). About sixty percent of IPF patients are current or former smokers or have been chronically exposed to inhaled toxic compounds such as metal dust and fumes. IPF is a lethal disease: Median survival in the absence of treatment is 3 to 5 years. Hopefully, the arrival of antifibrotic drugs changed the bail: Pirfenidone and nintedanib are able to slow disease course and prevent IPF-related exacerbations (although data on this latter point are more consistent for nintedanib).

For all these reasons, proper diagnosis and management are mandatory. The American (ATS), European (ERS), Latin American (ALAT) and Japanese (JRS) respiratory societies published joined updated guidelines for IPF diagnosis end of 2018 [1]. Those guidelines clearly highlight the role of a multidisciplinary discussion-based management. In the present chapter, we will discuss crucial aspects of IPF diagnosis and treatment, in line with recent recommendations.

IPF Diagnosis

ILD Classification and General Principles for Diagnosis

ILD are a heterogeneous group of diseases including about two hundred entities. Several ILD classifications have been published. The most commonly used was proposed by the European Respiratory Society (ERS) and the American Thoracic Society (ATS) in 2011 and was updated in 2013 [2]. ILD are divided in four groups: The first one gathers all ILD triggered by identified factors (drug-induced, connective tissue-disease-related, occupational ILD). The second group consists in all idiopathic interstitial pneumonia (IIP), the third one includes all granulomatosis and the last one gathers rare entities like alveolar proteinosis and lymphangioleyomyomatosis. The IIP group is further divided in three subgroups: Major IIP include six diseases: Idiopathic pulmonary fibrosis (by far the most frequent entity) and non-specific interstitial pneumonia (NSIP) are both progressive and fibrosing; respiratory bronchiolitis and ILD (RB-ILD) and desquamative insterstitial pneumonia (DIP) are smoking-related; acute interstitial pneumonia (AIP) and cryptogenic organizing pneumonia (COP) usually present with an acute onset. So-called minor IIP include idiopathic lymphocytic interstitial pneumonia and pleuro-parenchymal fibroelastosis (PPFE). Finally, unclassifiable ILD designates all IIP that do not fulfill criteria for a specific diagnosis.

Although it represents an interesting attempt to structure a group of various entities, this classification contains several flaws and lacks clinical applicability: For instance, hypersensitivity pneumonitis could be equally classified in the group if ILD of known cause, in granulomatosis and, in case the culprit antigen is not identified, in the IIP group.

Furthermore, the group of ILD of known cause is not further described and seems a bit like a catchall of very different entities.

Provided that most of ILD from known cause will benefit from a specific treatment (removal of the causative agent or treatment of the underlying condition) and that antifibrotic drugs are only used in IPF patients at this point, the whole ILD work-up will first aim at excluding a cause for the patient's ILD. Afterwards, it will be necessary to demonstrate whether it is IPF or not. Importantly, an experienced multidisciplinary team should conduct the whole process. Final diagnosis must be assessed during a multidisciplinary meeting and based on the conjunction of clinical, radiological and eventually histological findings.

Patient's Interrogation and Physical Examination

IPF usually present with progressive dyspnea and physical exhaustion. Half of patients report dry cough. Chest oppression is also classical, usually occurring after efforts.

The anamnesis should include a detailed description of past and current medical conditions and treatments. The physician should always interrogate about signs orienting towards a systemic disease: Did the patient experience arthralgia, Raynaud's phenomenon, mouth and/or eye dryness? Are there any skin lesions, scleroderma, ulcers, or lymph nodes swelling? Any systemic sign would constitute a strong argument against the diagnosis of IPF.

Past or current exposure to tobacco, smoke, toxic compound should be reported and, if possible, quantified. Significant smoking (above 20 pack-years) and long-term exposure to an occupational toxic are strongly related to IPF [3].

Familial anamnesis should not be neglected, as up to 10 percent of patients have at least one first-degree relative affected by IPF or another ILD [4]. Suspected monogenic lung fibrosis should be dealt with care in specialized centers.

Typical IPF signs are inspiratory Velcro crackles at the auscultation and clubbing, the latter affecting about half of patients. Central cyanosis might orientate the clinician towards hypoxemia, eventually requiring oxygen supplementation.

IPF Workup

The joint ATS-ERS-JRS-ALAT guidelines provide guidance for IPF diagnosis [1]. All patient should undergo, after complete interrogation and physical examination, a high resolution computed tomography (HRCT), lab testing for autoantibodies and pulmonary function tests. Depending on the situation and level of diagnosis certainty, patients could advocated for broncho-alveolar lavage (BAL) and/or lung biopsy. As previously stated, all findings should be integrated during a multidisciplinary meeting.

Interpretation of High-Resolution Computed Tomography

All ILD patients undergo HRCT (without contrast agent) for ILD characterization. The 2018 guidelines provide useful technical specifications for the quality of the CT. The radiologist's task is to describe parenchymal lesions and attest whether they fit in the definition of the "usual interstitial pneumonia (UIP)" pattern. The UIP pattern is defined by the presence of (1) subpleural reticulations presenting with a cranio-caudal distribution, (2) traction bronchiectasis (which are dilations of the small airway, presumably due to fibrosis and shrinking of the surrounding alveolar tissue) and (3) layers of subpleural cysts, best known as honeycombing. The absence of signs that are not compatible with the UIP pattern (micronodules, expiratory trapping, multiple enlarged lymph nodes) is also mandatory. Of note, UIP pattern may be associated with connective-tissue disease-associated ILD (CTD-ILD) or end-stage chronic hypersensitivity pneumonitis.

When all UIP features but honeycombing are present, the HRCT is labelled as "probable UIP". When some features are not compatible with a UIP pattern, the HRCT is labelled as "indeterminate". Finally, some HRCT features really point towards an alternate diagnosis (i.e., micronodules with a peribronchovascular distribution, consolidations); in this latter case the HRCT is labelled as "compatible with an alternate diagnosis".

HRCT grading is of crucial importance, as the presence of an UIP pattern in the adequate clinical setting is sufficient to assess the diagnosis of IPF. When an UIP pattern is not present, the multidisciplinary team should require broncho-alveolar lavage and lung biopsy to reach the final diagnosis.

Although radiological criteria appear quite straightforward, real-life experience shows that interobserver agreement for UIP pattern is poor [5]. The development of artificial intelligence-based software, such as CALIPER, developed by the MAYO clinic and the Royal Brompton Hospital, might help to overcome the diagnostic discordance between radiologists and could provide quantitative measures that could be used as predictors of disease-related outcomes [6].

When Should We Perform a Broncho-Alveolar Lavage?

Broncho-alveolar lavage (BAL) allows sampling of the alveolar cells, especially white blood cell profiling. The proportion of cell types may constitute a hint for an alternate diagnosis, although evidence in this peculiar matter is scarce. A normal BAL should be composed of 85 - 90% of macrophages, less than 15% lymphocytes, less than 1% eosinophils and less than 3% neutrophils. BAL from IPF patients may be enriched in eosinophils (up to 10%), neutrophils (up to 20%). Conversely, marked lymphocytosis

(>15%) or eosinophilia (>25%) should evoke an alternative diagnosis (lymphocytosis points towards LIP, sarcoidosis, hypersensitivity pneumonitis; strong eosinophilia is suggestive of eosinophilic pneumonia). Guidelines suggest to perform a BAL in suspected IPF when the differentiate diagnosis includes sarcoidosis, eosinophilic pneumonia or a chronic infection.

Conversely, it is recommended not to perform a BAL when the HRCT pattern is consistent with UIP. Another aspect to consider is local rules and regulations, as differences may exist in BAL procedure between countries or centers.

Integration of Lung Biopsy in the Diagnosis Process

Lung biopsy is required in suspected IPF when HRCT pattern is indeterminate or pointing towards an alternate diagnosis. For patients that display a UIP pattern, it is recommended not to perform a biopsy. For "probable UIP" pattern, the MDD team should weight downsides and outsides of the procedure in the clinical context. Surgical lung biopsy (SLB) is the gold standard to obtain lung samples. Transbronchial lung cryobiopsy is a recent endoscopic technique that may represent a valuable alternative to SLB.

However, conflicting results at this point preclude its use outside of experienced centers [7].

Like the radiologist, the pathologist should provide clear description of present features and integrate them in a pattern. Cardinal features of histological findings for a UIP pattern include dense fibrosis with heterogeneous distribution, subpleural thickening, histological honeycombing and the absence of features suggesting another diagnosis. Depending on the absence of some elements, the biopsy may be classified as "probable UIP", "indeterminate" or "suggestive of an alternative diagnosis".

Finally, a confident diagnosis of IPF may be achieved only with clinical and radiological features (in case of UIP pattern at HRCT) or with the input of BAL and/or biopsy findings.

Multidisciplinary Meeting

An experienced multidisciplinary team (MDT) should conduct workup, integration of results and treatment decision. The valuable input of the MDT in ILD management has been largely demonstrated by several studies since 2004 [8, 9].

Overall, MDT changes the diagnosis and treatment in more than 40 percent of cases [10]. MDT must include at least one pneumologist, one thoracic radiologist and one pathologist.

It is also recommended to include a rheumatologist or general internist in the team given the high frequency of CTD-ILD. MDT meetings are usually organized with a frequency ranging from once a month to once a week. The team should publish a report to be included in the patient's file.

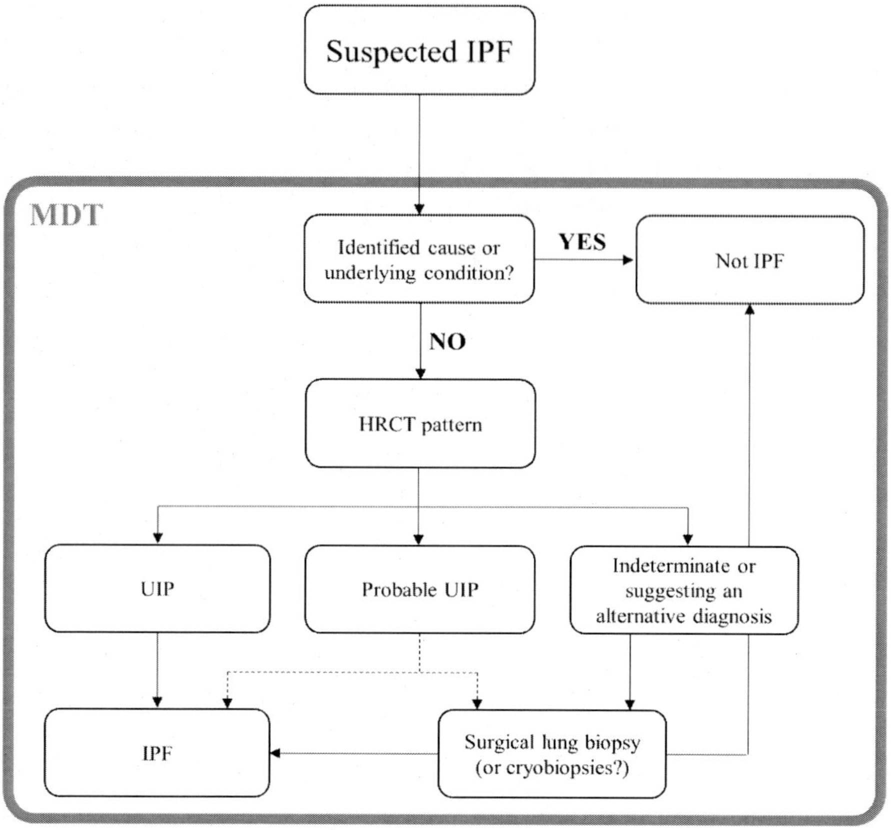

Figure 1. Overview of the diagnosis work-up for suspected idiopathic pulmonary fibrosis (MDT: multidisciplinary team).

IPF Treatment

Pharmacological Treatment

Antifibrotic Drugs

Until 2011, IPF patients were treated with immunosuppressive drugs (combination of prednisolone, azathioprine and N-acetylcycteine). However, a randomized trial evaluating this regimen was discontinued early due to a higher mortality in the treated arm, mostly related to immunosuppressive-induced adverse events [11]. Following studies demonstrated that IPF was an epithelial-derived fibrosing disease rather than an inflammatory one. This paradigm shift on the origins of IPF led to the development of new antifibrotic drugs: pirfenidone and nintedanib. Those drugs are now recommended for the treatment of IPF.

Pirfenidone is a pyridine molecule whose precise target and/or receptor are unknown. However, anti-fibrotic effects of pirfenidone have been extensively explored *in vitro* and *in vivo*: The molecule inhibits TGF-β gene expression in the lungs of bleomycin-induced models of lung fibrosis as well as fibroblast proliferation, migration, and differentiation in myofibroblasts. Pirfenidone also dampens TGF-β-induced collagen I expression on alveolar epithelial cells. Pirfenidone has some anti-inflammatory and antioxidant effects, as it inhibits TNF-α production by a macrophage-like murine cell line and reduces oxidative stress *in vitro*. The safety and efficacy of pirfenidone were evaluated in three double-blind randomized placebo-controlled phase III trials (CAPACITY 1 and 2 and ASCEND) [12, 13]. At week 52, there was a relative difference of 47.9% in the number of patients with an FVC decline of 10% or more in the ASCEND trial. Although none of the three trials showed significant difference regarding mortality, prespecified pooled analysis led to the conclusion that pirfenidone reduced all-cause mortality at 1 year by 48% (hazard ratio (HR), 0.52; 95% CI, 0.31 – 0.87; P = 0.01) and reduced IPF-related mortality by 68% (HR 0.32; 95% CI, 0.14 – 0.76; P = 0.006). This was also confirmed in a recent meta-analysis.

Nintedanib (former name BIBF1120) is a tyrosine kinase inhibitor targeting PDGF, VEGF, and FGF receptors, as well as non-receptor tyrosine kinases Src, Lck, and Lyn. It also inhibits TGF-induced collagen deposition in lung, fibroblast migration, fibroblast to myofibroblast differentiation, and possesses antiangiogenic properties in vitro. Furthermore, nintedanib downregulates protein and messenger RNA (mRNA) expression of extracellular matrix (ECM) proteins in IPF human lung fibroblasts in vitro. In two replicate phase III randomized control studies (INPULSIS-1 and 2) [14] including more than a thousand patients, there was a significant reduction in the annual FVC decline in the nintedanib-treated arm as compared to placebo (114.7 mL vs. 239.9 mL, P < 0.001). A significant difference in the time to first exacerbation and the number of reported exacerbations within time study (3.6% vs. 9.6%, HR0.38, P = 0.005) was found in INPULSIS-2 but not in INPULSIS-1 (HR 1.15, P = 0.67). However, a prespecified sensitivity analysis of pooled results from both trials showed a reduction of exacerbation risk in treated patients (HR 0.32; P = 0.001).

Antifibrotic drugs have adverse events that occur in about half of patients and may affect patient's quality of life: Pirfenidone may cause dyspepsia, nausea, photosensitivity and eczema. Its liver elimination imposes regular monitoring of liver enzymes. Forty to fifty percent of patients treated with nintedanib experience diarrhea and liver enzymes surveillance is also required. Therefore, close monitoring of adverse events is crucial: Symptomatic treatments may be prescribed for adverse events and adaptation of the dosage is possible for both drugs.

In some patients, IPF course is suddenly worsened by the occurrence of acute exacerbations (AE-IPF). These are events defined as a fast (less than a month) worsening of dyspnea and other symptoms, concomitant to the appearance of new infiltrates on chest X-ray or HRCT. The most recent definition of AE-IPF does no longer excludes events triggered by a known cause (infection, thromboembolism) but rather distinguishes

AE-IPF with an identified triggering factor and AE-IPF without any provoking factor. The prognosis of AE-IPF is dramatic, as intra-hospital mortality is above 50 percent and 3 months mortality up to 80 percent [15]. Current proposed treatment of AE-IPF includes a combination of systemic corticosteroids and broad-spectrum antibiotics, along with supportive care. AE-IPF management should be performed taking into account patient's age, comorbidities and potential for lung transplant.

Symptomatic Treatments for Cough

Cough affects a majority of IPF patients (prevalence ranges from 30 to 80 percent in series, depending on the definition used). Cough pathophysiology in IPF is still elusive and may include a lower threshold in response to irritant stimuli and mechanical distortion (due to fibrosis) of nerve fibers involved in cough. Furthermore, gastro-esophageal reflux and other comorbidities increase cough [16].

Cough may be evaluated with visual analogue scales or questionnaires like the Leicester Cough Questionnaire. Cough monitoring devices are also available and sometimes used in clinical trials.

To date, evidence regarding treatments that target cough in IPF is scarce. It is unfortunately often non-responsive to classical antitussive treatments. Non-randomized studies suggest a beneficial effect of low-dose prednisolone (from 5 to 10mg/day). Thalidomide has been also evaluated and was able to reduce cough, but at the price of serious adverse events, making its use difficult in clinical practice. Antifibrotic drugs may reduce IPF-related cough. In particular, an international prospective observational study evaluated the effect of pirfenidone on cough: The treatment was associated with a significant reduction of cough after 12 weeks in 20 of the 27 patients enrolled [17]. Regarding the perspectives, large randomized trials currently evaluate future treatments of IPF-related cough.

Non-Pharmacological Treatment of IPF

Rehabilitation

Exercise training is a safe intervention that has demonstrated benefits is many respiratory chronic diseases. Inclusion in a rehabilitation program should be proposed to all IPF patients. Recent trials have shown a clear benefit of rehabilitation in ILD patients, as demonstrated by improvements in six-minutes walking distance, symptoms (physical exhaustion) and health-related quality of life. As expected, the impact of rehabilitation on disease progression, mortality and lung function is marginal [18].

Most of studies evaluated rehabilitation in hospitals. Supervised exercise training based pulmonary rehabilitation programmes are part of the recommended treatment for IPF.

Oxygen Supplementation

As the disease progresses, patient might require oxygen supplementation at either exercise or both exercise and rest. The effect of oxygen supplementation on IPF was reviewed in a recent meta-analysis [19]. Current evidence suggest that although oxygen does not improve dyspnea at exercise, it increases exercise capacity. It does not seem to have any effect on survival or disease progression.

Lung Transplantation

IPF is a progressive and lethal disease. To date, lung transplantation is the only treatment that significantly increases life expectancy and IPF has become the most frequent indication of lung transplantation worldwide. The current challenge resides in the fact that as antifibrotic drugs slow the disease, it becomes more difficult to identify patients that are candidates for transplantation. One way to tackle this issue is to monitor disease progression during 6 to 12 months and refer patients that progress [20].

IPF comorbidities such as gastro-esophageal reflux, pulmonary hypertension and coronary artery disease must be taken into account prior to enlisting.

CONCLUSION

IPF is a progressive lethal disease. Diagnosis is based on the combination of clinical data, radiological aspect on the HRCT and histological features when a biopsy is required.

The role of multidisciplinary team is central in both diagnosis and management. Although antifibrotic drugs are the cornerstone of IPF treatment, a holistic approach, combining pharmacological and non-pharmacological interventions, is crucial. Patients' inclusion in therapeutic clinical trials (there are currently several compounds tested as add-on therapy in IPF) may also give early access to an effective and innovative treatment.

REFERENCES

[1] Raghu, G., Remy-Jardin, M., Myers, J. L., Richeldi, L., Ryerson, C. J., Lederer, D. J. et al. Diagnosis of Idiopathic Pulmonary Fibrosis. An Official ATS/ERS/JRS/ALAT Clinical Practice Guideline. *Am. J. Respir. Crit. Care Med.*, 2018; 198(5):e44 - e68.

[2] Travis, W. D., Costabel, U., Hansell, D. M., King, T. E., Jr., Lynch, D. A., Nicholson, A. G. et al. An official American Thoracic Society/European Respiratory Society statement: Update of the international multidisciplinary classification of the idiopathic interstitial pneumonias. *Am. J. Respir. Crit. Care Med.,* 2013; 188(6):733 - 48.

[3] Baumgartner, K. B., Samet, J. M., Stidley, C. A., Colby, T. V., Waldron, J. A. Cigarette smoking: a risk factor for idiopathic pulmonary fibrosis. *Am. J. Respir. Crit. Care Med.,* 1997; 155(1):242 - 8.

[4] Borie, R., Kannengiesser, C., Sicre de Fontbrune, F., Gouya, L., Nathan, N., Crestani, B. Management of suspected monogenic lung fibrosis in a specialised centre. *Eur. Respir. Rev.,* 2017; 26(144).

[5] Walsh, S. L., Calandriello, L., Sverzellati, N., Wells, A. U., Hansell, D. M., Consort, U. I. P. O. Interobserver agreement for the ATS/ERS/JRS/ALAT criteria for a UIP pattern on CT. *Thorax,* 2016; 71(1):45 - 51.

[6] Jacob, J., Bartholmai, B. J., Rajagopalan, S., Kokosi, M., Nair, A., Karwoski, R. et al. Mortality prediction in idiopathic pulmonary fibrosis: evaluation of computer-based CT analysis with conventional severity measures. *Eur. Respir. J.,* 2017; 49(1).

[7] Froidure, A., Pieters, T., Leduc, D., Bondue, B. Bad Performance of Lung Cryobiopsy in the Diagnosis of Interstitial Lung Diseases: Don't Throw the Baby out with the Bathwater. *Am. J. Respir. Crit. Care Med.,* 2019.

[8] Flaherty, K. R., King, T. E., Jr., Raghu, G., Lynch, J. P., 3rd, Colby, T. V., Travis, W. D. et al. Idiopathic interstitial pneumonia: what is the effect of a multidisciplinary approach to diagnosis? *Am. J. Respir. Crit. Care Med.,* 2004; 170(8):904 - 10.

[9] Walsh, S. L., Wells, A. U., Desai, S. R., Poletti, V., Piciucchi, S., Dubini, A. et al. Multicentre evaluation of multidisciplinary team meeting agreement on diagnosis in diffuse parenchymal lung disease: a case-cohort study. *Lancet Respir. Med.,* 2016; 4(7):557 - 65.

[10] Biglia, C. G. B., Reychler, G., Koenig, S., Yildiz, H., Lacroix, V., Tamirou, F., Hoton, D., Pieters, Th., Froidure, A. Multidisciplinary management of interstitial lung diseases: A real-life study. *Sarcoidosis Vasc. Diffuse Lung Dis.,* 2019; 36(2): 108 - 15.

[11] Uruga, H., Hanada, S., Kishi, K. Prednisone, azathioprine, and N-acetylcysteine for pulmonary fibrosis. *N Engl. J. Med.,* 2012; 367(9):870; author reply -1.

[12] King, T. E., Jr., Bradford, W. Z., Castro-Bernardini, S., Fagan, E. A., Glaspole, I., Glassberg, M. K. et al. A phase 3 trial of pirfenidone in patients with idiopathic pulmonary fibrosis. *N Engl. J. Med.,* 2014; 370(22):2083 - 92.

[13] Noble, P. W., Albera, C., Bradford, W. Z., Costabel, U., Glassberg, M. K., Kardatzke, D. et al. Pirfenidone in patients with idiopathic pulmonary fibrosis (CAPACITY): two randomised trials. *Lancet,* 2011; 377(9779):1760 - 9.

[14] Richeldi, L., du Bois, R. M., Raghu, G., Azuma, A., Brown, K. K., Costabel, U. et al. Efficacy and safety of nintedanib in idiopathic pulmonary fibrosis. *N Engl. J. Med.*, 2014; 370(22):2071 - 82.

[15] Collard, H. R., Ryerson, C. J., Corte, T. J., Jenkins, G., Kondoh, Y., Lederer, D. J. et al. Acute Exacerbation of Idiopathic Pulmonary Fibrosis. An International Working Group Report. *Am. J. Respir. Crit. Care Med.,* 2016; 194(3):265 - 75.

[16] van Manen, M. J., Birring, S. S., Vancheri, C., Cottin, V., Renzoni, E. A., Russell, A. M. et al. Cough in idiopathic pulmonary fibrosis. *Eur. Respir. Rev.,* 2016; 25(141):278 - 86.

[17] van Manen, M. J. G., Birring, S. S., Vancheri, C., Vindigni, V., Renzoni, E., Russell, A. M. et al. Effect of pirfenidone on cough in patients with idiopathic pulmonary fibrosis. *Eur. Respir. J.,* 2017; 50(4).

[18] Dowman, L. M., McDonald, C. F., Hill, C. J., Lee, A. L., Barker, K., Boote, C. et al. The evidence of benefits of exercise training in interstitial lung disease: a randomised controlled trial. *Thorax,* 2017.

[19] Bell, E. C., Cox, N. S., Goh, N., Glaspole, I., Westall, G. P., Watson, A. et al. Oxygen therapy for interstitial lung disease: a systematic review. *Eur. Respir. Rev.,* 2017; 26(143).

[20] George, P. M., Patterson, C. M., Reed, A. K., Thillai, M. Lung transplantation for idiopathic pulmonary fibrosis. *Lancet Respir. Med.,* 2019; 7(3):271 - 82.

In: Respiratory Ventilatory Strategies …
Editor: Antonio M. Esquinas
ISBN: 978-1-53617-847-0
© 2020 Nova Science Publishers, Inc.

Chapter 30

IDIOPATHIC PULMONARY FIBROSIS: CLINICAL BEHAVIOR AND AGING

Sara Campos Silva*, MD
Pulmonology Department, Hospital Santa Marta,
Centro Hospitalar Universitário Lisboa Central, Lisbon, Portugal

ABSTRACT

Idiopathic pulmonary fibrosis (IPF) is an age-associated, progressive, and irreversible disease of unknown etiology. IPF is typically diagnosed in the sixth decade, and its incidence significantly increases with age. It is characterized by a progressive decline in lung function from an irreversible process of destruction of pulmonary architecture, and currently approved antifibrotic agents, nintendanib and pirfenidone, only slow the progressive decline in lung function without improving survival. Early recognition allows referral to a multidisciplinary approach with consideration to lung transplantation.

Keywords: IPF, phenotypes, comorbidities, aging

INTRODUCTION

Idiopathic pulmonary fibrosis (IPF) is a chronic, and progressive fibrosing interstitial lung disease associated with the histopathologic pattern of usual interstitial pneumonia (UIP) [1]. IPF is considered a rare disease [2], but it is the most common form of

* Corresponding Author's E-mail: saracamposilva@gmail.com.

idiopathic interstitial lung diseases (ILD) [3, 4]. The precise incidence and prevalence of IPF remain challenging to determine. Raguh et al. [5], reported a prevalence of 14 and 42.7 per 100,000 persons and an incidence estimated at 6.8 and 16.3 per 100,000 persons for narrow and broad definitions, respectively. IPF incidence and prevalence increase with age, are higher among males, and appear to be increasing in recent years [3]. Mortality data is also difficult to determine. Retrospective longitudinal studies have suggested that median survival is 2 to 3 years from the time of diagnosis [6].

IPF remains without known pathogenesis. A few case-control observational studies have identified potential risk factors such as older age, gender, cigarette smoking, environmental exposures, gastro-esophageal reflux disease and viral infections [2, 3]. Despite the lack of clear causality, these risk factors may help to identify patients who are at higher risk of developing IPF.

Patients with IPF typically present with exertional dyspnea and a nonproductive cough. Dyspnea is the most prominent symptom, although it is often depreciate by patients, which lead to delay of medical attention [6]. The central issue is that the diagnosis of IPF is a diagnosis of exclusion and the accuracy of it increases with multidisciplinary discussion among pulmonologists, radiologists, and pathologists who are experienced in the diagnosis of ILD.

Since 2014, the first drugs for the treatment of IPF, nintendanib and pirfenidone, were approved. Both have shown to reduce disease progression in patients with IPF and mild or moderate impairment of lung function [3].

Lung transplant remains a treatment option for a minority of patients with IPF and demonstrated to improve survival in patients with IPF [3]. Referral shall be made from the time of diagnosis, given the unpredictable course of the disease.

Natural History of IPF

The natural history of IPF is not fully defined. It is felt like a progressive disorder of subjective and objective decline in pulmonary function, ultimately resulting in death. The diagnosis of IPF can be challenging. First, since patients develop IPF in the latter decades of life, they often attribute their symptoms to old age. Experts in IPF agree that patients usually have symptoms for 2 years or more before having a definitive diagnosis of IPF [6]. This situation may explain the fact that many older cohorts are enriched with advanced, late-stage of IPF. However, with the advent and more frequent use of high-resolution chest tomography (HRCT), which may detect interstitial markings and pick up the diagnosis of IPF at an earlier stage [6]. The other issue is that the clinical behavior is highly variable, and the individual course of the disease is difficult to predict. This heterogeneity has led to the consideration that there are several possible natural histories of IPF [6]. The majority of patients appear to follow a slowly progressive clinical course, though others appear to have a more rapid course. Selman et al., [7] described different clinical groups based on the length of symptoms prior to diagnosis. Some patients may present with a slow progression, others with a rapid decline and others with periods of relative stability interposed with acute deteriorations in respiratory function [2]. The patients who had symptoms <6 months (rapid progression) before the diagnosis had higher mortality than those who had symptoms for more than 24 months (slow progression). The rapid progression form is characterized by the rapid onset of respiratory failure, mainly in middle-aged patients (between 50-55 years of age) non-smokers [8, 9]. It was associated with alterations in the gene expression profile, as well as increased bronchoalveolar lavage active matrix metalloproteinase-9 and fibroblast migration [2, 7]. What influences these different clinical courses is not well known or understood [6].

The acute exacerbation of IPF (AE-IPF) can occur at any time being more often in a subset of patients with advanced disease and never smokers [3, 4]. It is estimated that it can occur in about 10-20% of patients each year [2, 5] and possibly initiate the terminal phase of the disease [2]. AE-IPF is distinguished by a sudden worsening of symptoms and has been associated with hypoxemic respiratory failure and new ground-glass opacities, consolidation or both [2] on the HRCT. The etiology of such episodes may be of unknown origin, or secondary to a recognizable cause such as viral infection, pulmonary embolism or heart failure among others [2, 4]. Acute exacerbations are the leading causes of hospitalization and death among IPF patients [8].

AGING

Aging is biologically defined by a progressive impairment in vital functions attached to a decreased capacity of organs to respond and adapt to environmental challenges. Age confers the greatest risk for IPF, and there is accumulating data showing how the biology of aging may influence the susceptibility to lung fibrosis among old people [10]. Several changes in the morphology and the physiology of the lung appear with age, even in the absence of any disease. Aging is associated with reduced muscle strength that modifies the inspiratory and expiratory movements [6, 11]; cough frequency is decreased among older people and particulate clearance from the lung is adversely affected and associated with ciliary dysfunction [12]. Aging lungs show increased lung compliance and reduction in the lung elastic recoil, which may be associated with structural and functional shifts in the extracellular matrix (ECM) of the lung parenchyma and loss of alveolar surface area [6, 12]. Lung diffusing capacity also declines as result of a reduction in the alveolar-capillary surface area available for gas exchange [6, 12]. The immune system changes with increased susceptibility to infections among older people [12].

The pathobiology of IPF is deeply linked to aging with rising evidence that cellular senescence has an important contribution. Various types of cells, including epithelial type II cells, fibroblasts, and endothelial cells, have shown to undergone senescence in IPF lungs [12]. Lung fibrosis develops as a result of uninterrupted insults associated with genetic and aging-related risk factors, leading to alveolar epithelial cell injuries. Injured epithelial cells then secrete an array of growth factors, chemokines/cytokines, and proteases that promote the activation of myofibroblasts and replacement of injured alveolar epithelium with fibrotic tissue, due to a decreased reparative capacity of the alveolar epithelium [12]. Clarification about cell senescence in lung cells, especially epithelial cells, may be a key to understand the disease pathogenesis and the development of effective treatments for this devastating disease.

López-Otín et al., [13] proposed nine hallmarks of aging including genomic instability, epigenetic alterations, telomere attrition, loss of proteostasis, deregulated nutrient sensing, mitochondrial dysfunction, cellular senescence, stem cell exhaustion and altered intercellular communication.

Genomic Instability

Throughout life, DNA is exposed to various endogenous and exogenous stimuli and the capacity of the cellular DNA repair system diminishes [14, 15]. The accumulation of errors can damage the genome and dysregulate homeostasis of the cell. For example, loss of heterozygosity (LOH), one of the markers of genomic instability, is located in key cell cycle genes such as p16, a marker of senescence [15]. Several studies have reported that genetic stability is impaired in IPF patients and may contribute to disease pathogenesis [15].

Epigenetic Changes

Epigenetic mechanisms are able to modulate gene activity in the absence of DNA sequence changes, including DNA methylation, histone modification, and expression of noncoding RNAs [12]. There is evidence that epigenetic alterations play a critical role in the biology of aging and pathophysiological of aging-related diseases as IPF [10]. Sanders et al., reported that senescence fibroblasts had global increases in histone (H4K20) trimethylation and decreases in fibrotic lung diseases [12]. These fibroblasts had marked enrichment of the Bcl-2 gene that was H4K20 acetylated and demethylated, suggesting that these epigenetic modifications led to active transcription of the Bcl-2 gene, which renders senescent fibroblasts an increased resistance to apoptosis [12]. Aging can also change the expression of sirtuins (SIRTs), a family of deacetylases that target both histone and nonhistone proteins [15]. For example, SIRT1 suppresses the expression of senescence-associated secretory phenotype (SASP) factors via histone deacetylation in their promoter regions and reduction in SIRT1 and SIRT3 has shown to promote pulmonary fibrosis. In contrast, SIRT3 upregulation has shown to rejuvenate hematopoietic stem cells that reverse aging-associated degeneration [15]. Standers et al., [17] reported that pharmacological regulation of histone acetylation should be a possible new therapeutic avenue for IPF.

Loss of Proteostasis

The autophagy-lysossomal system and the ubiquitin-proteosomal system are the two major proteolytic systems, both of which decline with aging, leading to increased accumulation of misfolded proteins, increased endoplasmic reticulum (ER) stress and defective autophagy [15]. For example, familial IPF has been linked to protein misfolding mutations in surfactant C and markers of ER stress are seen in IPF lungs from areas with dense fibrosis [15]. Autophagy is a catabolic process by which damage organelles and endogenous proteins are destroyed within lysosomes. Inhibition of autophagy accelerates cellular senescence in epithelial cells and promotes myofibroblast differentiation of lung fibroblasts [15]. In experimental studies, was shown that activation of autophafy can promote collagen turnover and resolve lung fibrosis [15]. Interestingly, pirfenidone has shown to induce noncanonical autophagy in lung fibroblasts that may, in part, contribute to its beneficial effects. These studies indicate that age-associated decline in autophagy may be a therapeutic target to maintain proteostasis in the aging lung.

Telomere Attrition

Telomeres are repetitive DNA sequences found at the end of chromosome that prevent chromosome fusion and confer protection to enconding DNA during chromosome replication. The telomeric DNA is incompletely replicated during each cell cycle by the telomerase complex, consisting of telomerase reverse transcriptase (TERT) and telomerase RNA (TERC) restores the telomere length [15]. IPF is the most common manifestation of telomere-related disorders [15]. Familial and sporadic IPF have been associated with mutations in the telomerase genes TERC and TERT. Around 8-15% of the familiar pulmonary fibrosis is associated with germline mutations in telomerase genes [15]. Genetic mutations related to telomerase (telomere elongating enzyme) are one of the common genetic defects found in patients with familial IPF. In addition to activating DNA damage pathways, shortened telomeres are also thought to contribute to fibrosis when exposed to an injurious stimulus, by impairing tissue repair. Chromosomal shortening resulting from telomere attrition activates checkpoint inhibitor p53, which in turn reduces mitochondrial biogenesis, increases ROS production and activates cellular senescent pathways [15].

Cellular Senescence

Diminution of the replicative capacity of lung cells is a well-known phenomenon in IPF. Cellular senescence is commonly defined as an irreversible state of stable growth arrest in association with high metabolic activity and secretory phenotype [12]. Alveolar epithelial cells and fibroblasts have been shown to assume senescent identities in IPF, contributing to the development of fibrosis. Established senescent markers such as p21, p16 and senescence-associated β-galactosidase activity are increased in both fibroblasts and epithelial cells in human IPF lung tissue as compared with controls [15]. IPF-derived fibroblasts exhibit accelerated replicative cellular senescence and increased resistance to oxidative stress-induced cytotoxicity as compared to normal lung fibroblasts. The secretome of both, IPF fibroblasts and alveolar epithelial cells, exhibits increased profibrotic and inflammatory makers and is thought to have a profound effect on the lung microenvironment by secretion of these mediators which perpetuate fibrotic scarring. Cellular senescence is being recognized as a therapeutic target in IPF. Based on the apoptosis-resistant phenotype of senescent fibroblast and myofibroblasts, strategies to increase their sensitivity to apoptosis by inhibition of antiapoptotic factors have been suggested. The antiapoptotic and prosenescent enzyme, NADPH oxidase 4 (NOX4) has been targeted in an aging murine model of persistent lung fibrosis with induction of apoptosis of interstitial myofibroblasts and marked improvement in lung fibrosis and survival [15]. Cellular senescence offers a potentially effective therapeutic target in IPF, and there is active research to determine the safety and efficacy of this approach [15, 12].

Mytochondrial Disfunction

Mytochondrial dysfunction is characterized by reduced mitochondrial biogenesis, release of reactive oxygen species (ROS), accumulation of NADH, and deregulated mitochondrial biogenesis and apoptosis [10, 15]. In IPF, dysfunctional mitochondria have been reported in AEC2 cells, lung fibroblasts and alveolar macrophages [15]. Evidence shown that in AEC2 cells the dysfunction is due to the reduced expression of PTEN-induced putative kinase 1 (PINK1) that is a master regulator of mitochondrial homeostasis with a key role in mitophagy [15]. Interestingly, PINK1 expression decreases with age, thus increasing the predisposition of older lungs to develop fibrosis. Mechanistically, decreased PINK1 expression in AEC2 leads to a senescent phenotype characterized by the secretion of pro-fibrotic TGFβ1 and other senescence-associated secretory phenotype (SASP) with higher expression of p16 and p21 and higher susceptibility to apoptosis. Further investigation is needed to learn about the role of mitochondrial dysfunction in the developing and maintenance of the pro-fibrotic conditions that drive IPF, regarding the interplay between mitochondrial and nuclear signaling in overall cellular dysfunction [17].

Extracellular Matrix

Alterations to the extracellular matrix (ECM) with aging have profound effects on the susceptibility to the development of lung fibrosis. ECM of aging lungs expresses a profibrotic phenotype characterized by increased Type I and III collagen and TGF- β1 expression along with enhanced fibronectin extracellular domain A (EDA) [15]. Old lungs also have an oxidizing extracellular environment as compared to young lungs, which has been shown to induce intracellular signals that stimulate proliferation and matrix expression in fibroblasts via upregulation of TGF- β 1 expression [15].

Future Perspectives

There is an emerging concept that impaired mucociliary clearance may represent a lung aging phenotype and contribute to IPF pathogenesis [15]. The progress in our understanding of IPF has dramatically advanced in recent years and has accelerated in part due to the incorporation of aging biology concepts in diseases pathogenesis. Critical gaps in understanding the pathogenesis include the role of epigenetic modifications, metabolic sensing, ECM alterations, and airway host defense mechanisms such as impaired mucociliary clearance. Further insights into these mechanisms will lead to the development of novel diagnostics and therapeutics for IPF and other age-associated lung diseases. Advances in imaging modalities and biomarkers that define/detect changes in the metabolic and inflammation-fibrosis related pathways would facilitate clinical translation [15, 16].

An integrated approach to these different pathways seen with aging and IPF is essential to determining therapeutic targets that are more likely to affect the natural history of IPF [18].

To future directions, it is imposed to understand the complex interplay between the genetic architecture, aging-associated processes, environmental factors, and the genome-environment interaction that impacts gene expression that finally results in the sequence of pathogenic mechanisms leading to the development of IPF [19].

CONCLUSION

Current efforts exist to integrate the normal physiology of aging with the pathobiology of age-related chronic diseases like IPF. A new understanding of how biological systems change with age offers novel pathways that might impact the course of IPF. As described above, multiple pathways associated with aging are activated in lung epithelial cells, fibroblasts, and progenitor cells in the IPF lung. One of the goals is to develop preventive and therapeutic approaches to multiple age-related diseases. In the future, innovative drugs may be able to prevent, delay, or reverse multiple or specific aging-related chronic diseases, including IPF.

REFERENCES

[1] Raghu G., Remy-Jardín M., Myers J. L., et al., Diagnosis of Idiopathic Pulmonar Fibrosis: An Official ATS/ERS/JRS/ALAT Clinical Practice Guideline. *Am J Resp Crit Care Med* 2018; 198:e44-e68.

[2] Sauleda J., Núñez B., Sala E., et al., Idiopathic Pulmonary Fibrosis: Epidemiology, Natural History, Phenotypes. *Med Sci* 2018; 110-14.

[3] Kim H. J., Perlman D., Tomic R. Natural history of idiopathic pulmonary fibrosis. *Resp Med.* 2015; 109:661-670.

[4] Hyldgaard C., Hilberg O., Bendstrup E. How does comorbidity influence survival in idiopathic pulmonary fibrosis? *Resp Med.* 2014; 108:647-653.

[5] Raghu G., Weycker D., Edelsberg J., et al., Incidence and prevalence of idiopathic pulmonary fibrosis. *Am J Respir Crit Care Med.* 2006; 174(7):810-816.

[6] Grippi M. A., Elias J. A., Fishman J. A., et al., Fishman's Pulmonary Diseases and Disorders. *McGraw-Hill Education.* 2015(5);842-858.

[7] Selman M., Carrillo G., Estrada A., et al., Accelerated variant of idiopathic pulmonary fibrosis: clinical behavior and gene expression pattern. 2007; *Plos One* e48.

[8] Buendía-Roldán I., Mejía M., Navarro C., et al., Idiopathic pulmonary fibrosis: Clinical behavior and aging associated comorbidities. *Resp Med.* 2017; 129:46-52.

[9] Bruminhent J., Yassir S., Pippim J. Acute Interstitial Pneumonia (Hamman-Rich Syndrome) as a Cause of Idiopathic Acute Respiratory Distress Syndrome. *Case Rep Med.* 2011; 2011:628743.

[10] Collard H. The Age of Idiopathic Pulmonary Fibrosis. *Am J Resp Crit Care Med.* 2010(8); 771-772.

[11] Lowery E. M., Brubaker A. L., Kuhlmann E., et al., The aging lung. *Clin Interv Aging.* 2013; 8:1489.96.

[12] Merkt W., Bueno M., Mora A. L., et al., Senotherapeutics: Targeting senescence in idiopathic pulmonar fibrosis. *Seminars in Cell and Developmental Biology.* 2019.

[13] López-Otín C., Blasco M. A., Patrtridge L., et al., The hallmarks of aging. *Cell.* 2013; 153(6):1194-1217.

[14] Liu R. M., Liu G., Cell senescence and fibrotic lung diseases. *Exp Geront.* 2020(132); 110836.

[15] Gulati S., Thannickal V. J., The aging lung and idiopathic pulmonary fibrosis. *Am J Med Sci.* 2019; 357(5):384-389.

[16] Mora A. L., Bueno M., Rojas M. Mitochondria in the spotlight of aging and idiopathic pulmonary fibrosis. *J Clin Invest.* 2017; 127(2):405-414.

[17] Sanders Y. Y., Hagood J. S., Liu H., et al., Histone deacetylase inhibition promotes fibroblast apoptosis and ameliorates pulmonary fibrosis in mice. *Eur Respir J.* 2014; 43(5):1448-1458.

[18] Zank D. C., Bueno M., Mora A. L., et al., Idiopathic Pulmonary Fibrosis: Aging, Mitochondrial Dysfunction, and Cellular Bioenergetics. *Front Med.* 2018; 5:10.

[19] Selman M., Pardo A. Revealing the Pathogenic and Aging-related Mechanisms of the Enigmatic Idiopathic Pulmonary Fibrosis. *Am J Resp Crit Care Med.* 2014(189); 1161:1172.

In: Respiratory Ventilatory Strategies …
Editor: Antonio M. Esquinas
ISBN: 978-1-53617-847-0
© 2020 Nova Science Publishers, Inc.

Chapter 31

PHARMACOLOGICAL MANAGEMENT OF PROGRESSIVE-FIBROSING INTERSTITIAL LUNG DISEASES

Kevin Lazo*[1,*]*, DO and Marwah Ibrahem*[2]*, DO
[1]Fellow in Pulmonary & Critical Care Medicine,
Memorial Sloan Kettering Cancer Center, New York, NY, US
[2]Attending Hospitalist, Division of Hospital Medicine,
Long Island Jewish Medical Center, New Hyde Park, NY, US

ABSTRACT

In 2011, clinical practice guidelines were established by a joint assembly of representatives from the American Thoracic Society (ATS), the European Respiratory Society (ERS), the Japanese Respiratory Society (JRS), and the Latin American Thoracic Association (LATA) to create recommendations for the treatment of Idiopathic Pulmonary Fibrosis (IPF). These guidelines were later updated in a 2015 statement published by the ATS [1]. These official joint statements, along with numerous other studies, continue to build upon current best practices to attenuate the progression of IPF. As of 2019, only two anti-fibrotic drugs have demonstrated clinical efficacy by significantly reducing decline in forced vital capacity - pirfenidone and nintedanib [2]. Current recommendations for the pharmacologic treatment of IPF are summarized in Table 1 [1, 2]. Other approaches to management seek to optimize patient's other comorbidities while providing symptom relief, pulmonary rehabilitation, and palliative care. In this chapter, we will discuss the pharmacologic therapies recommended for use in IPF, as well as discuss potential new therapies currently being investigated.

---

* Corresponding Author's E-mail: kgl823@gmail.com.

Keywords: pirfenidone, nintedanib

Molecular Pathophysiology of Idiopathic Pulmonary Fibrosis

Understanding the proposed molecular mechanisms of IPF help elucidate the choice of agents for drug therapy. It is believed that IPF is due to recurrent subepithelial injury of the alveoli superimposed on accelerated alveolar aging leads to abnormal repair of the alveoli and interstitial fibrosis by myofibroblasts in the alveolar space [3]. Protein synthesis, oxidative injury/mitochondrial dysfunction, and telomere shortening may contribute to fibroblast deposition and aberrant alveolar repair [3]. Genetic mutations of *MUC5B* have also been proposed to cause impaired responses to bacteria and impaired mucociliary clearance in the alveoli [3]. Figure 1 is a schematic representation of an alveolus in IPF.

In alveolar injury related to IPF, it is proposed that fibroblast proliferation is accompanied by myofibroblast differentiation, matrix deposition, reduction in apoptosis, senescence of the apoptotic phenotype, impaired autophagy, and downregulation of miRNA-29 [3]. The culmination of these factors leads to interstitial fibrosis. It is postulated that inhibition of the tyrosine kinase and serine-threonine kinase pathways, inhibition of the G-protein coupled receptor pathways, or inhibition of other numerous mechanisms would cause downregulation of this response and therefore halt progression of the disease.

Table 1. Current recommendations for the pharmacologic management of Idiopathic Pulmonary Fibrosis [1, 2]

Agent	**Strength of Recommendation**	**Confidence in effect estimates**
Recommendations for use		
Nintedanib	Conditional	Moderate
Pirfenidone	Conditional	Moderate
Anti-acid therapy	Conditional	Very low
Recommendations against use		
Imatinib	Strong	Moderate
Anticoagulation (warfarin)	Strong	Moderate
Prednisone + Azathioprine + N-acetylcysteine	Strong	Low
Selective endothelin receptor antagonists (ambrisentan)	Strong	Low
Dual endothelin receptor antagonists (macitentan, bosentan)	Conditional	Low
Phosphodiesterase inhibitor (sildenafil)	Conditional	Moderate
N-acetylcysteine monotherapy	Conditional	Low

Adapted from American Thoracic Society Guidelines 2015.

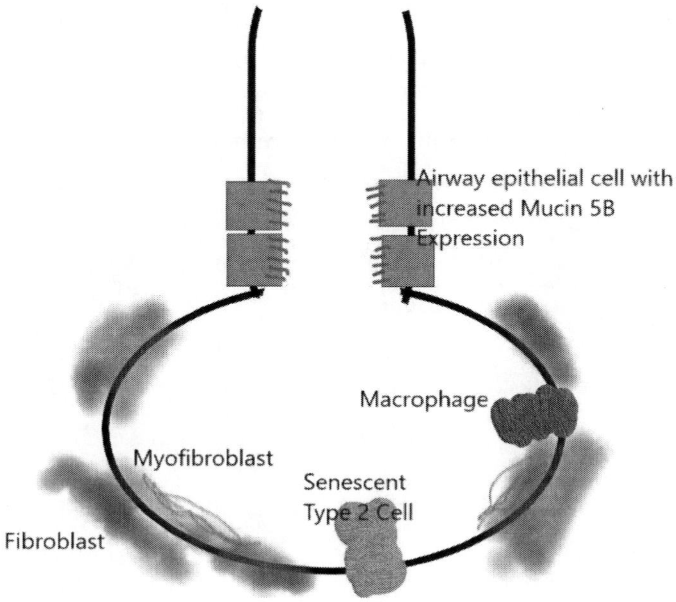

Figure 1. Molecular Pathophysiology of Idiopathic Pulmonary Fibrosis.

FDA APPROVED FOR PHARMACOLOGIC MANAGEMENT OF IDIOPATHIC PULMONARY FIBROSIS

Pirfenidone

Pirfenidone is an oral medication FDA approved in October 2014 for the treatment of idiopathic pulmonary fibrosis. While the exact mechanism of action of the drug is unknown, it is thought to have inhibitory effects on the expression of beta-1 transforming growth factor [4]. Pirfenidone's approved use for IPF was first established in Japan (October 2008) and Europe (February 2011). Evidence from the CAPACITY and ASCEND trials was analyzed for the 2015 ATS guidelines on IPF treatment [1].

The CAPACITY trial reported two independent study protocols that ultimately showed a reduction in decline of FVC in both study populations on high dose pirfenidone (2403 mg/day) compared to the placebo. The results of the low dose pirfenidone (1197 mg/day) in one of the study protocols was intermediate to the high dose group [5]. Furthermore, in the high dose pirfenidone group there was a higher incidence of adverse effects - nausea, vomiting, dyspepsia, photosensitivity, anorexia, and rash compared to placebo [5].

The ASCEND trial was a randomized, double-blind, placebo-controlled trial that randomly assigned 555 IPD patients oral pirfenidone (at a dose of 2403 mg per day) or placebo for 52 weeks. The primary endpoint was to assess for change in Forced Vital

Capacity (FVC) or death at week 52. The authors found that treatment with pirfenidone significantly reduced the decline in FVC from baseline to week 52 in the study population compared to the placebo group ($P < 0.001$) [6]. Furthermore, the proportion of patients with no decline in the percentage of the predicted FVC was increased by 132.5% in the pirfenidone group [6]. There was no statistically significant difference in death rate from any cause or IPF between treatment groups, nor was there any observed change in mortality rate due to other causes or IPF, and there was no observed effect on respiratory symptoms. Pooled results from the ASCEND and CAPACITY trials suggested improved mortality with pirfenidone, as well as reduced rate of FVC decline. These results led the 2015 ATS guidelines to use pirfenidone in patients with IPF on a conditional recommendation [1].

Nintedanib

Nintedanib is an oral medication that acts as an inhibitor of multiple tyrosine receptor kinases - including vascular endothelial growth factor, fibroblast growth factor, and platelet derived growth factor. By affecting these growth factor pathways, it is believed that there is a reduction in the rate of loss of lung parenchymal integrity and reduction of stiffening in the lungs - thereby inhibiting the progression of IPF [7]. The conditional recommendation by the 2015 ATS guidelines for the use of nintedanib was based on the evidence provided by the TOMORROW and INPULSIS 1 & 2 trials.

The INPULSIS-1&2 trials were two replicate randomized double blind trials that assessed the effect of 150 mg of Nintedanib twice a day versus placebo in 1066 total enrolled patients. The primary end point was assessing reduction in forced vital capacity over a 52 week study period [8]. Review of pooled data from the IMPULSIS 1&2 trials showed that there was a consistent treatment effect of reduced FVC across multiple subgroups [2]. As per the 2015 ATS summary of the evidence, there was no significant benefit of the drug on mortality or acute exacerbation of IPF, and more patients treated with nintedanib reported an adverse event - and had more frequent episodes of nausea and diarrhea compared to placebo [1].

The TOMORROW trial was a 12 month Phase 2 trial that randomized 432 patients to receive one of 4 doses of Nintedanib versus placebo. The group had found that Nintedanib at 150 mg twice a day slowed FVC decline at 0.06 liters for the year as opposed to 0.19 liters in the placebo group - or a 68.4% reduction in rate. They also had noticed a trend in fewer acute exacerbations of IPF ($P = 0.02$) and a small decrease in St. George's Respiratory Questionnaire Scores (SGRQ) in the treatment group as compared to increases in SGRQ scores in the placebo [5].

Optimization of Comorbidities in IPF

Arterial hypertension, diastolic dysfunction, arteriosclerosis, coronary artery disease, diabetes, pulmonary hypertension, lung cancer, COPD, and GERD are all comorbidities with a >10% prevalence in IPF [10]. Not surprisingly, the burden of the comorbidities in IPF patients contribute to a decrease in Health Related Quality of Life. Thus it stands to reason that in addition to attempting to slow progression of disease, control of comorbidities for these patients is paramount.

Anti-Acid Therapy

It has been previously described that up to 90% of patients with IPF also have concomitant Gastroesophageal Reflux Disease (GERD) [1]. It is proposed that GERD causes microaspirations that may induce lung injury or damage - which may cause or worsen IPF. The 2015 ATS Practice Guidelines noted that the recommendation of antiacid treatment (conditional recommendation, very low confidence in estimates of effect) is based off two studies - one retrospective analysis showing survival benefit of patients receiving antiacid medication, and another study that showed significantly smaller decrease in FVC in an aggregate analysis of three randomized controlled trials [1].

Cardiovascular Agents

Statins have been proposed to contribute anti-inflammatory effects that may be protective against smoking as well as decrease the rate of age-associated lung function. In a post hoc analysis of IPF patients - statins appear to be associated with better disease prognosis, less hospitalizations, and decreased mortality compared to IPF patients not taking statins [10]. Furthermore, ACE inhibitors (no ARBs) may be shown to have positive effects on mortality in IPF patients as well [10].

Novel Targets in IPF

Several phase II and III trials are being conducted to expand on treatments for IPF. As of 2019, there are multiple promising trials with positive outcomes. These include PRM 151 (Pentraxin-2 analogues), anti-connective tissue growth factor antibodies (pamrevlumab), PBI-4050, and autotaxin-LPA inhibitors [10].

PRM-151 refers to serum amyloid P. This is a protein that inhibits the differentiation of monocytes into pro-fibrotic fibrocytes and TGF-Beta producing macrophages. By inhibiting this differentiation of monocytes, the proposed mechanism would lead to a decrease in fibrosis. A phase 2 trial so far has demonstrated some effect in reducing pulmonary function test decline over 24 weeks compared to placebo [10].

Anti-connective tissue growth factor abnormalities seek to decrease expression of tissue growth factors which would usually cause upregulation of TGF-Beta and deposition of extracellular matrix and inhibition of degradation of extracellular matrix. A Phase III trial of the drug Pamrevlumab (FG3019) was shown to have a significant effect on reduction of lung function decline in 160 patients, but fully peer-reviewed data is still pending [10].

PBI-4050 is an analog of a medium-chain fatty acid that inhibits G-protein coupled receptor mediated pathways that promote endoplasmic reticulum stress and fibrocyte/fibroblast proliferation and migration. It has been shown in a phase II trial of 40 patients that this drug in combination with pirfenidone shows a statistically signicant greater decline in FVC than using pirfenidone or PBI-4050 alone [10].

GLPG1690 is an autotaxin-LPA inhibitor that helps to bind bioactive lysophphatidic acid (LPA) to decrease epithelial cell apoptosis and endothelial cell damage. A 12-week period study, phase IIa, has shown that patients with IPF have good tolerance to this experimental drug, with promising results towards halting FVC decline [10].

CONCLUSION

IPF is a progressive fibrosing lung disease without any known cure. Currently recommended therapies include Nintedanib and Pirfenidone, as well as optimization of comorbidities with antacid therapy or cardiovascular agents. Available drugs have demonstrated a slowing of pulmonary function decline however further trials are needed to discover novel therapies of the medication.

REFERENCES

[1] Raghu G, Rochwerg B, Zhang Y, et al. An official ATS/ERS/JRS/ALAT statement: idiopathic pulmonary fibrosis: evidence based guidelines for diagnosis and management an update of the 2011 clinical practice guideline, *Am. J. Respir. Crit. Care Med.* 192 (2015) e3ee19, http://dx.doi.org/10.1164/rccm.201506-1063ST.

[2] Raghu G, Richeldi L. Current approaches to the management of idiopathic pulmonary fibrosis. *Respiratory Medicine* 129 (2017); 24-30.

[3] Lederer DJ, Martinez FJ. Idiopathic pulmonary fibrosis. *N. Engl. J. Med.* 2018; 378: 1811-1823.

[4] Audibert C, Livoti C, Caze A. Idiopathic pulmonary fibrosis: Physicians' perceptions of patient treatment with recently approved drugs. *Contemporary Clinical Trials Communications* 3; 80-85. 2016.

[5] Noble PW, Albera C, Bradford WZ, et al. Pirfenidone in patients with idiopathic pulmonary fi brosis (CAPACITY): two randomised trials. *Lancet* 2011; 377: 1760-69.

[6] King TE, Bradford WZ, Castro-Bernardini S, et al. A Phase 3 Trial of Pirfenidone in Patients with Idiopathic Pulmonary Fibrosis. *N. Engl. J. Med.* 2014;370:2083-92. doi: 10.1056/NEJMoa1402582.

[7] Hajari CA, Johnson P. Clinical use of nintedanib in patients with idiopathic pulmonary fibrosis. *BMJ Open Respiratory Research* 2017;4:e000192. doi: 10. 1136/bmjresp-2017-000192.

[8] Richeldi L, du Bois RM, Raghu G, et al. Efficacy and Safety of Nintedanib in Idiopathic Pulmonary Fibrosis. *N. Engl. J. Med.* 2014;370:2071-82. doi: 10.1056/ NEJMoa1402584.

[9] Richeldi L, Costabel U, Selman M. et al. Efficacy of a Tyrosine Kinase Inhibitor in Idiopathic Pulmonary Fibrosis. *N. Engl. J. Med.* 2011;365:1079-87.

[10] Somogyi V, Chaudhury N, Torrisi SE, Kahn N, Muller V, Kreuter M. The therapy of idiopathic pulmonary fibrosis: what is next? *Euro. Respi. Rev.* 2019; 28:190021.

In: Respiratory Ventilatory Strategies …
Editor: Antonio M. Esquinas

ISBN: 978-1-53617-847-0
© 2020 Nova Science Publishers, Inc.

Chapter 32

LONG TERM MANAGEMENT OF IDIOPATHIC PULMONARY FIBROSIS USING NON-INVASIVE AND CPAP OXYGEN THERAPY

Zuhal Karakurt[1*], MD and Meltem Ağca[2], MD

[1]Pulmonary and Critical Care Department,
Pulmonology and Intensivist, Dean in Hospital,
University of Health Sciences Istanbul Sureyyapaşa Chest Diseases and Thoracic Surgery Teaching and Research Hospital, İstanbul-Turkey
[2]Pulmonary Department, Pulmonology Specialist
University of Health Sciences Istanbul Sureyyapaşa Chest Diseases and Thoracic Surgery Teaching and Research Hospital, İstanbul-Turkey

ABSTRACT

Over the last decade advances in pulmonary radiology have led to an increased familiarity of interstitial lung disease (ILD). Among the ILDs, idiopathic pulmonary fibrosis (IPF) is the most studied *in terms of basic* pharmaceutical research. Following diagnosis, disease progression can be slowed and quality of life can be improved, however, despite the availability of promising new drugs, life expectancy is still 3 to 5 years after diagnosis. There is still no definitive evidence regarding the effect of long term oxygen therapy (LTOT) on prolonged survival of patients with IPF although patients mostly opt to use LTOT as it improves their level of comfort. Even acute state, high flow oxygen with a nasal cannula (HFO-NC) provides promising results with respect to patient's comfort and allowing them to feel better in their last days of life in hospital. Domiciliary continuous positive airway pressure (CPAP) and non-invasive mechanical ventilation (NIV) can provide respiratory support in the advanced stages of IPF. CPAP with LTOT shows a similar effect to that of HFO-NC. NIV can be helpful if in cases with hypercapnia. Regardless of this respiratory support, the involvement of lung parenchyma determines the outcome. In this review, the long term management of IPF with LTOT and CPAP/NIV are evaluated.

Keywords: interstitial lung disease, prognosis, management of idiopathic pulmonary fibrosis, domiciliary non-invasive ventilation, CPAP, high flow oxygen, long term oxygen therapy

INTRODUCTION

With the advancements in tomography imaging techniques, familiarity of interstitial lung diseases (ILDs) has increased, and it has been observed that heterogeneity of the radiological pattern can determine the response to treatment. Among the ILDs, the most common and most studied is idiopathic pulmonary fibrosis (IPF). In this review, we evaluate the use of oxygen, non-invasive mechanical ventilation (NIV), and continuous positive airway pressure (CPAP) for the long term management of IPF. The impact of oxygen therapy on mortality is discussed in another chapter (Chapter 44).

OXYGEN THERAPY

The need for supportive oxygen use is seen in the advanced stages of IPF. Acute exacerbation of IPF results predominantly in refractory hypoxemia [1]. On a long-term basis, international guidelines strongly recommend long term oxygen therapy (LTOT) for IPF patients [2]. Oxygen therapy is generally prescribed by physicians, however, the impact of oxygen therapy on dyspnea, exercise tolerance, health- related quality of life (HRQoL), and mortality is not clear. Long term supplemental oxygen treatment is recommended if the resting hypoxemia pulse oxygen saturation is below 88% in room air [2].

Reasons for Oxygen Therapy in Patients with Interstitial Lung Diseases

1. Hypoxemia at rest
2. Hypoxemia during exertion
3. Dyspnea during exertion
4. Improved physical activity
5. Better health-related quality of life
6. Prevention of secondary pulmonary hypertension and right heart failure
7. Improved survival

A recent systematic review analyzed 12 studies to evaluate the impact of oxygen therapy on dyspnea, HRQoL, exercise tolerance and mortality in all ILDs [3]. Most physicians believe that LTOT improves dyspnea and HRQoL, and there are two studies that support this belief [4, 5]. A possible mechanism is that LTOT may positively stimulate a chemoreceptor that diminishes the respiratory drive and decreases the respiratory rate. A second potential mechanism is stimulation of signaling within the upper airway by oxygen flow [6]. However, in a randomized control trial [7], LTOT did not result in a satisfactory improvement in exercise capacity, namely the six minute walk distance (6MWD) [8]. Nonetheless, the systematic review determined that oxygen therapy is helpful to eliminate dyspnea and improve physical activity [3]. Long term "ambulatory oxygen" use is crucial for IPF patients to control "dyspnea" on exertion and increase physical activity. Very recently a randomized study showed that supplementary ambulatory oxygen had further benefits on HRQoL and hypoxia during exertion [9]. However, ambulatory oxygen supply devices are expensive and not often provided or covered by insurance companies. Short term oxygen therapy has not demonstrated satisfactory supportive effects in patients with ILD, the benefit of LTOT has not been conclusively shown, and the high cost of oxygen therapy is a further issue. In cases of acute exacerbation of IPF the use of HFO-NC has shown promising results in improving oxygenation and decreasing mortality, however, elevated serum C-reactive protein levels are a negative predictor of short term outcome [10]. While oxygen treatment is clearly recommended by international guidelines for patients with IPF [2], and ambulatory oxygen can provide further freedom with respect to physical activity and an improved HRQoL, further convincing evidence is needed to support the use of supplemental oxygen therapy for IPF patients [11].

Long Term Non Invasive Mechanical Ventilation and Continuous Positive Airway Pressure

Long term NIV use in patients with ILD is not well documented. NIV is the preferred option in acute respiratory failure in patients with ILD, including IPF, due to the poor prognosis associated with invasive mechanical ventilation (IMV) by physicians in the emergency department and intensive care unit [12-14]. Early NIV initiation prevents potential intubation for IMV in IPF patients with acute respiratory failure [15-17]. There are no reports on the effect of long term NIV use on ILD/IPF patients with chronic respiratory failure (CRF), however, a study last decade demonstrated that NIV resulted in improvement in patients with ILD [18]. In that study, the higher respiratory rate (i.e., 23.5 breaths per minute) and higher inspiratory pressure (i.e., 28 cmH_2O) with a pressure controlled NIV mode, successfully decreased the patient's $PaCO_2$ and increased the PaO_2

[18]. Meanwhile the absence of NIV use in CRF patients with ILD/IPF, physicians deal with NIV and prescribe domiciliary NIV can assure the effectivity of NIV for patients with ILDs/IPF. However, further definitive evidence is needed for long term NIV use in cases of ILD with CRF. CPAP is the preferred first option in acute settings of exacerbations of ILD, and it can prevent the need for intubation [17]. On a long term basis, CPAP can be helpful in those patients with non-hypercapnic ILD. HFO-NC can provide a similar response to CPAP and will be compared and studied in a randomized control trial. Clinical sensibility tells us that the long term use of NIV will be better for nearly all ILD/IPF patients, particularly in end stage ILD [20]. This is in concordance with other diseases that lead to hypercapnia and respiratory deterioration, i.e., obesity, sleep disorders, chronic obstructive lung diseases, and lung cancer. Current domiciliary NIV devices are small, have better respiratory triggering, higher pressure settings, an ambulatory battery system and an ambulatory oxygen supplement system. These facilities allow ILD patients to have an improved HRQoL. The primary concern is the timing of prescribing long term NIV and ambulatory oxygen systems and insurance reimbursement.

REFERENCES

[1] Marchioni A, Tonelli R, Ball L, Fantini R, Castaniere I, Cerri S, Luppi F, Malerba M, Pelosi P, Clini E. Acute exacerbation of idiopathic pulmonary fibrosis: lessons learned from acute respiratory distress syndrome? *Crit. Care.* 2018 Mar 23;22(1):80. doi: 10.1186/s13054-018-2002-4. Review.

[2] Raghu G, Rochwerg B, Zhang Y, Garcia CA, Azuma A, Behr J, et al.; American Thoracic Society; European Respiratory society; Japanese Respiratory Society; Latin American Thoracic Association. An Official ATS/ERS/ JRS/ALAT Clinical Practice Guideline: Treatment of Idiopathic Pulmonary Fibrosis. An Update of the 2011 Clinical Practice Guideline. *Am. J. Respir. Crit. Care Med.* 2015 Jul; 192(2):e3–19.

[3] Bell EC, Cox NS, Goh N, Glaspole I, Westall GP, Watson A, Holland AE. Oxygen therapy for interstitial lung disease: a systematic review. *Eur. Respir. Rev.* 2017 Feb 21;26(143).

[4] Swigris JJ, Gould MK, Wilson SR. Health-related quality of life among patients with idiopathic pulmonary fibrosis. *Chest* 2005; 127: 284–294.

[5] Duck A, Spencer LG, Bailey S, et al. Perceptions, experiences and needs of patients with idiopathic pulmonary fibrosis. *J. Adv. Nurs.* 2015; 71: 1055–1065.

[6] Parshall MB, Schwartzstein RM, Adams L, et al. An official American Thoracic Society statement: update on the mechanisms, assessment, and management of dyspnea. *Am. J. Respir. Crit. Care Med.* 2012; 185: 435–452.

[7] Nishiyama O, Miyajima H, Fukai Y, et al. Effect of ambulatory oxygen on exertional dyspnea in IPF patients without resting hypoxemia. *Respir. Med.* 2013; 107: 1241–1246.

[8] Holland AE, Spruit MA, Troosters T, et al. An official European Respiratory Society/American Thoracic Society technical standard: field walking tests in chronic respiratory disease. *Eur. Respir. J.* 2014; 44: 1428–1446.

[9] Visca D, Mori L, Tsipouri V, Fleming S, Firouzi A, Bonini M, et al. Effect of ambulatory oxygen on quality of life for patients with fibrotic lung disease (AmbOx): a prospective, open-label, mixed-method, crossover randomized controlled trial. *Lancet Respir. Med.* 2018 Oct; 6(10): 759–70.

[10] Vianello A, Arcaro G, Molena B, Turato C, Braccioni F, Paladini L, Vio S, Ferrarese S, Peditto P, Gallan F, Saetta M. High-flow nasal cannula oxygen therapy to treat acute respiratory failure in patients with acute exacerbation of idiopathic pulmonary fibrosis. *Ther. Adv. Respir. Dis.* 2019 Jan-Dec;13:1753466619847130.

[11] Wuyts WA, Wijsenbeek M, Bondue B, Bouros D, Bresser P, Robalo Cordeiro C, Hilberg O, Magnusson J, Manali ED, Morais A, Papiris S, Shaker S, Veltkamp M, Bendstrup E. Idiopathic Pulmonary Fibrosis: Best Practice in Monitoring and Managing a Relentless Fibrotic Disease. *Respiration.* 2019 Dec 12;99(1):1-10. doi: 10.1159/000504763. [Epub ahead of print] Review. PubMed PMID: 31830755.

[12] Güngör G, Tatar D, Saltürk C, Cimen P, Karakurt Z, Kirakli C, Adıgüzel N, Ediboglu Ö, Yılmaz H, Moçin ÖY, Balcı M, Yılmaz A: Why do patients with interstitial lung diseases fail in the ICU? A 2-center cohort study. *Respir. Care* 2013, 58:525–531.

[13] Fernandez-Perez ER, Yilmaz M, Jenad H, Daniels CE, Ryu JH, Hubmayr RD, Gajic O: Ventilator settings and outcome of respiratory failure in chronic interstitial lung disease. *Chest* 2008, 133:1113–1119.

[14] Aliberti S, Messinesi G, Gamberini S, Maggiolini S, Visca D, Galavotti V, Giuliani F, Cosentini R, Brambilla AM, Blasi F, Scala R, Carone M, Luisi F, Harari S, Voza A, Esquinas A, Pesci A. Non-invasive mechanical ventilation in patients with diffuse interstitial lung diseases. *BMC Pulm. Med.* 2014 Dec 5;14:194.

[15] Yokoyama T, Kondoh Y, Taniguchi H, Kataoka K, Kato K, Nishiyama O, Kimura T, Hasegawa R, Kubo K: Noninvasive ventilation in acute exacerbation of idiopathic pulmonary fibrosis. *Intern. Med.* 2010, 49:1509–1514.

[16] Tomii K, Tachikawa R, Chin K, Murase K, Handa T, Mishima M, Ishihara K: Role of non-invasive ventilation in managing life-threatening acute exacerbation of interstitial pneumonia. *Intern. Med.* 2010, 49:1341–1347.

[17] Yokoyama T, Tsushima K, Yamamoto H, Koizumi T, Kubo K: Potential benefits of early continuous positive pressure ventilation in patients with rapidly progressive interstitial pneumonia. *Respirology* 2012, 17:315–321.

[18] Koschel D, Handzhiev S, Wiedemann B, Höffken G. Acute effects of NPPV in interstitial lung disease with chronic hypercapnic respiratory failure. *Respir. Med.* 2010 Feb;104(2):291-5.

[19] Nishiyama O, Taniguchi H, Kondoh Y, et al. Health-related quality of life in patients with idiopathic pulmonary fibrosis. What is the main contributing factor? *Respir. Med.* 2005; 99:408–414.

[20] Gifford AH. Noninvasive ventilation as a palliative measure. *Curr. Opin. Support Palliat. Care*. 2014 Sep;8(3):218-24. doi: 10.1097/SPC.0000000000000068. Review.

In: Respiratory Ventilatory Strategies …
Editor: Antonio M. Esquinas

ISBN: 978-1-53617-847-0
© 2020 Nova Science Publishers, Inc.

Chapter 33

EXACT RESULTS FOR TWO-DIMENSIONAL ISING MODELS OBTAINED BY TRANSFORMATION METHODS

Viktor Urumov *
Faculty of Natural Sciences and Mathematics,
Saints Cyril and Methodius University, Skopje, Macedonia

ABSTRACT

Several transformations are used to reduce more complex Ising models on two-dimensional lattices to known exact solutions. In this way one can greatly extend the variety of systems that could be analyzed without any approximation. The systems discussed are based on the standard square lattice, the more elaborate 4-6 lattice and the triangular lattice. Four examples of solvable models are studied that include pairwise interactions with nearest neighbours and also with some more distant spins, competing and frustrated interactions, higher spins and crossing bonds. One observes models with disordered ground states showing coexistence of order and disorder, a model with critical surface with singular critical point that affects the behaviour in the proximity of the neighbouring regular critical points in the parameters space. Re-entrance phenomenon is quite common and manifests itself in two different forms. Its appearance does not require minimal coordination number of four. One model mapped to the eight-vertex displays three transitions each of them having different sets of critical exponents. The same system has an ordered phase at higher temperatures while its ground state is disordered. Two ordered and two partially ordered phases are observed on a decorated triangular lattice.

* Corresponding Author's E-mail: v.urumov@gmail.com.

Keywords: two-dimensional models, exact solutions, multiple transitions, re-entrance, crossing bonds, frustration

INTRODUCTION

The Ising model in its initial formulation deals with particles with spin distributed on some regular lattice and interacting in some determined manner with their nearest neighbours. The model was proposed with the aim to understand the behaviour of magnetic materials, but over the decades the applications have spread in various directions. It has received particular attention in statistical physics in connection with phase transitions. Abundant amount of literature is devoted to the model and the number of published papers now exceeds several tens of thousands. A distinctive field of study is dedicated to two-dimensional models. Onsager (1944) was the first to obtain an exact analytic expression of the partition function for the two-dimensional Ising model on a square lattice that demonstrates existence of a transition between ordered and disordered phase. Yang (1952) published derivation of the magnetization of the same system. Exact solution for the proper Ising model in three dimensions has not been found, as is the case when an external magnetic field is present, both in two and three dimensions. This is also true already in two dimensions when the lattice contains crossing bonds or consists entirely of higher spins.

There are many applications of the model in physics related problems, but also in quite different fields. The most natural problems in two dimensions are surface phenomena at the boundary layers or adsorbed monolayers. Applications in three dimensions are related to rare earth compounds, alloys, structural transitions, lattice gases, liquid mixtures and other systems. One-dimensional systems, chains of spins have been also of interest. The model has been applied in the study of helix-coil transition of DNA molecules, polymers in general and other medical topics, in particular to neuroscience.

From the enormous number of references a few selected to be mentioned are the following, a monograph by Baxter (1982), series of books that were published since 1972 and dedicated to phase transitions, edited by Domb and other coeditors, and a collection edited by Diep and Giacomini (2013) on frustrated systems. As introductory papers one may use the articles published by Fisher (1959), Brush (1967), Barber (1980), Vaks et al. (1983), Strečka and Jaščur (2015). Stanley (1973) edited a selective bibliography with abstracts and reprints of representative articles.

In this chapter it is shown how by using transformation methods one can obtain some new exact analytic results. The dual transformation related the partition function of two lattices that are dual to each other, like honeycomb and triangular lattices, or square lattice with itself. The dual lattice is composed by single spins added to each polygon of the original lattice. There is a limitation that the original lattice should be without crossing bonds. Another transformation, the star-triangle transformation provides relationship between interaction parameters of star configuration with central spin surrounded by three neighbouring spins and the triangle of these three mutually interacting spins. The consecutive application of these transformations permits to determine the critical points of honeycomb and triangular lattices. More general transformation was established by Rojas et al. (2009).

Syozi (1951) proposed a transformation to eliminate a spin that is connected only to two neighbours. It is known as decoration-iteration transformation. With some extensions, this is the main tool to be used in the chapter. In the first example it will be shown that a decorated square lattice can have several transitions and that below the critical temperature a coexistence of order and disorder is possible. The next model demonstrates a critical surface with partially folded structure that creates a singularity on the surface with reflections on the critical behaviour and the behaviour in the neighbourhood of the nearby critical points. The 4-6 lattice that consists of squares and hexagons can be dealt with in similar manner even in the case with some crossing bonds present. Finally a decorated triangular lattice with next-nearest neighbours crossing bond interactions is resolved without any approximations.

DECORATED SQUARE LATTICE WITH HIGHER SPINS

In this section we consider an Ising models on a decorated square lattice. The model is presented in Figure 1. On each bond of the square lattice one additional spin is introduced. These additional sites are known as decorating sites in distinction from the sites of the ordinary square lattice. Spins on the decorating sites interact with their nearest neighbours. All additional spins are of the same magnitude S and may have $2S + 1$ orientations $(-S, -S+1, \ldots, S-1, S)$, whereas the spins s on the sites of the underlying square lattice may have only one of the two possible orientations of $+1$ or -1. The interaction parameters between spins on each single bond are indicated in the figure. The contribution to the Hamiltonian of the system from a single bond is given by

$$H_{\text{bond}} = -JS_1(s_1 + s_2)/S - aJs_1s_2, \tag{1}$$

where a is a parameter. Positive J favours parallel orientation of the neighbouring spins, while negative J leads preferably to antiparallel orientation of the interacting pair.

Equilibrium properties of statistical systems are determined by the partition function. It is defined by

$$Z(K, a) = \sum \exp\left(-\beta \sum H_{\text{bond}}\right), \tag{2}$$

$K = \beta J$, $\beta = 1/k_B T$, k_B is the Boltzmann constant and T is the absolute temperature. The summation in the exponent takes into account every decorated bond of the lattice while the other summation runs over all possible orientations of all spins, those on the decorating sites and those on both ends of each bond.

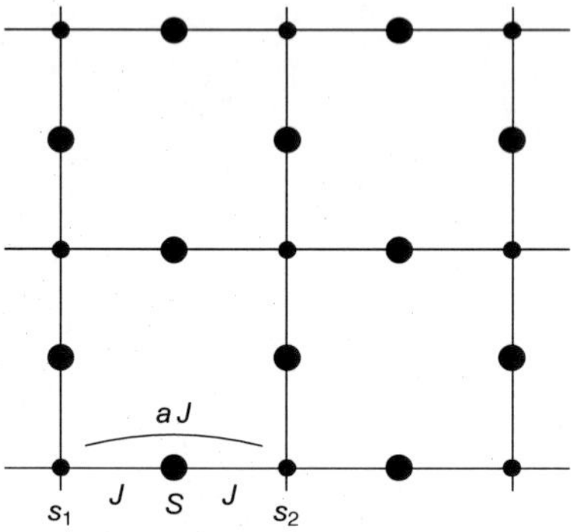

Figure 1. Square lattice decorated with higher S spins.

The transformation method used in this section is known as decoration-iteration method. For the first time it was applied by Syozi (1951, 1972). It is based on the observation that the contribution to the partition function from each decorated bond can be represented as a simple undecorated bond between the corner spins interacting with some effective interaction which depends on temperature, magnitude of the decorating spins and interaction parameters. Each decorating spin enters the partition function individually without direct connection with other decorating spins. Therefore, the sum over its orientations expressed with a geometric series, can be calculated separately, leading to

$$\sum_{S_1=-S}^{S} \mathrm{e}^{K(s_1+s_0)S_1/S} = \frac{\sinh[K(S+1/2)(s_1+s_0)/S]}{\sinh[K(s_1+s_0)/2S]} = A\mathrm{e}^{Qs_1s_0}. \tag{3}$$

The latter equation becomes an identity with A and Q determined from

$$A\mathrm{e}^{Q} = \frac{\sinh[(2S+1)K/S]}{\sinh(K/S)}, \qquad A\mathrm{e}^{-Q} = 2S+1. \tag{4}$$

Last relations are obtained from (3) for $s_1 = s_0 = \pm 1$ and $s_1 = -s_0 = \pm 1$. It follows that

$$A^2 = (2S+1)\frac{\sinh\{(2S+1)K/S\}}{\sinh(K/S)}, \qquad \mathrm{e}^{2Q} = \frac{\sinh\{(2S+1)K/S\}}{(2S+1)\sinh(K/S)}. \tag{5}$$

As a result the decorating spins are eliminated and the partition function for the decorated lattice Z_d is expressed with the partition function of the ordinary square lattice

Z_{sq} as a function of the effective interaction between the remaining spins on the square lattice

$$Z_d(K, S, a) = A^{2N_{sq}} Z_{sq}(Q + aK), \quad (6)$$

where N_{sq} is the number of sites of the square lattice.

The Ising model on the square lattice undergoes second order phase transition from paramagnetic to ferromagnetic or antiferromagnetic state, when the argument of the partition function becomes equal to $K_c = \pm (1/2) \ln(1 + \sqrt{2})$, respectively. To find the critical conditions of the decorated model we have two equations

$$y(K, a) = Q(K) + aK = \pm(1/2) \ln(1 + \sqrt{2}). \quad (7)$$

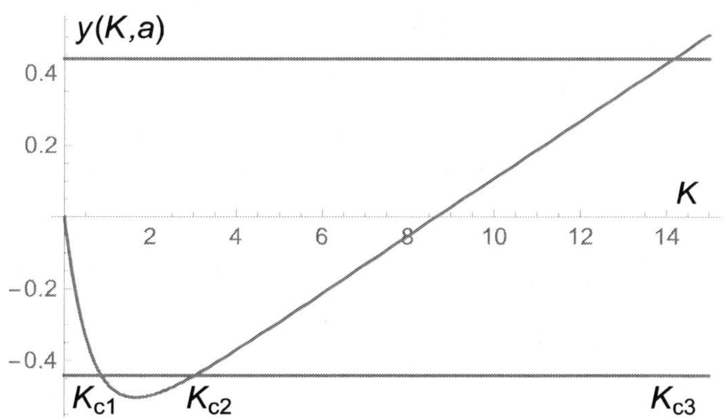

Figure 2. Intersections of the effective interaction $y(K, a)$ between spins at the ends of a bond with $y = \pm K_c = \pm\, 0.0440686794$, for $S = 3/2$ and $a = -0.92$.

Graphical illustration of the solutions is shown in Figure 2 for the case of decorating spins $S = 3/2$ and $a = -0.92$. Depending on the parameter a, the equations (7) can have one or three solutions. There is only one phase transition when $a > -0.88$ or $a \leq -1$. In the first case at the critical temperature $T_c = J/k_B K_c$, the system undergoes a transition to ferromagnetic state and all spins, on decorating and nondecorating sites, tend to have identical orientation with further decreasing of temperature. When $a \leq -1$, spins on the underlying square lattice are ordered antiferromagnetically, while spins on decorating sites are oriented randomly. This is the simplest example of coexistence of order and disorder that persists also in the ground state. In the interval $-1 < a < -0.88$ three transitions occur and the system passes through four states, namely paramagnetic at high temperatures ($K < K_{c1}$), hybrid state with antiferromagnetic order and disorder on the decorating sites ($K_{c1} < K < K_{c2}$), paramagnetic state ($K_{c2} < K < K_{c3}$) and ferromagnetic state at low temperatures ($K_{c3} < K$). For decorating spins of magnitude $S = 1$, 3/2, 2, 5/2 and 3, the corresponding bounds for the parameter a are -1 on the lower side and -0.94, -0.88, -0.84, -0.81 and -0.79, respectively on the upper side. Multiple transitions occur on isotropic square lattice with multiple decorating sites on each bond with ± 1 spins and also on anisotropic square lattice when only vertical or only horizontal bonds are decorated (Syozi, 1972).

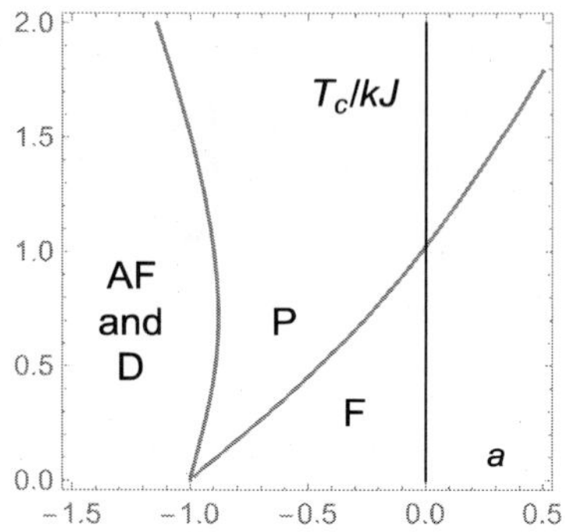

Figure 3. Phase diagram of the system defined with H_{bond} in (1) for $S = 3/2$.

In Figure 3 the phase diagram of the system is presented in the plane of temperature versus parameter a. Two curves delineate the three phases: ferromagnetic (F), paramagnetic (P) and hybrid phase with coexisting antiferromagnetic order and disorder (AF and D). Three transitions materialize in a narrow interval of the parameter a. For $-1 < a < -0.88$, one observes the phenomenon of re-entrance, establishment of a disordered paramagnetic phase at lower temperature than that of the partially ordered antiferromagnetic phase in coexistence with random ordering of spins at the decorating sites. Other models exhibiting re-entrance have much more narrow area of embeded paramagnetic phase (Vaks et al, 1965; Diep and Giacomini, 2013). This example shows that the randomly oriented spins do not need to have four neighbours in order to observe the re-entrance phenomenon as it was previously assumed. The increase of the magnitude S contributes to weak reduction of the area of F-phase and some enlargement of the domain for the hybrid state.

CRITICAL SURFACE WITH SINGULAR POINT

The next model to be discussed is defined again on a decorated square lattice, but now each bond has three additional spins, two of them of higher magnitude S. Their dispositions and interaction parameters are shown in Figure 4. The interaction energy of the spins along each bond is expressed as

$$H_{\mathrm{bond}} = -J[S_1(s_1 + s_0)/S + S_2(s_0 + s_2)/S] - aJs_0(s_1 + s_2) - bJs_1s_2. \quad (8)$$

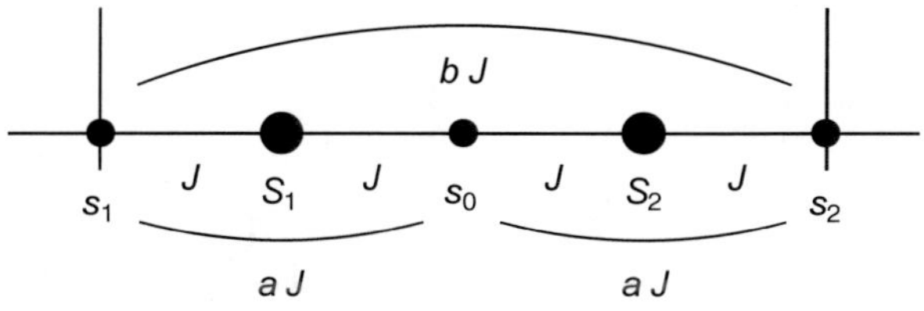

Figure 4. Triply decorated bond of a square lattice.

The elimination of the internal decorating spins could be made in two stages. At the beginning the *S*-spins are eliminated by repeating the steps shown in equations (3-5) and afterward the same procedure is applied to discard the central s_0-spin. As a result, the partition function of the decorated lattice is determined by

$$Z_{\mathrm{d}}(K,a,b) = A^{4N_{\mathrm{sq}}}B^{2N_{\mathrm{sq}}}\,Z_{\mathrm{sq}}(P+bK), \tag{9}$$

$$B^2 = 4\cosh[2(Q+aK)], \qquad \mathrm{e}^{2P} = \cosh[2(Q+aK0]. \tag{10}$$

with *A* and *Q* given in (5).

The same condition for the determination of the critical temperature applies again. Using the definitions for *P* and *Q*, expressed by the equations (10) and (5), the critical temperature can be obtained from the equation,

$$z(K,\ a,b) = P(K,a) + bK = \pm(1/2)\ln(1+\sqrt{2}). \tag{11}$$

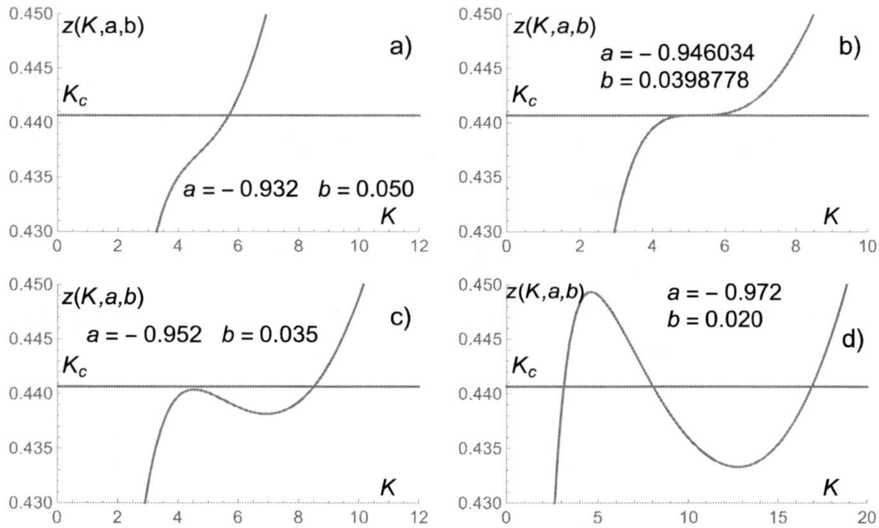

Figure 5. The effective interaction and critical points on the critical surface for $S = 2$ and for the singular point and three points on the line $b = 3a/4 + 0.749$.

Having more parameters and three decorating sites, the equation for determination of the critical temperature is more involved. Solutions indicating singular critical surface were obtained only for the equation (11) with positive right hand side. Depending on the parameters *a* and *b*, for given *S*, there is either single critical value for *K* or three critical conditions. This bears similarity to the re-entrance phenomenon discussed in the previous section, but now there is only one ordered phase, the ferromagnetic phase and all three transitions are between ferromagnetic and paramagnetic phase. The existence of multiple transitions suggests that at some stage there is a transition from the situation with one phase transition to a state when their number increases to three. In Figure 5 this evolution is illustrated on the graphs a, c and d. In the first two cases the equation (11) has single solution, but the behaviour of the effective interaction $z(K, a, b)$ already changes from monotonous to non-monotonous. Further change of the parameters gives rise to the appearance of two additional solutions for the critical temperature. The selected parameters *a* and *b* used for the graphs a, c and d belong to the line $b = (3/4)a + 0.749$. The appearance of three transition points is due to the folding of the critical surface $K_c(a, b)$. The folding, at least in the beginning develops approximately along the above line connecting parameters *a* and *b*. The graph in Figure 5b shows the effective interaction that determines the singular point *C* of the critical surface. The singular point is a point of inflection of $z(K, a, b)$. In *a*-*b* parameters plane the singularity is positioned slightly above the mentioned straight line. For $S = 2$, the three distinct critical points coalesce into a single point for $a = -0.94603406190$ and $b = 0.03987777729$, when $K_c = J/k_BT_c = 5.2395493473$. The critical temperature and the parameters *a* and *b* determining the singular point are obtained from the system of equations

$$z(K, a, b) = (1/2)\ln\left(1 + \sqrt{2}\right), \quad \partial z/\partial K = 0, \quad \partial^2 z/\partial K^2 = 0. \tag{12}$$

According to the topological theory devised by Thom and known as catastrophe theory, the observed critical surface is the only possible type of a singular surface dependent on two parameters (Zeeman, 1976). It appears quite commonly in various phenomena. The critical parameters for square lattices for some values of the decorating *S*-spins are given in Table 1. It is interesting to observe what are the consequences for the critical behaviour in the vicinity of the singular point.

Table 1. Critical parameters for different magnitudes of decorating spins

S	*a*	*b*	K_c
2	-0.946034061900	0.039877777292	5.239549347290
5/2	-1.120366129255	0.079173042401	3.394265812182
3	-1.302463579206	0.108183865765	2.653817020737
7/2	-1.486372805907	0.133922880278	2.210946279718

The magnetization for the Ising model on a square lattice was derived by Yang (1952) and the expression is given by

$$M = (1 - 16u^4(1 - u^2)^{-4})^{1/8}, \tag{13}$$

$$u = \exp(-2K_{\text{eff}}) = \text{e}^{-2bK}/\cosh(2Q + 2aK). \tag{14}$$

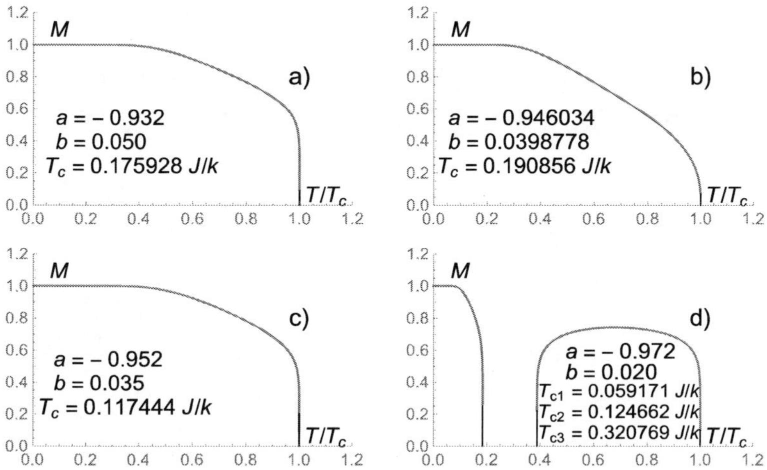

Figure 6. Magnetization versus reduced temperature for the same parameters as those used in the previous figure.

The magnetization of the lattice is shown in Figure 6 for the same sets of parameters as in Figure 5. In the vicinity of the singular point, Figure 6b, it is evident that the magnetization dependence on temperature is quite different from the universal behaviour for the two-dimensional Ising model characterized by the critical exponent $\beta = 1/8$ that describes the asymptotic behaviour when the temperature approaches from below the critical temperature of the system. Instead, in this case the exponent β is three times larger. This is a result of typical singularity of cusp catastrophe surface. It is evident from (12) that the effective interaction around the singular point has Taylor expansion that after the constant term continues with powers of order three and higher terms, in contrast with all other ordinary points of the critical surface where the expansion continues with linear terms. As an outcome, the temperature dependence of magnetization, sucseptibility and correlation length will have modified three times larger critical exponents. But this is not the only consequence of the existence of singularity on the critical surface. When a critical point is close to the singularity, as can be seen in Figure 6a and c, the shape of the magnetization curve, except in the proximity of the critical temperature is similar to Figure 6b, the magnetization curve corresponding to the singular point. In addition there are two characteristic curves in the *a*-*b* plane that correspond to the projection of the curves on the critical surface representing the sets of its folding points. These points are defined by the minima or maxima of the effective interaction. In the vicinity of the points of the lower folding of the critical surface the magnetization will have two times larger critical exponent. This characteristic behaviour has been observed previously (Urumov, 1982) in the case of triangular lattice with ordinary spins, but then at least seven decorating spins were required. Projections of the folding curves in horizontal and vertical plane are shown in Figure 7. Re-entrance happens for points (*a*,*b*) in Figure 7a enclosed between the curves *l* and *u*. Finally, it should be mentioned that the decorating *S*-spins remain in a disordered state below the critical temperature, as it was the case in the example of the previous section. Spins at the end of each bond have preferably parallel orientation, while spins in the middle of the bond have opposite orientation. This is due to the negative value of parameter *a* defining the singular critical point, as a reflection of competing interactions among the spins.

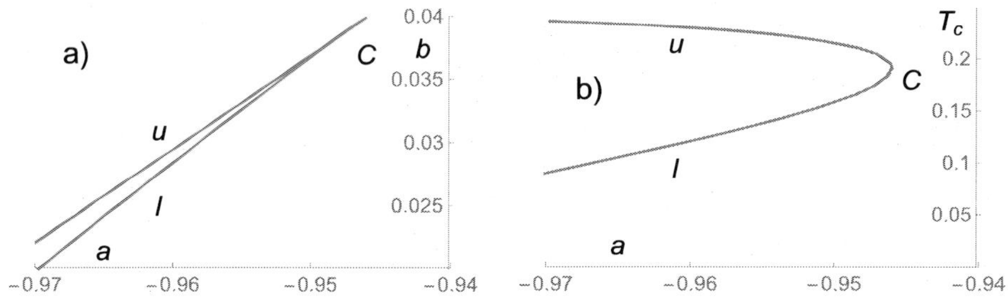

Figure 7. Projections of the folding lines of the critical surface, *C* is the singular point, *u* and *l* are projections of the upper and lower folding curves: a) projection in the plane of parameters *a* and *b*; b) projection in the vertical plane a-T_c.

FRUSTRATED ISING MODEL ON A 4-6 LATTICE

It is well known that the triangular lattice with isotropic antiferromagnetic interaction does not sustain a phase transition as all three pairs of spins from a single triangle are unable to achieve simultaneously antiparallel ordering. This provided an early example of the concept of frustration in the context of statistical physics. Given spin system is frustrated if it is not possible to achieve a configuration with all the interacting entities having their lowest possible energy. Here an Ising model is considered on a lattice built from squares and hexagons. Exact results are available for two topologically different 4-6 lattices (Lin and Wang, 1988, Oitmaa and Keppert, 2002). One of them, including some additional elements is shown in Figure 8. There are a few modifications to the original 4-6 lattice. First, the internal squares have diagonal crossing bonds. Second, the interactions of the spins on the internal squares change sign alternatively. Finally, the larger external squares, neighbouring elementary plaquettes of the lattice, are rotated with respect to each other by 90°. Such structures were used to obtain solutions for Ising models on the pentagonal and 3-7 lattices (Urumov, 2012, 2016). In this way each hexagons obtain five ferromagnetic bonds and one antiferromagnetic, making it impossible to reach specific ground state.

The Hamiltonian of a single square plaquette is defined as

$$H_{\rm pl} = - J_1\,(s_1\sigma_1 + s_2\sigma_2 + s_3\sigma_3 + s_4\sigma_4) - J_2\,(\sigma_1\sigma_2 - \sigma_2\sigma_3 + \sigma_3\sigma_4 - \sigma_4\sigma_1) - J_3\,(\sigma_1\sigma_3 + \sigma_2\sigma_4), \qquad (15)$$

where $s_{\rm i}$ and $\sigma_{\rm i}$ stand for the external and internal spins respectively (Figure 9).

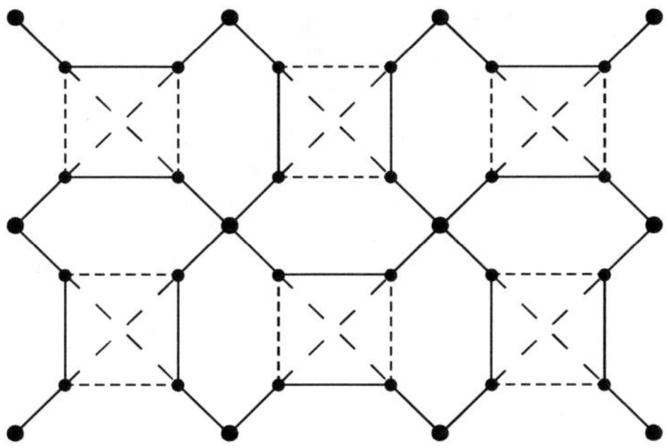

Figure 8. Ising model on a 4-6 lattice with additional crossing bonds.

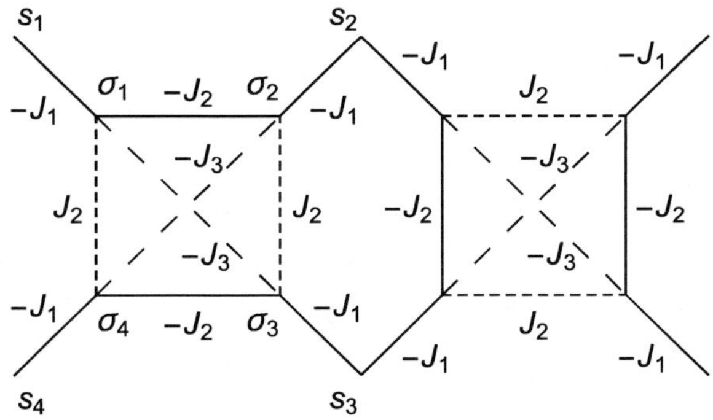

Figure 9. Two neighbouring plaquettes of 4-6 lattice with interaction parameters.

The goal is to transform the problem to another lattice with partition function that is known. As it was done in the previous sections, some effective interactions are introduced eliminating the internal spins σ_i, i = 1, 2, 3, 4 by partial summation in the partition function

$$w(K_1, K_2, K_3, s_1, s_2, s_3, s_4) = \sum_{\sigma_i=\pm 1} \exp(-\beta H_{\rm pl}) =$$

$$A\exp[K'(s_1 s_2 + s_3 s_4) + K''(s_2 s_3 + s_1 s_4) + L(s_1 s_3 + s_2 s_4) + M s_1 s_2 s_3 s_4], \qquad (16)$$

where $K_i = J_i/kT$.

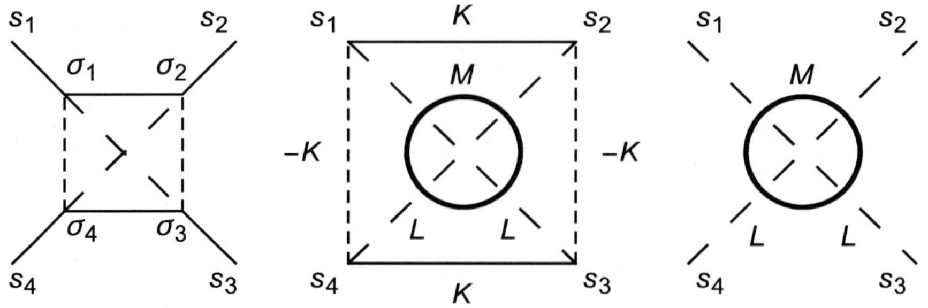

Figure 10. Transformation steps of the 4-6 lattice.

Taking into account all 16 possible different orientations of the set of four external spins s_i, due to the present symmetries, one finds only four different values for the weighting factors w. They are

$$w_1 = 8\cosh 2K_1 + 4\exp(-2K_3)\cosh 4K_2 + 2\exp(2K_3) + 2\exp(2K_3)\cosh 4K_1,$$

$$w_2 = 6 + 2\cosh 4K_1 + 4\left[\exp(-2K_3)\cosh 4K_2 + \exp(2K_3)\right]\cosh 2K_1,$$

$$w_3 = 8\cosh 2K_1 + 2\exp(4K_2 - 2K_3)\cosh 4K_1 + 2\exp(-4K_2 - 2K_3) + 4\exp(2K_3)$$

$$w_4 = 8\cosh 2K_1 + 2\exp(-4K_2 - 2K_3)\cosh 4K_1 + 2\exp(4K_2 - 2K_3) + 4\exp(2K_3)$$

$$w_5 = w_1, \tag{17}$$

and they correspond to the following spin orientations around the larger squares: (+,+,+,+), (+,+,+,−), (+,+,−,−), (−,+,+,−) and (+,−,+,−). The weighting factors have the following equivalent expressions

$$w_1 = Ae^{2K'+2K''+2L+M}, \qquad w_2 = Ae^{-M}, \qquad w_3 = Ae^{2K'-2K''-2L+M},$$
$$w_4 = Ae^{-2K'+2K''-2L+M}, \qquad w_5 = Ae^{-2K'-2K''+2L+M}. \tag{18}$$

The factor A and functions defining the effective interactions in the identity (16) are expressed as

$$A^8 = w_1^2 w_2^4 w_3 w_4,$$

$$e^{8K'} = {w_3}/{w_4}, \qquad e^{8L} = {w_1^2}/{w_3 w_4}, \qquad e^{8M} = {w_1^2 w_3 w_4}/{w_2^4} \tag{19}$$

and $K'' = -K'$.

After the elimination of the internal spins, the remaining spins interact with their nearest neighbours with equal strength but different signs in horizontal and vertical direction, identical interactions persist along the diagonals and in addition there is an interaction connecting all four spins in the corners of larger squares. Due to the specific arrangement of elementary plaquettes, the interactions between remaining nearest neighbour spins vanish. The transformation steps are shown in Figure 10, where the circle stands for the four-spin interaction. The initial 4-6 lattice is reconstructed into two square lattices with the former diagonals as sides of the squares interconnected with four-spin interactions.

This new adapted form of the initial problem on the 4-6 lattice is equivalent to the eight-vertex model expressed in terms of an Ising model (Wu, 1971, Kadanoff and Wegner, 1971). The eight-vertex model has the unusual property that its critical exponents are continuous functions of the parameters defining the system in contradiction with the universality hypothesis. Therefore this is also the case with the 4-6 model under consideration. The equation for determination of the critical temperature is given by (Wu, 1971)

$$\exp(2M)\sinh(2L) = 1 \qquad \text{or} \qquad w_1 - \sqrt{w_3 w_4} = 2w_2\,. \tag{20}$$

Equation (20) is symmetric with respect to change of signs of K_1 or K_2. In Figure 11, the critical conditions are depicted for each pair of critical parameters for some particular value of the remaining critical parameter. In-built frustration in the system does not allow for a phase transition until some boundary value of the interaction parameter J_3 is reached. The phase transition occurs only when the parameter J_3 is positive and sufficiently large. It is remarkable that this minimal value for the interaction parameter J_3 at criticality is defined by the critical point for the square lattice $K_c = (1/2)\ln(1+\sqrt{2})$.

The critical exponent α for the specific heat is expressed with the relations (Wu, 1971)

$$\alpha = 2 - \frac{\pi}{\mu_+}, \qquad \mu_+ = \frac{\pi}{2} + \sin^{-1}(\tanh 2M)\,, \tag{21}$$

where M takes its value at the critical point. One should note that the whole evaluation is valid also in the case when all spins at the internal squares of the 4-6 lattice have magnitude S.

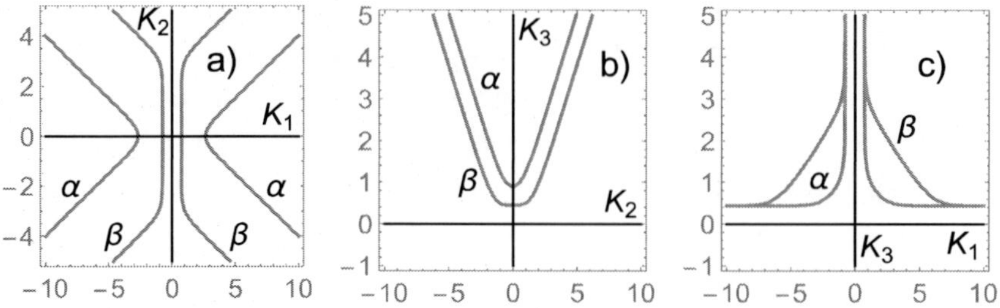

Figure 11. Interdependence between interaction parameters at the critical point obtained from equation (20): a) $K_3 = 0.45\ (\alpha),\ K_3 = 3\ (\beta)$; b) $K_1 = 1\ (\alpha),\ K_1 = 3\ (\beta)$; c) $K_2 = 1\ (\alpha)$, $K_2 = 3\ (\beta)$.

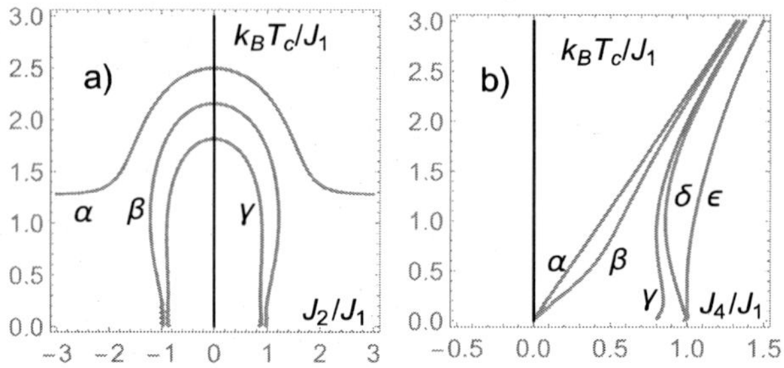

Figure 12. Interdependence between interaction parameters at the critical point obtained from equation (22): a) $J_4/J_1 = 1.1\ (\alpha)$, $J_4/J_1 = 0.95\ (\beta)$, $J_4/J_1 = 0.8\ (\gamma)$; b) $J_2/J_1 = 0.1\ (\alpha)$, $J_2/J_1 = 0.5\ (\beta)$, $J_2/J_1 = 0.9\ (\gamma)$, $J_2/J_1 = 1\ (\delta)$, $J_2/J_1 = 2\ (\varepsilon)$.

The same approach can be applied to a modification of the Hamiltonian (15) obtained by replacement of its last term $-J_3(\sigma_1\sigma_3 + \sigma_2\sigma_4)$ with $-J_4(s_1s_3 + s_2s_4)$, that is by displacing the diagonal interactions from the internal to the external squares of elementary plaquettes. The elimination of the internal spins (16) is still valid but in the weighting factors w_i, the interaction term K_3 becomes 0, which is further reflected in changes of the expressions (19) for A, K', K'', L and M. The equation for the critical point (20) becomes ($K_4 = J_4/kT$)

$$\exp(2M)\sinh 2(L + K_4) = 1 \text{ or } e^{2K_4}w_1 - e^{-2K_4}\sqrt{w_3w_4} = 2w_2. \tag{22}$$

In this second version of extended 4-6 Ising model with additional diagonal bonds, the transition occurs always without any requirement on the strength of the diagonal interaction. In two limiting situations when the parameters J_1 or J_2 tend to zero, the model is reduced to the ordinary square lattice. As can be seen from Figure 12a and b, the re-entrance phenomenon is present in this model. This means that the same system can undergo two or three transitions each characterized with its own critical exponents. Selecting the parameters defining curve γ in Figure 12b ($J_2/J_1 = 0.9$), for $J_4/J_1 = 0.83$ three transitions occur, at $T_{c1} = 0.08948\ J_1/k_B$, $T_{c2} = 0.41053\ J_1/k_B$ and $T_{c3} = 1.27754\ J_1/k_B$. The corresponding critical exponents of the specific heat are $\alpha_{c1} = 0.999916$, $\alpha_{c2} = 0.865507$

and $\alpha_{c3} = 0.300059$. Change of the magnitude of the internal spins σ_i to some higher value S, will result in similar change of the critical exponents. Comparable behaviour has been observed in a model on a Union Jack with triplet spin interactions (Urumov, 1980). Besides dependence on the spin magnitude, the same model demonstrates critical exponents dependence on the magnitude of an external magnetic field.

There is one additional feature concerning behaviour similar to re-entrance observed in Figure 12a and 12b, curves β and δ, respectively. In both cases for certain range of corresponding parameters there is an ordered state between two critical temperatures, while the ground states of both systems are disordered. Such behaviour clearly differs from what is known as re-entrance phenomenon when the system has defined ground state and disordered phase limited by two ordered regions on the sides of lower and higher temperatures.

DECORATED TRIANGULAR LATTICE WITH CROSSING BONDS

In this last section an Ising model on the triangular lattice shown in Figure 13 is examined. All the interactions are concentrated in the shaded triangles. The interaction parameters are introduced in Figure 14. Each edge of the triangles is decorated with one spin. These additional spins interact among themselves within a given triangle and also with all vertices. This means that besides interactions with the nearest neighbours, interactions with next nearest neighbours are also present. The latter interactions are crossing each other.

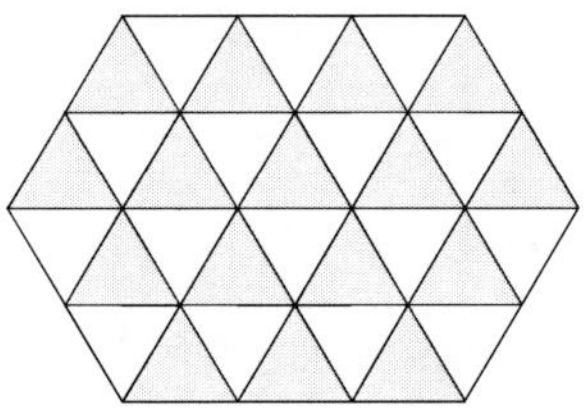

Figure 13. Triangular lattice.

The Hamiltonian of the system is determined by the interactions in each shaded triangle

$$H_{tr} = -J_1[s_1(\sigma_2 + \sigma_3) + s_2(\sigma_3 + \sigma_1) + s_3(\sigma_1 + \sigma_2)] - J_2(s_1\sigma_1 + s_2\sigma_2 + s_3\sigma_3) - J_3(\sigma_1\sigma_2 + \sigma_2\sigma_3 + \sigma_3\sigma_1). \quad (23)$$

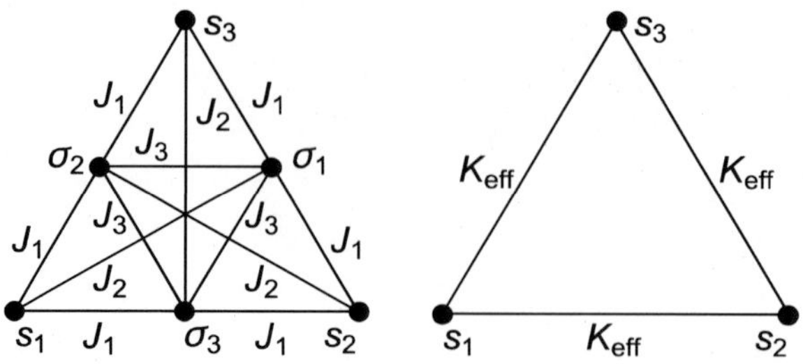

Figure 14. Substitution of all internal interactions with one effective interaction.

Repeating the main theme of the chapter, elimination of internal spins from the smallest entities of the system, one can reduce the problem to a simple triangular lattice with effective interaction K_{eff} along each bond (Figure 14). The effective interaction is determined with the expression

$$\exp(4K_{\text{eff}}) = \frac{3\cosh(2K_1+K_2)+\exp(4K_3)\cosh 3(2K_1+K_2)}{\cosh(2K_1-3K_2)+2\cosh(2K_1-K_2)+\exp(4K_3)\cosh(2K_1+K_2)} \tag{24}$$

where $K_i = J_i/k_BT$. It does not change when both K_1 and K_2 alter their signs. The same method can be applied also in the case when the decorating spins have higher magnitude. Moreover they can have different magnitudes and then the transformation leads to the anisotropic Ising model on a triangular lattice.

The critical temperature for the ordinary triangular lattice (Syozi, 1972) is determined from the equation $\exp(4K_{\text{eff}}) = 3$, while the magnetization is expressed as

$$M_{\text{tr}} = [1 - 16e^{4K_{\text{eff}}}/(e^{4K_{\text{eff}}}+3)(e^{4K_{\text{eff}}}-1)^3]^{1/8}. \tag{25}$$

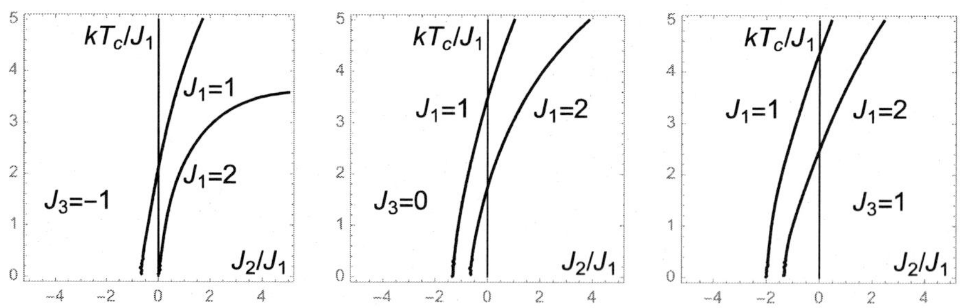

Figure 15. Critical temperature as a function of J_2/J_1 for $J_1 = 1$ and 2, $J_3 = -1, 0$ and 1.

Figure 15 depicts the dependence of the critical temperature obtained from the equation $\exp(4K_{\text{eff}}) = 3$, as a function of J_2/J_1 for $J_1 = 1$ and $J_1 = 2$, and three values of J_3.

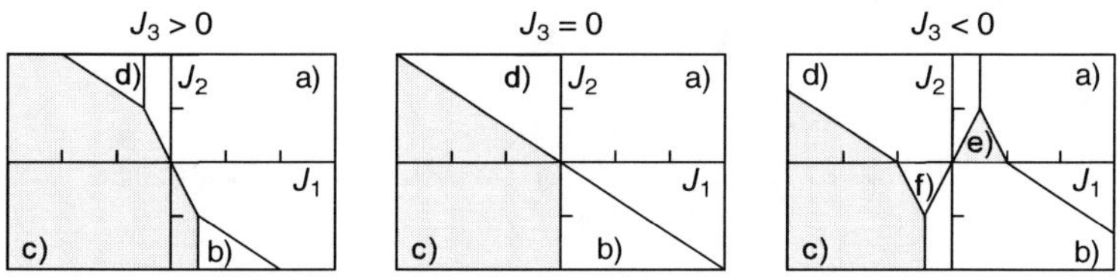

Figure 16. Ground state phase diagrams for the decorated triangular lattice.

a)	b)	c)	d)	e)	f)
+	+	+	+	+	+
+ +	− −	− −	+ +	+ +	− −
+ + +	− + −	+ − +	− − −	+ − +	+ + +

Figure 17. Spin ordering in triangles for a given phase.

In Figure 16 the phase diagrams of the system are shown at its lowest energy for three different cases determined by the interaction parameter J_3. The possible orderings of spins in the triangles are indicated in Figure 17. Lowest energy states are obtained in two cases. Case a, when all interaction parameters J_i are positive and case c, when $J_3 > 0$, and $J_{1,2} < 0$. These two cases correspond to the regions a and c in the phase diagrams in Figure 16, with ferromagnetic and ferrimagnetic order respectively. When the system is defined with parameters corresponding to the regions b and d, it remains disordered at all temperatures. In the remaining two cases e and f, the equation for the critical temperature has unique solutions, but disorder persists to the lowest temperatures. This can be seen from Figure 18 where the orientation of spins is indicated by black disks (+1) and open circles (-1). There are four spins that are additionally encircled with larger circles. If their orientations are changed, the ordering becomes broken, although the energy of the system remains constant. Similar situation arises in case e.

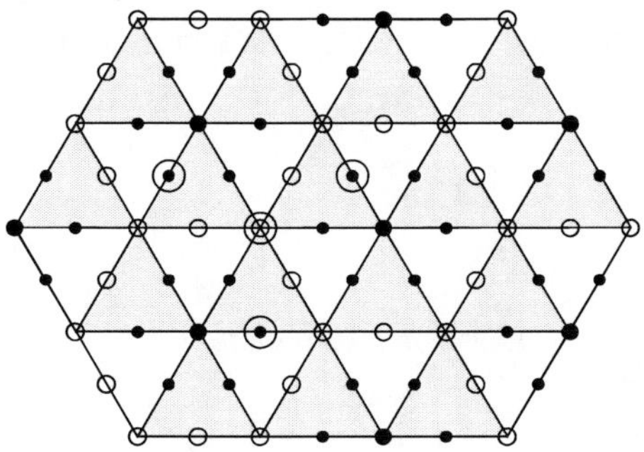

Figure 18. Up and down oriented spins represented as black disks and open circles.

CONCLUSION

Hundred years ago Lenz (1920) published a paper that discusses ideas that are the basis of what is widely known as Ising model (Brush, 1967). Ising (1925) solved the model in one dimension. The study of the model continues until today and appears, to say the least, not to diminish in its intensity. Theoretical studies are intriguing from mathematical point of view, but they can provide also insight into new territories. Exact solutions can also serve as benchmark for validation of approximate methods.

Here the solutions of four two-dimensional models are presented. Solutions were obtained by mapping the problems onto already known exact solutions. The transformation method has been shown to be applicable also in some particular three-dimensional case (Urumov, 1980).

In the first model it is demonstrated that re-entrance can happen when the sites that are responsible for the phenomenon are interacting with two neighbours only and not with four that was meant previously to be a necessary condition. The second model has a critical surface of cusp singularity type. The critical behaviour of the system at the singular point of the critical surface is modified and differs from the universal behaviour. Some consequences are visible in the shape of the magnetization curves for critical points on the critical surface in the vicinity of its singular point. The third model, a variation of the 4-6 lattice, has an in-built geometric frustration and is disordered at all temperatures. With additional crossing interactions with further neighbours it is possible to transform the model to the exactly solved eight-vertex model. In one case one observes a necessity of minimal crossing interaction strength to achieve phase transition. In the other case for some particular values of the interaction parameters one finds three consecutive transitions with three different sets of critical exponents for the same model. All three models have some form of re-entrance behaviour as a result of frustrations and/or competing interactions. The last model on a triangular lattice includes crossing interactions and has several phases showing order, disorder or coexistence of order and disorder.

REFERENCES

Barber, Michael N. 1980. "Phase Transitions in Two Dimensions." *Physics Reports* 59:375-409.

Baxter, Rodney J. 2007. *Exactly Solved Models in Statistical Mechanics*. New York: Dover Publications. First published by Academic Press, 1982.

Brush, Stephen J. 1967. "History of the Lenz-Ising Model." *Reviews of Modern Physics* 39:883-893.

Diep, H. T., and Hector Giacomini. 2013. “Frustration – Exactly Solved Frustrated Models.” In *Frustrated Spin Systems*, edited by H. T. Diep, 1 – 58. Singapore: World Scientific.

Fisher, Michael E. 1959. “Transformations of Ising Models.” *Physical Review* 113:969-981.

Ising, Ernst. 1925. “Beitrag zur Theorie des Ferromagnetismus,” *Zeitschrift für Physik* 31: 253-258. Contribution to the Theory of Ferromagnetism.

Kadanoff, Leo P., and Franz J. Wegner. 1971. “Some Critical Properties of the Eight-vertex Model.” *Physical Review B* 4:3989-3993.

Lenz, Wilhelm. 1920. “Beiträge zum Verständis der magnetischen Eigenschaften in festen Körpern”, *Physikalische Zeitschrift* 21: 613. Contributions to the Understanding of Magnetic Properties of Solids.

Lin, K. Y., and S. C. Wang. 1988. “Spontaneous Magnetization of the Ising Model on the Union Jack and 4-6 Lattices.” *Physics Letters A*, 128:143-145.

Oitmaa, J., and M. Keppert. 2002. “Exact Solution of the Ising Model on a 4-6 Lattice.” *Journal of Physics A: Mathematical and General,* 35:L219-L224.

Onsager, Lars. 1944. “Crystal Statistics. I. A Two-dimensional Model with an Order-disorder Transition.” *Physical Review*, 65:117-149.

Rojas, Onofre, J. S. Valverde, and S. M. de Souza. 2009. “Generalized Transformation for Decorated Spin Models.” *Physica A: Statistical Mechanics and its Applications*, 388:1419-1430.

Stanley, H. Eugene. 1973. *Cooperative Phenomena near Phase Transitions, A Bibliography with Selected Readings*. Edited by H. Eugene Stanley. Cambridge: MIT Press.

Strečka, Jozef, and Michal Jaščur. 2015. “A Brief Account of the Ising and Ising-like Models: Mean Field, Effective-field and Exact Results.” *Acta Physica Slovaca* 65:235-367.

Syozi, Itiro 1951. “Statistics of Kagome Lattice.” *Progress of Theoretical Physics* 6:36-308.

Syozi, Itiro. 1972. “Transformation of Ising Models.” In *Phase Transitions and Critical Phenomena* vol. 1, edited by Cyril Domb and Melville S. Green, 269 - 329. London: Academic Press.

Urumov, Viktor. 1980. “Exact Solution of “Three-dimensional” Ising Model with Four-spin Interaction.” *Physics Letters*, 78A: 95-97.

Urumov, Viktor. 1980. “Examples of Spin and External Field Dependent Critical Exponents”. In *Ordering in Two Dimensions*, edited by Sunil K. Sinha, 361-364. New York: Elsevier North Holland.

Urumov, Viktor. 1982. “Decorated Ising Model with Singular Critical Surface and Modified Critical Exponents.” *Journal of Physics C: Solid State Physics,* 15:777-781.

Urumov, Viktor. 2002. "Exact Solution of the Ising Model on a Pentagonal Lattice." *Journal of Physics A: Mathematical and General*, 35:7317-7321.

Urumov, Viktor. 2016. "Ising Model on a 3-7 Lattice: Order and Disorder." *AIP Conference Proceedings*, 1722:020004.

Vaks, V., A. Larkin and Y. Ovchinnikov. 1965 and 1966. "Ising Model with Interaction between Non-nearest Neighbours." *Zhurnal eksperimental'noy i teoreticheskoy fiziki*, 49:1180-1189, *Soviet Physics – JETP*, 22:820-826.

Vaks, V., V. I. Zinenko and V. E. Schneider. 1983. "Microscopic theories of order-disorder structural phase transitions in crystals." *Uspekhi fizicheskih nauk* 141:629.

Wu, Fa Yueh. 1971."Ising Model with Four-spin Interactions." *Physical Review B* 4:2312-2314.

Yang, Zhenning (Chen-Ning). 1952. "The Spontaneous Magnetization of a Two-dimensional Ising Model." *Physical Review*, 85:808-815.

Zeeman, Erik Christofer. 1976. "Catastrophe Theory." *Scientific American*, 234:65-70, 75-83.

In: Respiratory Ventilatory Strategies …
Editor: Antonio M. Esquinas
ISBN: 978-1-53617-847-0
© 2020 Nova Science Publishers, Inc.

Chapter 34

HOMECARE PLATFORM FOR REMOTE MONITORING OF PATIENTS WITH IDIOPATHIC PULMONARY FIBROSIS

Carolina Cabo**, MD, Vânia Fernandes, MD and Margarida Afonso, MD
Pneumology Unit, Coimbra University Hospital, Coimbra, Portugal

ABSTRACT

Chronic respiratory diseases represent a burden for healthcare systems, demanding new solutions in monitoring and treating these patients. New technologies may have a role in this setting.The present chapter describes the main telemedicine platforms used in monitoring patients with respiratory diseases and the experience with idiophatic pulmonary fibrosis.

Keywords: idiophaticpulmonaryfibrosis, telehealth, homecareplatform

INTRODUCTION

Chronic respiratory diseases represent an increasing challenge and burden for healthcare systems. In the face of that, new diagnostic, therapeutic and follow-up options emerged in the last years. Telehealth has been defined as the use of information and communication technologies to deliver healthcare services and transmit medical data over long and short distances [1].

* Corresponding Author's E-mail: carolinapmatoscabo@gmail.com.

These technologies have been used in multiple areas, including chronic heart failure(CHF), diabetes, cystic fibrosis and chronic obstructive pulmonary disease (COPD) with promising results in terms of reducing hospitalisations, improving self-care and improving quality of life [2, 3]. In idiopathic pulmonary fibrosis (IPF) and other interstitial lung diseases the data are scarce.

PLATFORMS AND INTERVENTIONS FOR REMOTE MONITORING

A variety of devices, systems and modalities have been used in different studies for telehealth interventions in respiratory disease, including [4]:

- Biological sensors of patient's vital signs and physiological data such as: spirometry, respiratory and heart rate, oxygen peripheral saturation, capnography;
- data from medical equipment such as tidal volume and pressures of mechanical ventilators;
- devices for transmission of data from those sensors and equipments such as: phone calls, sms, email, videophones, websites or mobilephones, video conferencing;
- medical devices programmed at distance;
- dedicated internet softwares.

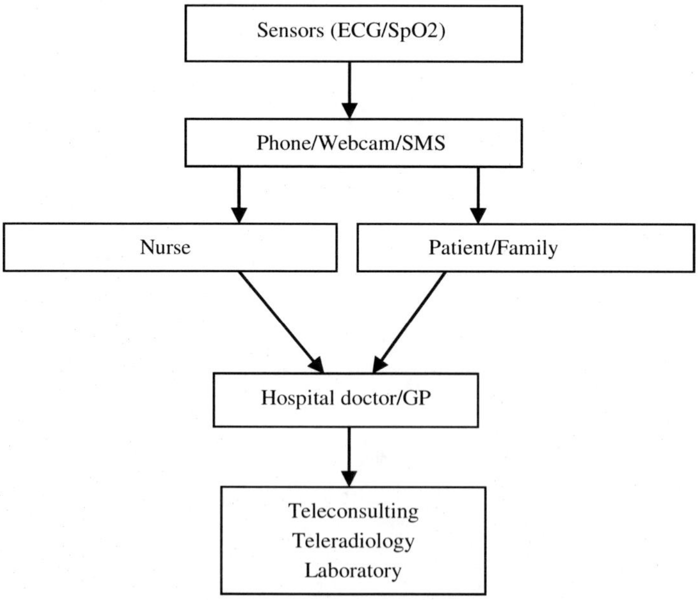

Figure 1. An example of eHealth platform. SpO2: oxygen saturation measured by pulse oximetry; ECG: electrocardiogram; GP: general practitioner. Adapted from [2].

The main telehealth interventions in respiratory medicine are based on the above technologies by video or telephone links with healthcare professionals in real time or using store-and-forward technologies, pulmonary rehabilitation programmes with home-based, video conferencing-supervised exercise and counseling (telerehabilitation) and telemonitoring of patients on home mechanical ventilation (HMV) [2]. Figure 1 shows an example of a telehealth platform.

EXPERIENCE INIDIOPATHIC PULMONARY FIBROSIS

IPF is an interstitial lung disease, described first in 1933 by Hamman and Rich [5], as a progressive and fatal disease characterized by extreme dyspnea and cough. Since then, investigations havebeen made in this field improving diseases diagnostic and treatment, but these patients still have a poor prognosis and progressive, incapacitating symptoms.

Outpatient management in this disease is a challenge and some good results in other respiratory diseases lead to implementation of telehealth programs in these patients. Still the evidence is limited.Two pilot studies were published using different approaches.The first, with a six-month duration, used a commodity hardware [3].The system enables daily monitoring of a patient's vital signs, includes communication features that facilitate doctor-patient contact and provides emergency response [3].The second, with a four-week duration, used a pre-developed home monitoring program in IPF, integrated with real-time, wireless home spirometry [6]. Both showed that home monitoring in these patients is feasible (even in older patients). Patients were able to use the implemented system, integrate it in their daily routines and consider it useful in monitoring their disease [3, 6]. Families understood the purpose of the project and doctors were also easily adapted to proposed technologies [3]. In spirometry study, home-based measurements were slightly lower than hospital-based FVC but home and hospital readings were highly correlated [6]. These findings suggest that homespirometry may be a useful in remote monitoring of IPF patients. Early detection of alert signs may improve treatment and quality of care in IPF.

Other projects are still in progress in various centers in this area, including in authors reffering hospital[1]. Developments in this field are expected at short-term.

---

[1]Telehealthprogram supported by a Portuguese telehealth company and developed since 2014 with COPD patients. In October 2018, 3 patients with IPF were integrated in this project.

Conclusion

Telehealth represent a wide area of technologies aimed to improve outcomes in different diseases. Several studies were developed in CHF, COPD and CF, with some promising and conflicting results.

Data on IPF are limited but represent a line of investigation in improving prognosis and quality of life in these patients. Some pilot studies reveal feasible results with these technologies in IPF regarding early detection of exacerbations and disease progression.

Key Messages

- Chronic respiratory diseases represent an increasing challenge and burden for healthcare systems, demanding new monitoring solutions.
- Telehealth has been defined as the use of information and communication technologies to deliver healthcare services and transmit medical data
- The main telehealth interventions in respiratory medicine are based in store-and forward technologies, telerehabilitation, and telemonitoring of patients on home mechanical ventilation (HMV).
- Idiophatic pulmonary fibrosis is a chronic, progressive disease and one of the fields of investigation in telehealth. Some pilot-projects showed already some benefits.

References

[1] International Organisation for Standardization (2016). *ISO strategy for services: case study 1 – International SOS* (ISO/TS 13131, Telehealth Services), https://www.iso.org/publication/PUB100386.html.

[2] Ambrosino N., Vagheggini G., Mazzoleni S., et al., (2016). Telemedicine in chronic obstructive pulmonary disease. *Breathe*, 12:350-356.

[3] Panagopoulos C., Malli F., Menychtas A., et al., (2017). Utilizing a Homecare Platform for Remote Monitoring of Patients with Idiopathic Pulmonary Fibrosis. GeNeDis 2016, *Advances in Experimental Medicine and Biology,* 989:177-18.

[4] Ambrosino N., Makhabah D. and Sutanto Y. (2017). Tele-medicine in respiratory diseases. *Multidisciplinary Respiratory Medicine,* 12:9.

[5] Hamman L. and Rich A. (1933). Clinical pathologic conference. *Int Clin,* 1:196-231.

[6] Moor C., Wapenaar M. and Miedema J. (2018). A home monitoring program including real-time wireless home spirometry in idiopathic pulmonary fibrosis: a pilot study on experiences and barriers. *Respiratory Research,* 19:105.

In: Respiratory Ventilatory Strategies …
Editor: Antonio M. Esquinas
ISBN: 978-1-53617-847-0
© 2020 Nova Science Publishers, Inc.

Chapter 35

MORTALITY IN ACUTE AND CHRONIC MANAGEMENT OF IDIOPATHIC PULMONARY FIBROSIS

Zuhal Karakurt*[1,*], *MD and Özlem Soğukpınar*[2,†], *MD
[1]Pulmonology and Critical Care Specialist,
University of Health Sciences Istanbul Sureyyapaşa Chest Diseases and Thoracic Surgery Teaching and Research Hospital, Istanbul, Turkey
[2]Pulmonology Specialist,
University of Health Sciences Istanbul Sureyyapaşa Chest Diseases and Thoracic Surgery Teaching and Research Hospital, Istanbul, Turkey

ABSTRACT

Idiopathic pulmonary fibrosis (IPF) is a well-known interstitial lung disease (ILD) and has the worst prognosis of all the ILDs. The median life expectancy is approximately 3-5 years after diagnosis. In the last decade new anti-fibrotic drugs have led to an improvement in the health-related quality of life (HRQoL) and a slowing of IPF disease progression. Despite advances in diagnostic technology and medical treatment there is still a high mortality rate, i.e., nearly 50%, in cases of acute exacerbation of IPF or infectious conditions due to immunosuppression therapy, which require intubation for mechanical ventilation in the intensive care unit. As IPF progresses, supplemental oxygen treatment is required (when pulse oxygen saturation is below 88% at rest and in room air) and these IPF patients' have a decreased life expectancy. IPF patients 60 years or older and with acute respiratory failure have a shorter survival and a higher mortality rate. IPF

* Corresponding Author's E-mail: zuhalkarakurt@hotmail.com.
† Corresponding Author's E-mail: ozlemsogukpinar@yahoo.com.

is a crucial health problem that requires further research and attention to prevent mortality.

Keywords: interstitial lung diseases, prognosis, management of idiopathic pulmonary fibrosis, mortality of idiopathic pulmonary fibrosis

INTRODUCTION

Idiopathic pulmonary fibrosis (IPF) is a rare, progressive and fatal interstitial lung disease. IPF is, however, a relative unknown, making it difficult to prevent and treat. At present there are no curative treatment approaches [1]. Following diagnosis, the survival is 3-5 years, and lung transplantation should be considered. However, even after lung transplantation, survival is nearly 5 years [2, 3]. Mortality of acute respiratory failure (ARF) patients with IPF is observed in nearly 50% of all intubated and invasively ventilated patients, for whom the reasons for intubation are exacerbation of IPF, immune suppressive pneumonia, or progression of underlying chronic diseases (i.e., pulmonary hypertension, cardiovascular disease, chronic obstructive pulmonary disease, and emphysema) in the intensive care unit (ICU) [4, 5-7]. Non-invasive mechanical ventilation (NIV) has a better outcome in terms of ICU survival and long term survival following discharge [4, 8, 9].

MORTALITY AND ACUTE RESPIRATORY MANAGEMENT OF IPF

ARF due to the acute exacerbation of IPF has a high mortality rate of nearly 40% [10], and if intubation is required in the ICU, the mortality rate is even higher (>50%) [4-6]. In one study that had a large ILD patient series (n = 120; 96 with IPF), ILD patients that were admitted to the ICU and required invasive mechanical ventilation (IMV) had a 90% mortality rate [4]. In that study, an Acute Physiology and Chronic Health Evaluation (APACHE II) score over 20, intolerance to respiration with supplemental oxygen, and a requirement for continuous NIV in the ICU, were significant predictors for a worse prognosis [4]. Intubation is not a lifesaving approach in this setting and NIV confers an increased chance of survival in the ICU. High flow nasal cannula oxygen treatment with small doses of opioid infusion can control the dyspnea, give time for a treatment response, and decrease the work-off breath.

Higher ICU mortality in patients with IPF is associated with:

- APACHE II over 20
- The need for intubation for IMV

- Older age
- Uncontrolled, advanced stage co-morbid diseases
- Pneumonia with resistant infections
- Intolerance to feeding, and/or speaking due to respiratory insufficiency
- Refractory hypoxemia.

Acute respiratory failure requiring ventilator support has a high risk of mortality for patients with IPF and the physician should inform patients and their relatives. In the initial stages of the disease following diagnosis, the patients and their family should be informed of the prognosis, the potential need for a lung transplant, and the 3-5 year mortality. The management approach for acute respiratory failure should be planned once the diagnosis is made.

MORTALITY AND CHRONIC RESPIRATORY MANAGEMENT AF IPF

Survival with IPF is 3-5 years [1], and following an acute exacerbation of IPF, the mean survival decreases to less than a year; a 90-day mortality has even been observed in half the IPF patients observed [10]. Management of acute exacerbation is important as the frequency of exacerbation is nearly 9.6% over a two year period. New anti-fibrotic drugs help to prolong acute exacerbation intervals [11-13], however, they do not yet prolong survival.

In chronic cases the approach for patients with IPF during follow-up are:

- Medical treatment (anti-fibrotic drugs), if necessary.
- Supplementary ambulatory oxygen.
- Continuous positive airway pressure (CPAP) device use, given normocapnia.
- Bi-level positive airway device use if hypercapnia present.
- Pulmonary rehabilitation.

All these approaches can increase the HRQoL and decrease dyspnea. The end of life care should be planned and the palliative approach should be explained to the patient and their family. Home based end of life is crucial. The hospital, especially the ICU, is not a suitable place for IPF patients to die. Despite new anti-fibrotic drugs, life expectancy is still 3-5 years after dyspnea symptoms begin and, unfortunately, each year, the IPF mortality rate increases worldwide [15-17]. In Europe, the number of IPF deaths has increased and is higher than in the United States [16]. The question is whether this increase in the number of deaths is due to an increasing population, an increased rate of diagnosis, or something else? Nowadays, IPF and ILD are hot topics for international congresses, and there are many studies regarding anti-fibrotic drugs are really hard to follow-up. Nonetheless, long term survival is still 3-5 years and the mortality rate is increasing worldwide. Although the rate of mortality is increasing each year, dyspnea and HRQoL has improved with the use of anti-fibrotic drugs, supplemental ambulatory oxygen treatment, and a NIV approach without intubation in cases of acute exacerbation.

REFERENCES

[1] Raghu G., Rochwerg B., Zhang Y., Garcia C. A., Azuma A., Behr J., et al., American Thoracic Society; European Respiratory society; Japanese Respiratory Society; Latin American Thoracic Association. An Official ATS/ERS/JRS/ALAT Clinical Practice Guideline: Treatment of Idiopathic Pulmonary Fibrosis. An Update of the 2011 Clinical Practice Guideline. *Am J Respir Crit Care Med.* 2015 Jul; 192(2):e3-19.

[2] Yusen R. D., Edwards L. B., Dipchand A. I., Goldfarb S. B., Kucheryavaya A. Y., Levvey B. J., et al., The registry of the International Society for Heart and Lung Transplantation: thirty-third adult lung and heart-lung transplant Report - 2016; focus theme: primary diagnostic indications for transplant. *J Heart Lung Transplant.* 2016; 35:1170-84.

[3] Hutchinson J. P., T. M. McKeever, A. W. Fogarty, V. Navaratnam, R. B. Hubbard, Increasing global mortality from idiopathic pulmonary fibrosis in the twenty first century, *Ann. Am. Thorac. Soc.* 11 (8) (2014) 1176e1185.

[4] Güngör G., Tatar D., Saltürk C., Cimen P., Karakurt Z., Kirakli C., Adıgüzel N., Ediboglu Ö., Yılmaz H., Moçin Ö. Y., Balcı M., Yılmaz A.: Why do patients with interstitial lung diseases fail in the ICU? A 2-center cohort study. *Respir Care* 2013, 58:525-531.

[5] Fernandez-Perez E. R., Yilmaz M., Jenad H., Daniels C. E., Ryu J. H., Hubmayr R. D., Gajic O.: Ventilator settings and outcome of respiratory failure in chronic interstitial lung disease. *Chest* 2008, 133:1113-1119.

[6] Saydain G., Islam A., Afessa B., Ryu J. H., Scott J. P., Peters S. G. Outcome of patients with idiopathic pulmonary fibrosis admitted to the intensive care unit. *Am J Respir Crit Care Med.* 2002 Sep 15; 166(6):839-42.

[7] Aliberti S., Messinesi G., Gamberini S., Maggiolini S., Visca D., Galavotti V., Giuliani F., Cosentini R., Brambilla A. M., Blasi F., Scala R., Carone M., Luisi F., Harari S., Voza A., Esquinas A., Pesci A. Non-invasive mechanical ventilation in patients with diffuse interstitial lung diseases. *BMC Pulm Med.* 2014 Dec 5; 14:194.

[8] Yokoyama T., Kondoh Y., Taniguchi H., Kataoka K., Kato K., Nishiyama O., Kimura T., Hasegawa R., Kubo K.: Noninvasive ventilation in acute exacerbation of idiopathic pulmonary fibrosis. *Intern Med* 2010, 49:1509-1514.

[9] Tomii K., Tachikawa R., Chin K., Murase K., Handa T., Mishima M., Ishihara K.: Role of non-invasive ventilation in managing life-threatening acute exacerbation of interstitial pneumonia. *Intern Med* 2010, 49:1341-1347.

[10] Natsuizaka M., Chiba, H., Kuronuma, K., Otsuka, M., Kudo, K., Mori, M., Bando, M., Sugiyama, Y., Takahashi, H. Epidemiologic survey of Japanese patients with idiopathic pulmonary fibrosis and investigation of ethnic differences. *Am. J. Respir. Crit. Care Med.* 2014, 190, 773-779.

[11] Richeldi L., Cottin, V., du Bois, R. M., Selman, M., Kimura, T., Bailes, Z., Schlenker-Herceg, R., Stowasser, S., Brown, K. K. Nintedanib in patients with idiopathic pulmonary fibrosis: Combined evidence from the Tomorrow and Inpulsis(®) *trials. Respir. Med.* 2016, 113, 74-79.

[12] Azuma A., Taniguchi, H., Inoue, Y., Kondoh, Y., Ogura, T., Homma, S., Fujimoto, T., Sakamoto, W., Sugiyama, Y., Nukiwa, T. Nintedanib in Japanese patients with idiopathic pulmonary fibrosis: A subgroup analysis of the INPULSIS® randomized trials. *Respirology* 2017, 22, 750-757.

[13] Furuya K., Sakamoto, S., Shimizu, H., Sekiya, M., Kinoshita, A., Isshiki, T., Sugino, K., Matsumoto, K., Homma, S. Pirfenidone for acute exacerbation of idiopathic pulmonary fibrosis: A retrospective study. *Respir. Med.* 2017, 126, 93-99.

[14] Kalluri M., Claveria F., Ainsley E., Haggag M., Armijo-Olivo S., Richman-Eisenstat J. Beyond idiopathic pulmonary fibrosis diagnosis: multidisciplinary care with an early integrated palliative approach is associated with a decrease in acute care utilization and hospital deaths. *J Pain Symptom Manag*. 2018; 55:420-6.

[15] Olson A. L., Swigris J. J., Lezotte D. C., Norris J. M., Wilson C. G., Brown K. K. Mortality from pulmonary fibrosis increased in the United States from 1992 to 2003. *Am J Respir Crit Care Med.* 2007 Aug 1; 176(3):277-84.

[16] Hutchinson J. P., McKeever T. M., Fogarty A. W., Navaratnam V., Hubbard R. B. Increasing global mortality from idiopathic pulmonary fibrosis in the twenty-first century. *Ann Am Thorac Soc*. 2014 Oct; 11(8):1176-85.

[17] Wuyts W. A., Dahlqvist C., Slabbynck H., Schlesser M., Gusbin N., Compere C., Maddens S., Lee Y. C., Kirchgaessler K. U., Bartley K., Bondue B. Longitudinal clinical outcomes in a real-world population of patients with idiopathic pulmonary fibrosis: the PROOF registry. *Respir Res.* 2019 Oct 24; 20(1):231. doi: 10.1186/s12931-019-1182-z.

In: Respiratory Ventilatory Strategies …
Editor: Antonio M. Esquinas
ISBN: 978-1-53617-847-0
© 2020 Nova Science Publishers, Inc.

Chapter 36

REHABILITATION IN PATIENTS AFTER LUNG TRANSPLANTATION

Annalisa Fui[1], Guido Vagheggini[2], Antonella Fossi[1], Behar Cekorja[1,2] and Elena Bargagli[1,*]
[1]Pulmonary Medicine Unit, University of Siena, Siena, Italy
[2]Cardiac and Pulmonary Rehabilitation Unit,
Auxilium Vitae Rehabilitation Centre, Volterra, Italy

ABSTRACT

Lung transplantation (LTX) is an established treatment for patients with end-stage lung disease. Since the first combined heart and lung transplants we assessed to an amelioration of survival rates in solid organ transplantation and for this reason an evaluation on long-term outcomes following transplant is needed. Pulmonary Rehabilitation (PR) is an exercise-based treatment that improves walking endurance, muscle strength, and functional recovery: it has been demonstrated that PR is beneficial for patients with Chronic Pulmonary Diseases.

After lung transplant it has been observed that despite an improvement in lung function, exercise intolerance and reductions in quality of life could persist up to years after transplantation. Literature reported that Pulmonary Rehabilitation post-LTx increases physical exercise capacity and health-related quality of life (HRQL), but few studies are available and a clear consensus is needed.

Lung transplantation is an established treatment for patients with end-stage lung diseases. The primary clinical aim of lung transplantation is to improve survival and to

---

* Corresponding Author's E-mail: bargagli2@unisi.it.

ameliorate the quality of life (QOL) of these patients [1]. In the past years an improvement on survival rate in solid organ transplantation has been obtained, and actually an evaluation on long-term outcomes (including physical function, health-related quality-of-life and cardiovascular mortality) of lung transplantation is needed. Exercise training is necessary in lung transplanted patients but unfortunately research on the optimal timing, type, dose of exercise, mode of delivery and relevant outcomes is limited [2]. It has been observed that despite an improvement in lung function parameters, the exercise intolerance could persist up to years after transplantation [3]. Post-transplantation QOL is increased in comparison with pre-transplant values but limitations in daily physical activities still persist after lung transplantation [4], for example the limitations in maximal exercise capacity between 40-60% of predicted values have been reported and mostly unrelated to ventilatory or cardiovascular problems [5, 6]. Candidates for lung transplantation show physiological changes consequent to their severe and chronic lung diseases associated with limb muscle dysfunction, deconditioning, nutritional depletion and reduced exercise capacity and tolerance [2]. After transplantation, the prolonged hospital stay and sedentary time of inactivity, the immunosuppressive treatments and the acute and chronic episodes of organ rejections may affect exercise tolerance and QOL in lung transplant recipients [2]. In these patients leg fatigue is one of the main symptom limiting exercise tolerance and endurance, as reported by Williams et al., [7]. These authors demonstrated the long persistence of exercise limitation after lung transplantation without improvement during time [7]. Exercise capacity persists limited in these subjects due to an early and pathologic lactate threshold associated with peripheral muscle weakness [8]; reduced muscle mass and quadriceps strength compared with pre-transplant period. These alterations have been shown to persist up to 3 years after lung transplantation [9]. Regarding pharmacological medications, the long-term use of high dose corticosteroids has been associated with limb muscle atrophy and myopathy [10, 11]. The concomitant use of immunosuppressant therapies including calcineurin inhibitors has a negative impact in mitochondrial respiration and muscle remodelling [12] inducing limb muscle dysfunction and impairment in exercise capacity after transplantation. As a result of medications, debilitation, inactivity and other peripheral factors, the exercise capacity after lung transplantation is generally limited to approximately 50-60% of the predicted values [1, 13].

After lung transplant the participation of the patient in daily activities are increased both after 3 and 6 months from the surgical intervention compared to the pre transplant phase [14] but it persist reduced in comparison with healthy controls up to 1 year after transplantation. In fact, steps, standing time and moderate-intensity activity score are reduced by 42%, 29% and 66%, respectively in lung recipients than healthy controls [15]. Randomized controlled trials are needed to examine whether physical activity can be assessed in these patients and to verify how to improve functional recovery after lung transplantation.

Moreover, increased participation in daily physical activity after transplantation might be useful to prevent the development of comorbidities after solid organ transplantation. In fact, it has been demonstrated that 30-50% of patients develop comorbidities such as osteoporosis, hyperlipidemia and diabetes in the years after lung transplantation [5]. The prevalence of hypertension in 5-year survivors of lung transplantation is described to be around 90% [5], associated with other cardiovascular diseases and to weight gain that is a real common problem and all these negative conditions can be modifiable by physical activity and exercise training [16, 17].

Literature reported that pulmonary rehabilitation (PR) post-lung transplantation increases physical exercise capacity and health-related quality of life (HRQL) [18]. Moreover, it seems that pulmonary rehabilitation outcomes are similar regardless of single or double lung transplant [19] and a recent retrospective cohort study, conducted to quantify the outcomes of multidisciplinary inpatient rehabilitation following cardiopulmonary transplants, concluded that for debilitated transplanted patients, the multidisciplinary inpatient rehabilitation allowed to improve physical function, mobility and independence of patients [20]. Randomized controlled trials evaluated the impact of defined exercise programs on outcomes but, despite the general belief that exercise training has potential for both short- and long-term benefits in this population, the number of studies regarding this argument is too limited, and available data is insufficient [19]. ATS/ERS statement [18] on pulmonary rehabilitation recommended pulmonary rehabilitation in the management of individuals both before and after lung transplantation. Pre-transplant pulmonary rehabilitation has been demonstrated to be useful to optimize and maintain the functional status of the lung transplant recipients before surgery.

A recent systematic review on randomized controlled trials and prospective cohorts on functional outcomes of lung transplantation recipients [21] concluded that although the overall quality of the studies was fair to moderate, positive outcomes of pulmonary rehabilitation were demonstrated regarding maximal and functional exercise capacity, skeletal muscle function, and lumbar bone mineral density. Further research is needed to study the potential role of exercise training in increasing functional outcomes and to identify optimal guidelines for exercise prescription in the lung transplant patients. Fuller et al., in a recent randomized controlled trial to investigate the effects of a supervised longer- versus shorter-duration rehabilitation program after lung transplantation showed that 6MWT increased in both groups with no significant differences. They concluded that shorter duration of rehabilitation achieves comparable outcomes with 14 weeks of supervised rehabilitation for functional exercise capacity, lower limb strength, and quality of life evaluated 6 months after transplantation [22].

The importance of early (starting 24 h postoperatively) mobilization is recognized [23]: rehabilitation in the first 24-48 hours after surgery is based on optimizing lung expansion and secretion clearance, breathing pattern efficiency, upper and lower extremity mobility, strength, and basic transfer [18].

Although a formal study about this argument is still lacking, an immediate mobilization after surgery is probably very useful in lung-transplanted population with pre- and post-transplant limb muscle dysfunction. Intensive Care Unit-acquired weakness is a highly prevalent complication due to the duration of mechanical ventilation, use of sedative drugs, neuromuscular blockers, corticosteroids, and immobilization [3]. In the early postoperative period some patients are unable to participate in any active mobilization. Neuromuscular electrical stimulation might be an alternative treatment strategy to prevent deterioration of muscle function in this kind of patients [24].

Suggested elements of rehabilitation during hospitalization after lung transplantation also include breathing exercises, secretion clearance control, and posture improvement exercise. In the early postoperative period rehabilitation, it is useful to improve breathing retraining, optimizing supplemental oxygen need, balancing activities, building upper and lower extremity range of motion, and managing eventual neuropathic pain [25]. Patients should also be encouraged to cough. At a later stage, begin with transfers from bed to chair and start ambulation using a specialized walker, paying attention on chest tubes and pain. Exercise progression should gradually include lower limb resistance training. It should also be imperative to ensure that lower extremity strength and balance to minimize the risk of falls and patients safety [3, 25].

Regarding the Immediate Post-transplant Phase, in a range of 12 months at discharge, there is a lack of randomized controlled trials (RCTs) on exercise training for transplant recipients. All data derived from small monocentric studies that suggest how supervised exercise training might be useful to improve clinically relevant outcomes in the immediate post-transplant phase [3].

In a clinical randomized controlled trial, Langer et al., evaluated a 3-month supervised exercise training program performed on 76 patients (40-65 years old), who experienced no major perioperative complications after lung transplant. The rehabilitant intervention included three weekly sessions of education and cycling, walking, stair climbing and lower-extremity resistance exercises. Forty subjects were randomized; 34 patients were enrolled (18 included in the intervention group and 16 in the control group). The intervention group reported significantly higher peak work rate during a maximal incremental cardiopulmonary cycle exercise test, with increased 6-min walking distance, quadriceps' strength thanks to the participation in daily physical activity. Their QOL significantly improved up to 1 year after lung transplantation [14].

In another randomized controlled study, Mitchell et al., analized the effects of a supervised 6-month lumbar extension exercise training program (started 8 weeks after hospital discharge) on bone mineral density of the lumbar vertebrae in comparison with a usual care group. In this study, bone mineral density significantly improved and mechanical loading associated with progressive resistance exercise was demonstrated to be useful in preventing steroid-induced osteoporosis in lung transplanted patients [26]. The effects of a 6-week formal exercise training program was described by Ross et al., reporting an improvement in peak oxygen consumption by incremental cycle ergometer activity performed before and after lung translant [27]. Another cohort study investigated the impact of outpatient pulmonary rehabilitation after lung transplantation on skeletal muscle function and exercise tolerance, finding significant improvement in 6-min walking distance and limb muscle strength in a combined endurance and resistance training [28]. Analogously another cohort study revealed a significant improvement in 6-min walking distance, limb muscle strength and QOL after 12 weeks of standard outpatient post-LT PR program [29]. The recommendation of rehabilitation in the immediate post-transplant phase is that functional capacity (e.g., 6-min walking distance or cardiopulmonary exercise testing) and strength measurements should be monitored to establish a postoperative baseline. Patients should wear face masks during group outpatient PR sessions. It is important to disinfect the hands as well as handles of exercise training equipment before and after each exercise, balancing the exercise training to higher intensity and duration over time. It's also important to monitor comorbidities such as diabetes and osteoporosis; activities that include excessive flexion and rotation should be avoided to reduce the risk of possible vertebral compression fracture [3, 25]. Since lung recipients are prone to developing tendinopathies [30] these symptoms should be closely investigated, avoiding overburdening tendons by repetitive tasks against high resistances. Make use of interval exercises, sufficient warm-up and stretching procedures to avoid injuries [3, 25].

Regarding the Long-Term Post-transplant Phase, the effect of a rehabilitation program on health-related quality of life and exercise capacity in long-term survivors of lung transplantation had been established comparing the effects of a 4-week inpatient pulmonary rehabilitation program with an outpatient physiotherapy group [31]. In this study no significant differences between-the two groups in exercise capacity or QOL were reported and both groups achieved significant increase in 6-min walking distance and HRQOL [31]. The positive effects of physical activity training on muscle function and exercise capacity in the long-term post-transplant patients were further established also through a study demonstrating that the exercise training can also improve the alterations in the intracellular organization in energy cellular metabolism through improvement in mitochondrial functions [32]. An interesting study concluded that training program led to significant improvements in endurance time, QOL and increased muscle strength also after only 3 months of rehabilitation [33].

The effects of 6 weeks of aerobic endurance exercise on a cycle ergometer in 9 transplanted patients were reported demonstrating that the patients achieved statistically significant improvements in maximal exercise capacity and minute ventilation at iso-work rate [34].

Since Bronchiolitis Obliterans Syndrome (BOS) is a debilitating disease with limited treatment options that threatens both the quality of life and long-term survival of lung transplant recipients, prospective studies should be provided to explore whether rehabilitative interventions might be useful to improve symptoms and slow down deterioration of exercise capacity in these patients developing BOS [35]. This is a novel and interesting topic for future researches.

In conclusion, pulmonary rehabilitation seems to be a positive therapeutic intervention improving the quality of life and preventing many comorbidities in lung transplant recipients. Further clinical studies are needed to establish correct international guidelines to standardize the therapeutic rehabilitative intervention pre- and post-lung transplantation. It has been demonstrated that not all transplant recipients achieve expected results in muscle strength or exercise capacity after rehabilitation. The real effectiveness of pulmonary rehabilitation on preventing the risk of organ rejection, survival and comorbidities need to be clearly established through randomized multicentre trials.

REFERENCES

[1] Singer J. P., Singer L. G. Quality of life in lung transplantation. *Semin Respir Crit Care Med.* 2013; 34(3):421-30.

[2] Mathur S., Janaudis-Ferreira T., Wickerson L., Singer L. G., Patcai J., Rozenberg D., et al., Meeting report: consensus recommendations for a research agenda in exercise in solid organ transplantation. *Am J Transplant.* 2014; 14(10):2235-45.

[3] Langer D. Rehabilitation in patients before and after lung transplantation. *Respir Int Rev Thorac Dis.* 2015; 89(5):353-62.

[4] Myaskovsky L., Dew M. A., McNulty M. L., Switzer G. E., DiMartini A. F., Kormos R. L., et al., Trajectories of change in quality of life in 12-month survivors of lung or heart transplant. *Am J Transplant Off J Am Soc Transplant Am Soc Transpl Surg*. 2006; 6(8):1939-47.

[5] Studer S. M., Levy R. D., McNeil K., Orens J. B. Lung transplant outcomes: a review of survival, graft function, physiology, health-related quality of life and cost-effectiveness. *Eur Respir J.* 2004; 24(4):674-85.

[6] Mathur S., Reid W. D., Levy R. D. Exercise limitation in recipients of lung transplants. *Phys Ther.* 2004; 84(12):1178-87.

[7] Williams T. J., Patterson G. A., McClean P. A., Zamel N., Maurer J. R. Maximal exercise testing in single and double lung transplant recipients. *Am Rev Respir Dis* 1992; 145(1):101-5.

[8] Reinsma G. D., ten Hacken N. H. T., Grevink R. G., van der Bij W., Koëter G. H., van Weert E. Limiting factors of exercise performance 1 year after lung transplantation. *J Heart Lung Transplant Off Publ Int Soc Heart Transplant* 2006; 25(11):1310-6.

[9] Rozenberg D., Wickerson L., Singer L. G., Mathur S. Sarcopenia in lung transplantation: a systematic review. *J Heart Lung Transplant Off Publ Int Soc Heart Transplant.* 2014; 33(12):1203-12.

[10] Schakman O., Kalista S., Barbé C., Loumaye A., Thissen J. P. Glucocorticoid-induced skeletal muscle atrophy. *Int J Biochem Cell Biol.* 2013; 45(10):2163-72.

[11] Schakman O., Gilson H., Thissen J. P. Mechanisms of glucocorticoid-induced myopathy. *J Endocrinol.* 2008; 197(1):1-10.

[12] Sakuma K., Yamaguchi A. The functional role of calcineurin in hypertrophy, regeneration, and disorders of skeletal muscle. *J Biomed Biotechnol.* 2010; 2010:721219.

[13] Bartels M. N., Armstrong H. F., Gerardo R. E., Layton A. M., Emmert-Aronson B. O., Sonett J. R., et al., Evaluation of pulmonary function and exercise performance by cardiopulmonary exercise testing before and after lung transplantation. *Chest.* 2011; 140(6):1604-11.

[14] Langer D., Burtin C., Schepers L., Ivanova A., Verleden G., Decramer M., et al., Exercise training after lung transplantation improves participation in daily activity: a randomized controlled trial. *Am J Transplant Off J Am Soc Transplant Am Soc Transpl Surg* 2012; 12(6):1584-92.

[15] Langer D., Gosselink R., Pitta F., Burtin C., Verleden G., Dupont L., et al., Physical activity in daily life 1 year after lung transplantation. *J Heart Lung Transplant Off Publ Int Soc Heart Transplant.* 2009; 28(6):572-8.

[16] Forli L., Bollerslev J., Simonsen S., Isaksen G. A., Godang K., Pripp A. H., et al., Disturbed energy metabolism after lung and heart transplantation. *Clin Transplant.* 2011; 25(2):E136-143.

[17] Savioli G., Surbone S., Giovi I., Salinaro F., Preti P., Meloni .F, et al., Early development of metabolic syndrome in patients subjected to lung transplantation. *Clin Transplant* 2013; 27(3):E237-243.

[18] Spruit M. A., Singh S. J., Garvey C., ZuWallack R., Nici L., Rochester C., et al., An official American Thoracic Society/European Respiratory Society statement: key concepts and advances in pulmonary rehabilitation. *Am J Respir Crit Care Med.* 2013; 188(8):e13-64.

[19] Schneeberger T., Gloeckl R., Welte T., Kenn K. Pulmonary rehabilitation outcomes after single or double lung transplantation in patients with chronic obstructive pulmonary disease or interstitial lung disease. *Respir Int Rev Thorac Dis.* 2017; 94(2):178-85.

[20] Shiner C. T., Woodbridge G., Skalicky D. A., Faux S. G. *Multidisciplinary inpatient rehabilitation following heart and/or lung transplantation - examining cohort characteristics and clinical outcomes.* PM R. 2019; in press.

[21] Wickerson L., Mathur S., Brooks D. Exercise training after lung transplantation: a systematic review. *J Heart Lung Transplant Off Publ Int Soc Heart Transplant.* 2010; 29(5):497-503.

[22] Fuller L. M., Button B., Tarrant B., Steward R., Bennett L., Snell G., et al., Longer versus shorter duration of supervised rehabilitation after lung transplantation: A randomized trial. *Arch Phys Med Rehabil.* 2017; 98(2):220-226.e3.

[23] Burtin C., Clerckx B., Robbeets C., Ferdinande P., Langer D., Troosters T., et al., Early exercise in critically ill patients enhances short-term functional recovery. *Crit Care Med.* 2009; 37(9):2499-505.

[24] Segers J., Hermans G., Bruyninckx F., Meyfroidt G., Langer D., Gosselink R. Feasibility of neuromuscular electrical stimulation in critically ill patients. *J Crit Care* 2014; 29(6):1082-8.

[25] Rochester C. L., Fairburn C., Crouch R. H. Pulmonary rehabilitation for respiratory disorders other than chronic obstructive pulmonary disease. *Clin Chest Med.* 2014; 35(2):369-89.

[26] Mitchell M. J., Baz M. A., Fulton M. N., Lisor C. F., Braith R. W. Resistance training prevents vertebral osteoporosis in lung transplant recipients. *Transplantation.* 2003; 76(3):557-62.

[27] Ross D. J., Waters P. F., Mohsenifar Z., Belman M. J., Kass R. M., Koerner S. K. Hemodynamic responses to exercise after lung transplantation. *Chest.* 1993; 103(1):46-53.

[28] Maury G., Langer D., Verleden G., Dupont L., Gosselink R., Decramer M., et al., Skeletal muscle force and functional exercise tolerance before and after lung transplantation: a cohort study. *Am J Transplant Off J Am Soc Transplant Am Soc Transpl Surg*. 2008; 8(6):1275-81.

[29] Munro P. E., Holland A. E., Bailey M., Button B. M., Snell G. I. Pulmonary rehabilitation following lung transplantation. *Transplant Proc.* 2009; 41(1):292-5.

[30] Chhajed P. N., Plit M. L., Hopkins P. M., Malouf M. A., Glanville A. R. Achilles tendon disease in lung transplant recipients: association with ciprofloxacin. *Eur Respir J.* 2002; 19(3):469-71.

[31] Ihle F., Neurohr C., Huppmann P., Zimmermann G., Leuchte H., Baumgartner R., et al., Effect of inpatient rehabilitation on quality of life and exercise capacity in long-term lung transplant survivors: a prospective, randomized study. *J Heart Lung Transplant Off Publ Int Soc Heart Transplant.* 2011; 30(8):912-9.

[32] Guerrero K., Wuyam B., Mezin P., Vivodtzev I., Vendelin M., Borel J. C., et al., Functional coupling of adenine nucleotide translocase and mitochondrial creatine

kinase is enhanced after exercise training in lung transplant skeletal muscle. *Am J Physiol Regul Integr Comp Physiol*. 2005; 289(4):R1144-1154.

[33] Vivodtzev I., Pison C., Guerrero K., Mezin P., Maclet E., Borel J. C., et al., Benefits of home-based endurance training in lung transplant recipients. *Respir Physiol Neurobiol.* 2011; 177(2):189-98.

[34] Stiebellehner L., Quittan M., End A., Wieselthaler G., Klepetko W., Haber P., et al., Aerobic endurance training program improves exercise performance in lung transplant recipients. *Chest.* 1998; 113(4):906-12.

[35] Cebrià I Iranzo M. À., Vos R., Verleden G. M., Gosselink R., Langer D. Evolution of functional exercise capacity in lung transplant patients with and without bronchiolitis obliterans syndrome: A longitudinal case-control study. *Arch Bronconeumol*. 2018.

In: Respiratory Ventilatory Strategies …
Editor: Antonio M. Esquinas
ISBN: 978-1-53617-847-0
© 2020 Nova Science Publishers, Inc.

Chapter 37

Pulmonary Rehabilitation in Fibrosing Interstitial Lung Diseases and Idiopatic Pulmonary Fibrosis: Key Practical Aspects

Guido Vagheggini[1,2,*], Elena Bargagli[3], Behar Cekorja[1,3] and Eugenia Panait[1,2]

[1]Cardiac and Pulmonary Rehabilitation Unit, Auxilium Vitae Rehabilitation Centre, Volterra, Pisa, Italy

[2]Fondazione Volterra Ricerche ONLUS, Volterra, Pisa, Italy

[3]Department of Medicine, Surgery and Neurosciences, Respiratory Diseases and Lung Transplantation Section, University of Siena, Siena, Italy

Abstract

Idiopathic pulmonary fibrosis (IPF) and other forms of fibrosing interstitial lung diseases (F-ILD) induce a very severe limitation to exercise, due to changes in mechanical lung properties, impaired gas exchange and vascular pulmonary disruption. Disease progression is associated with a progressive impairment of exercise capacity and mobility, as a consequence of dyspnoea and exercise-induced hypoxaemia. Deconditioning and muscle wasting contribute to the inactivity of these patients, worsening the age-related loss of muscle mass quality and strength (Holland, 2010).

Pulmonary rehabilitation is recognized as a core component in the management of individuals with chronic respiratory disease, able to alleviate respiratory and psychological symptoms in different fibrosing interstitial lung disease. Improvement in exercise tolerance, walking capacity and quality of life scores following rehabilitation have been described, as well as improvement in dyspnoea and anxiety (Swigris, 2011; Spagnolo, 2015; Vainshelboim, 2016).

* Corresponding Author's E-mail: guidovagheggini@libero.it.

Clinically relevant improvements in exercise capacity, symptoms and quality of life have been observed in F-ILD of different aetiologies following pulmonary rehabilitation, as well as after lung transplantation. Given the positive impact on patient-centred outcomes, irrespective of disease severity, efforts should be made to increase the accessibility of symptomatic ILD patients to pulmonary rehabilitation.

Keywords: pulmonary rehabilitation, interstitial lung disease, pulmonary fibrosis, idiopathic pulmonary fibrosis, exercise training, dyspnoea, quality of life, self-management, lung transplant, pulmonary hypertension

INTRODUCTION

The group of interstitial lung diseases (ILD) includes idiopathic pulmonary fibrosis (IPF) and a large group of parenchymal pulmonary disorders characterised by the development of progressive lung fibrosis. The definition of "progressive-fibrosing" or "fibrosing ILD" (F-ILD) has recently been adopted, to emphasize the clinical and pathological overlapping with hypersensitivity pneumonitis (HP), rheumatoid arthritis-associated ILD (RA-ILD) and other unclassifiable diseases. Disease progression is associated with worsening of respiratory symtoms and progressive impairment of exercise capacity and mobility. Deconditioning and muscle wasting are due to dyspnoea and exercise-induced hypoxaemia, worsening an underlying age-related loss of muscle mass quality and strength (Holland, 2010).

A potential common treatment pathway has been hypothesized for F-ILDs, as a combination of inflammation and fibrosis has been found, albeit in varying proportions, in almost all of these diseases. Immunomodulatory therapies result more effective in nonspecific interstitial pneumonia, fibrosing HP and connective tissue associated ILD (CT-ILD). In recent years two anti-fibrotic agents have been introduced in IPF treatment. Pirfenidone, a compound with anti-fibrotic, anti-oxidant and anti-inflammatory properties, and nintedanib, a tyrosine kinase inhibitor selective for vascular endothelial growth factor, platelet-derived growth factor and fibroblast growth factor receptors. Antifibrotic therapy is currently under investigation for other F-ILDs, preliminary results seem to confirm their effectiveness in delaying pulmonary function decline and disease progression. Despite these therapeutic options, IPF and other F-ILDs are still considered as untreatable and progressive diseases; quality of life and palliation of symptoms remain therefore the key issues in the management of these patients.

Pulmonary rehabilitation is recognized as a core component of the management of individuals with chronic respiratory diseases, even if symptoms (dyspnoea, exercise intolerance, impaired quality of life, muscle weakness) are sustained by different pathophysiological mechanisms (Spruit, 2013; Vainshelboim, 2016). Respiratory and psychological symptoms improve after pulmonary rehabilitation in different fibrosing interstitial lung diseases, as well as exercise tolerance, 6MWD and quality of life (QOL) scores. Improvement in dyspnoea and anxiety scores after PR has been reported (Swigris, 2011; Spagnolo, 2015; Vainshelboim, 2016).

Exercise Limitation in F-ILD

Exercise limitation is one of the most important symptoms in F-ILD, mainly due to the severe exertional dyspnoea and fatigue that worsen with disease progression, affecting quality of life. During exercise, lung mechanics and gas exchange abnormalities limit pulmonary reserve and lead to severe hypoxaemia through the following main mechanisms:

Rapid Shallow Breathing

Early physiological studies conducted in subjects with diffuse pulmonary fibrosis showed that most patients develop a low tidal volume and a high frequency pattern of breathing. This rapid, shallow breathing pattern is present at rest and worsens during exercise and is seen as an adaptation for small, stiff lungs (Burdon, 1983). During exercise, tidal volume (Vt) response to increases in ventilation has been reported lower than in normal subjects matched for size. Despite this, a large ventilatory reserve can be observed in many subjects with low peak VO2 values at the end of exercise. Therefore, changes in respiratory mechanics and ventilatory pattern are not thought to have a primary role in limiting exercise capacity.

Circulatory Limitation

The reduced peak VO2 during incremental cardiopulmonary exercise test (CPET) is strongly correlated with the impairment of lactic acidosis threshold (LAT), extended 02 pulse, and oxygen uptake/work rate relationship (ΔVO2/ΔWR), strongly supporting the hypothesis that impaired O2 transport (circulatory impairment) may represent the main factor contributing to exercise limitation in most patients (Marciniuk, 1994).

Circulatory impairment has been described as the primary limitation to exercise also in patients with systemic sclerosis and restrictive lung disease (Sudduth, 1993). It is primarily due to pulmonary vascular disease and the accompanying gas exchange impairment, and correlates with the severity of the underlying lung disease and the extent of lung fibrosis. Pulmonary capillary destruction and hypoxic pulmonary vasoconstriction are the main mechanisms of circulatory dysfunction, and may lead to pulmonary hypertension and cardiac dysfunction in some patients (Agustì, 1991).

V/Q Mismatch

Studies conducted with multiple inert gas exchange technique highlighted the role of pulmonary vascular tone in resting and exercise-induced mismatch of pulmonary ventilation and perfusion. After oxygen administration, the release of hypoxic pulmonary vasoconstriction increase the percentage of blood flow perfusing low ventilation-to-perfusion (V/Q) lung units. Higher vascular tone, that is higher vascular reactivity to oxygen, is associated to less V/Q mismatching at rest and during exercise, and higher arterial p02 during exercise (Hansen, 1996). Patients with more severe anatomic derangement of the pulmonary vasculature lose vascular reactivity to oxygen. A relationship has been found between the extent of fibrosis on imaging and the worsening of pulmonary gas exchange, with greater hypoxemia induced by exercise (Risk, 1984). As well as V/Q mismatch, diffusion limitation also contributes to exercise induced hypoxemia, as do reduction in mixed venous oxygen content and hypoxic pulmonary vasoconstriction as well (McDonald, 2018; Troy, 2016).

Ventilatory Inefficiency

Patients suffering from pulmonary hypertension have impaired exercise tolerance and poor ventilatory efficiency. In addition, in these patients, the increased ventilatory requirements significantly contribute to dyspnoea. Ventilatory inefficiency, expressed as the VE vs. VCO2 slope, has been found significantly higher in patients with pulmonary hypertension, and has been considered as a factor in the impairment of exercise capacity (Glaser, 2009).

Peripheral Muscle Dysfunction

A relationship between peak VO2 and quadriceps force has been described in sarcoidosis patients who reported fatigue, and an impairment in quadriceps muscle force has been described also in IPF, and other F-ILD. Whereas in sarcoidosis patients these findings can be explained by the well-known muscular involvement, systemic muscular damage needs yet to be defined in IPF. Physical deconditioning, and the influence of corticosteroid treatment on peripheral and respiratory muscle strength should be taken into account in F-ILD, as in other chronic lung diseases (Kabitz, 2006; Spruit, 2005).

EXERCISE TESTING

Clinical exercise testing may help to understand the role of the different mechanisms contributing to exercise limitation. The evaluation of exercise capacity and exercise-induced hypoxaemia may have prognostic value. The choice of which exercise test should be guided by the purpose of the test, and by the clinical characteristics of the patient. Cardiopulmonary exercise testing (CPET) is used to determine peak oxygen consumption, and to quantify the level of disability; it is also useful to identify determinants of dyspnoea and exercise limitation, as well as the role of concomitant clinical conditions. Exercise tolerance, peak oxygen uptake and other CPET variables have proven useful in evaluating the prognosis of patients with pulmonary and cardiac diseases, e.g., chronic pulmonary artery disease (COPD), cystic fibrosis (CF), interstitial lung diseases (ILD), heart failure (HF) and pulmonary hypertension (PH). Peak oxygen uptake, adjusted for lung function, age, gender and smoking status, has been reported to be related to survival in patients with ILD referred for lung transplant, and a value of less than 8.3 mL/kg/min has been associated to a threefold greater hazard of death (Fell, 2009). A lower survival rate in IPF patients has been associated with a distance walked lower than 207 meters and with desaturation $\leq$ 88% on six-minute walking test (6MWT) (Lederer, 2006; Lama, 2003).

Cardiopulmonary exercise test and 6-minute walk test are the most commonly used exercise tests in ILD to plan individualized exercise training and to evaluate the impact of therapeutic interventions (i.e., oxygen, pharmacological therapy, exercise training). Other tests, including incremental shuttle test, 4-min and 6-min step tests, and endurance treadmill tests have been reported to monitor changes in exercise capacity over time and after therapeutic interventions. Nonetheless, while CPET is frequently used in F-ILD as a tool for diagnosis and staging, 6-minute walk test is commonly used to monitor progression over time.

PULMONARY REHABILITATION IN F-ILD

"Pulmonary rehabilitation (PR) is a comprehensive intervention (...) designed to improve the physical and psychological condition of people with chronic respiratory disease and to promote the long-term adherence to health-enhancing behaviours"(Spruit, 2013).

Growing evidence is supporting short term benefits of PR for ILD. A Cochrane review analysed nine RCTs of PR in ILD, of which for three only the abstracts were available (Dowman, 2014). Studies differed for setting, components and duration of the programme. Most studies included participants with several types of ILD; four studies examined predominantly individuals with IPF. No adverse effects of PR were reported. Exercise capacity significantly improved following PR, with a weighted mean change in 6MWD of 44.34 m and 1.24 ml/kg/minute in peak oxygen consumption (VO2). Similar improvements were observed in the subgroups of patients with IPF (35.63 m and 1.46 ml/kg/min, respectively).

Beneficial effects of PR in F-ILD seem to be related to: chest expansion during deep-breathing exercises; stretching of thoracic muscles resulting in a more efficient breathing pattern; improvement of respiratory muscle strength; enhanced pleural elasticity and pulmonary compliance (Kenn, 2013).

Large studies of PR are difficult to conduct in rare ILDs, and few data are available regarding PR in nonspecific interstitial pneumonia, hypersensitivity pneumonia and connective tissue disease (CTD) ILD (Holland, 2015). Nonetheless, existing studies suggests that PR is effective across the spectrum of ILD, regardless of underlying diagnosis, and should probably be offered to all patients who are symptomatic on exertion.

Components of PR Programme

According to the American Thoracic Society and European Respiratory Society (ATS/ERS) definition, comprehensive rehabilitation programmes should be patient tailored, and based on exercise training, both resistance and endurance training, and non-exercise components. Education, psychological support and nutritional therapy should be included in PR programmes, along with behavioural education and training in self-management of the disease, early recognition and treatment of acute exacerbations (Spruit, 2013).

No clear recommendations exist for the ideal duration of PR programmes for people suffering from ILD, and a standard length of PR programme, ranging from 6 to 12 weeks for outpatient programmes has been adopted in the currently published studies associated with clinically relevant positive outcomes.

Current evidence does not identify the ideal timing of PR for ILD, but symptomatic patients referred to PR early may be more likely to achieve greater benefits (Holland, 2012).

Greater improvements in exercise capacity have been reported in patients with a higher forced vital capacity, less desaturation on exertion and less disability before PR (Kozu, 2011). Larger improvements of dyspnoea at 6 months after PR have been reported in patients with more severe baseline breathlessness, and higher improvement in 6MWD was reported in subjects with worst baseline walking distance (Ryerson, 2014). A clinically improvement in physical activity and health-related quality of life after PR have been observed at any stage of IPF and in patients awaiting lung transplantation (Kenn, 2015).

TRAINING STRATEGIES

Exercise training has proven to be a safe and effective intervention for prevention and rehabilitation of COPD and other chronic respiratory diseases. Despite the heterogeneity of clinical presentation, supervised exercise training represents a feasible and effective treatment also in IPF and F-ILD. Emerging data show significant improvement in exercise capacity, dyspnoea and quality of life after exercise training interventions. However, due to the severity of exertional dyspnoea, exercise-induced oxyhaemoglobin desaturation and the rapid disease progression in some patients, exercise prescription in ILD patients requires careful planning and adaptation (Nakazawa, 2017).

The majority of studies on pulmonary rehabilitation in IPF combined aerobic activity (walking and/or cycling) with resistance and flexibility exercises for peripheral skeletal muscles. Short-term effects of pulmonary rehabilitation on IPF outcomes are supported by several retrospective and prospective studies, but its long-term effects have not been extensively studied. Systematic investigation in this regard is needed, also considering the different clinical progression of some F-ILD (Dowman, 2017). Overall, supervised exercise training programs appear to provide the best results in terms of compliance and maintenance of physical activity, while home-based programs seem to be associated with lower improvements (Vainshelboim, 2017).

OXYGEN ADMINISTRATION

Supplemental oxygen is commonly prescribed in COPD and ILD to improve symptoms (breathlessness, fatigue, cough) survival and quality of life. Supplemental oxygen can be provided: at rest continuously (15-24 hours a day), on exertion, overnight. In COPD patients with PaO2 $\leq$ 55 mHg or PaO2 = 56-59 mmHg with concomitant pulmonary hypertension or right heart failure, long term continuous oxygen therapy showed to improve survival if administered for $\geq$ 15h daily, compared to no oxygen supplementation or to 12hrs daily (NOTT, 1980; MRCWP, 1981).

Despite limited evidence, the same guidelines for long-term continuous oxygen therapy are applied to other chronic pulmonary diseases determining respiratory failure.Long-term oxygen therapy is also recommended in patients suffering from F-ILD with resting hypoxaemia (Raghu, 2011). Placebo controlled trials of long term oxygen in chronically hypoxic ILD pts would be unethical because ILDs are rapidly progressive and characterized by severe breathlessness that oxygen is able to relieve. Table 1 summarizes current recommendations of oxygen therapy.

Table 1. Recommendations on oxygen therapy

Guidelines	Type of oxygen therapy	Oxygen recommendation
BTS 2015	Long-term oxygen therapy (LTOT)	Resting hypoxaemia (Pa_{O2} < 55 mmHg [7.3 kPa] or < 60 mmHg [< 8 kPa] if clinical evidence of pulmonary hypertension)
	NOCTURNAL oxygen	Nocturnal oxygen therapy should not be given to patients with ILD with nocturnal hypoxaemia alone, who do not fulfil LTOT criteria (Grade B)
	Ambulatory oxygen	AOT should not be routinely offered to patients who are not eligible for LTOT. However, if severe breathlessness and all other interventions optimised, ambulatory oxygen could be considered
ATS/ERS/JRS/ALA T 2011	LTOT	Clinically significant resting hypoxaemia
Australia and NZ 2017	LTOT	Resting hypoxaemia (Pa_{O2} < 55 mmHg [7.3 kPa] or < 60 mmHg [< 8 kPa] if clinical evidence of pulmonary hypertension)
	NOCTURNAL oxygen	Consider in patients who desaturate below 88% for at least one-third of total sleep time, in the absence of concomitant OSAS
	Ambulatory oxygen	In patients with isolated exertional hypoxia, placebo air vs oxygen controlled 6MWT: consider if improvement in dyspnoea or exercise capacity

6MWT, 6-minute walk test; ALAT, Latin American Thoracic Society; AOT, ambulatory oxygen therapy; ATS, American Thoracic Society; BTS, British Thoracic Society; ERS, European Respiratory Society; JRS, Japanese Respiratory Society; NZ, New Zealand; OSAS, obstructive sleep apnoea syndrome.

Isolated exertional hypoxia, without hypoxemia at rest is a negative prognostic factor and a significative determinant of symptoms and quality of life both in ILD and COPD. For similar levels of physiological impairment, exertional hypoxaemia is more profound and more frequent in ILD than COPD, and may obstacle exercise and daily life activities. Supplemental oxygen during exercise training is recommended in ILD patients by the ATS/ERS statement for PR to ensure safety in case of profound desaturation, and usual practice is to deliver oxygen therapy for any patient who desaturates to less than 85% during training, with the aim of maintaining SpO2 above 88% (Spruit, 2013).

Daily use of supplemental oxygen in patients with isolated exertional hypoxia is not supported by current guidelines, and although the 2015 British Thoracic Society guidelines stated that ambulatory oxygen should not be routinely offered to patients who are not hypoxic at rest, no specific considerations for patients with interstitial lung disease were made (except mentioning the possible benefit of ambulatory oxygen for individual patients with severe exertional breathlessness). Supplemental oxygen improved exercise performance and/or symptoms in several studies of acute effects of high-flow supplemental oxygen on exercise, conducted in laboratory setting. Long-term benefits of ambulatory oxygen in day-to-day life need to be further investigated (Schaeffer, 2017; Dowman, 2017). Recently, a prospective, open-label, crossover randomised controlled clinical trial evaluated the effect of ambulatory oxygen on QOL in patients with interstitial lung disease not hypoxic at rest but with fall in oxygen saturation ≤88% during 6MWT (Visca, 2018). Compared with no treatment, ambulatory oxygen improved day-to-day health-related QOL, and scores in the activity and breathlessness subdomains. Large longer-term prospective randomised trials in fibrotic ILD are needed to determine long-term effects on quality of life, predictors of benefit and potential impact on oxidative stress, pulmonary vasculature.

Frequently in F-ILD, nocturnal hypoxemia may occur also in the absence of daytime resting hypoxemia and has been linked to pulmonary hypertension (PH) and early mortality (Schiza, 2015; Corte, 2012). Correction of nocturnal hypoxemia could prevent development of pulmonary hypertension, and some guidelines suggest to consider nocturnal oxygen in patients who desaturate below 88% for at least one-third of total sleep time, in absence of concomitant obstructive sleep apnea (Jo, 2017).

HOW TO BUILD A COMPREHENSIVE PR PROGRAMME

Exercise Training Strategies

General principles of exercise training suitable for healthy individuals can be also applied to patients suffering from ILD (Garber, 2011). To be beneficial, training must be based upon an individual's specific requirements and capacities, exceeding in effort the activities of daily living and progressing as physiological adaptations occur. Training methods will be addressed to the cardiovascular, pulmonary and peripheral muscle metabolic limitations of the individual patient.

Training strategies adopted in the studies have used aerobic exercise alone or a combination of aerobic and resistance training; Even though the most effective exercise training strategy for patients has yet to be confirmed, training intensities of 60–80% of peak work capacity for continuous exercise have been used in published studies. Exercise sessions of 20-60 min, 3 to 5 days per week have been used in outpatient programmes lasting 8-12 weeks (Dowman, 2014).

Comprehensive Supportive Care

Idiopathic pulmonary fibrosis and other forms of fibrosing interstitial lung disease (F-ILD) may induce relevant changes in patients' life and have a very great impact on the quality of life of patients and their caregivers. A comprehensive supportive care approach is required to achieve a strong partnership between patients, caregivers and the healthcare team. Patients' needs and wishes should be identified and the principal aim should be to help patients to maintain their quality of life at the highest level possible, to prevent or alleviate suffering, and ensure a dignified end of life.

As symptoms are the most determinants of patient's quality of life, a comprehensive care should encompass interventions aimed to deal with dyspnea, cough, and fatigue. Disease-related education, and emotional support should be included in the care plan, with timed discussions and implementation of end-of-life care, as the disease progresses (Wijsenbeek, 2019).

Dyspnoea Management

Dyspnea is a term used to characterize a subjective experience of breathing discomfort, and is usually the most important symptom of chronic respiratory diseases. Some disease-specific issues make the experience of breathlessness different in COPD and IPF. Breathlessness in COPD develops gradually and patients adapt their everyday routines, often reducing overall daily life activities. Patients suffering from ILD/IPF reports higher impact of dyspnoea in limiting their activities, most frequently described as: "unsatisfactory inspiratory effort," "inspiratory difficulty,' "rapid breathing" (Parshall, 2012).

The patient's experience of breathlessness involve multiple physiological, psychological, and relational factors, and may induce secondary physiological and behavioural responses.

Pharmacological treatment of dyspnoea may include symptom relief with benzodiazepines and/or opioids, but possibly due to safety concerns, their use is limited in common clinical practice. However, no association between opioid use and either hospitalisation or mortality was found in a recent study of over 1600 patients with F-ILD with long term oxygen therapy, while benzodiazepines were associated with increased risk for hospitalisation only at higher doses (Bajwah, 2018).

Multidisciplinary interventions, first of them pulmonary rehabilitation, represent the most successful approaches to dyspnea management in ILD, addressing patients' physical, emotional and psychological needs. Maintaining the benefits of PR may be a challenge, and breathlessness services have been recently proposed in the long term management of F-ILD patients. Improved breathlessness mastery and a survival advantage was found in F-ILD patients with refractory breathlessness included in a six-months patient-centred programme combining multidisciplinary assessment and care (Higginson, 2014).

Cough Control

Cough is a common symptom in F-ILD, is reported by up to 87% of patients and may greatly affect patient QOL (van Manen, 2016). Gastro-oesophageal reflux is a frequent concomitant condition in patients with F-ILD, but the effect on cough of the anti-acid therapy is still debated. In IPF, pirfenidone has shown a positive effect on objective cough measurements and cough-related QOL (van Manen, 2017a). High dose corticosteroids have shown a positive effect of cough in ILD, but this practice may cause a potential harmful immunosuppression. Thalidomide showed a positive effect on patient-reported cough and cough-related QOL in patients with IPF, but further studies have not been conducted (Horton, 2012).

In patients with scleroderma-related lung disease, treatment with mycophenolate mofetil or oral cyclophosphamide was associated with a decrease in reported cough frequency, but neither had an effect on cough-related QOL (Tashkin, 2017).

Other drugs tested for cough treatment in F-ILD were inhaled sodium cromoglicate, and other drugs targeting the cough reflex (e.g., gabapentin, amitriptyline), but further confirmation studies are needed to support their wide clinical use (Wijsenbeek, 2019).

Disease Education and Psychosocial Support

Specialist ILD centres and ILD nurses usually have a relevant role as sources of information and patient support. Attending pulmonary rehabilitation programmes and meeting other patients has reported to be very helpful, through peer support groups, and online forums (van Manen, 2017b).

The main goals of comprehensive disease management programs for patients suffering from F-ILD include disease education and emotional support. Some trials are ongoing to evaluate long-term effects on well-being of patients and caregivers (Lindell, 2018).

Psychological Outcomes

A great part of people suffering from F-ILD reports anxiety and depression, although very few of them receive pharmacotherapy for this (Carvajalino, 2018). Whereas dyspnoea and cough may contribute to anxiety and depression, these mood alterations may themselves worsen dyspnoea and affect QOL (Holland, 2014).

Screening of emotional well-being and mood disturbance should be considered in the comprehensive management of patients with F-ILD, and regular re-assessment along the clinical course of the disease should be done, in order to include in the programme a dedicated psychological or pharmacological treatment. Cognitive behavioral psychological intervention has been shown to be beneficial, an improvement in anxiety and depression was observed in patients and care-givers participating in a palliative care programme which included comprehensive assessment, a care plan and a series of community case conferences (Heslop-Marshall, 2018; Bajwah, 2015).

Exacerbations of ILD

The ATS/ERS definition of acute exacerbation in IPF incorporates unexplained worsening of dyspnoea, evidence of hypoxaemia, new radiographic alveolar infiltrates, in the absence of an alternative diagnosis (Raghu, 2011). Although PR has been recommended after an acute exacerbation of COPD, no recommendation was given for patients with acute exacerbation of IPF (Bolton, 2013; Spruit, 2013). Recently, a large study including 21 ILD patients showed negative effects of exercise rehabilitation after an exacerbation of chronic respiratory disease (Greening, 2014). Further studies are needed to evaluate possible risks associated with exercise rehabilitation following an acute exacerbation of ILD. Early mobilization may help to improve autonomy in activties of daily life and promote earlier discharge from hospital, but we should be cautious in starting PR early after an IPF exacerbation.

Lung Transplantation

The worldwide frequency of the lung transplant procedure is around 4,000 cases per year, with 5-year survival rates ranging from 50 to 60%, and 10-year survival is around 30%. An increasing number of patients with F-ILD receive lung transplant during the course of the disease, and in the last ten years, IPF has become the most common indication for lung transplantation, accounting for a proportion of 49.6% of cases in 2015 (Yusen, 2014). The median survival of patients with ILD after lung transplant is 4.7 years, significantly lower than patients with chronic obstructive pulmonary disease (COPD) and cystic fibrosis (CF) (5.5 and 8.3 years, respectively) (Valapour, 2015). The trend in transplanting older patients may further increase in the future due to greater experience of transplant centers and the raising awareness of IPF patient advocacy groups, pointing out that age restrictions for lung transplantations actually exclude many healthy, viable patients (Bonella, 2016).

Some studies evaluating pulmonary rehabilitation effectiveness in lung transplant recipient suffering from F-ILD reported favourable outcomes in exercise capacity and

QOL. In a prospective study conducted in patients with baseline forced vital capacity (FVC) 49% ± 13% of predicted; 64.5% of patients successfully completed PR (31/48). A clinically relevant improvement in 6MWD (58 ± 63 m) and in several domains of the HRQL questionnaire was observed irrespectively from disease severity (FVC, DLCO, and dyspnea) and improvement in clinical outcomes (Kenn, 2015). Similar improvements in 6MWD and QOL were observed in another retrospective study, after a short-term comprehensive PR programme (de Fontoura, 2018). A large retrospective study analyzed PR outcomes of 722 pts after lung transplantation (389 ILD) included in a 6-week inpatient PR programme. All lung transplant (LTx) patients achieved clinically relevant improvement in exercise capacity and QOL after an inpatient PR programme performed within 1 year after transplant. PR outcomes were similar, irrespective of diagnosis and both aftersingle or double LTx (Schneeberger, 2017).

Conclusion

Clinically relevant improvements in exercise capacity, symptoms and QOL have been observed in F-ILD of different aetiologies following pulmonary rehabilitation, as well as after lung transplantation. Although PR should be considered an important part of comprehensive care, current evidence does not suggest that impacts on patient's prognosis. Exercise training is a key component of PR for ILD and should include endurance and resistance training.

Other components may include education, psychological support, dyspnoea and cough management, education to ambulatory oxygen and self-care plan. Given the positive impact of PR on patient-centred outcomes, irrespective of disease severity, efforts should be made to increase the accessibility of symptomatic ILD patients to PR programmes.

References

Agusti AG, et al. 1991. "Mechanisms of gas-exchange impairment in idiopathic pulmonary fibrosis." *Am Rev Respir Dis*; 143:219-225.

Bajwah S, et al. 2015. "Palliative care for patients with advanced fibrotic lung disease: a randomised controlled phase II and feasibility trial of a community case conference intervention." *Thorax;* 70(9):830-9.

Bajwah S, et al. 2018. "Safety of benzodiazepines and opioids in interstitial lung disease: a national prospective study." *Eur Respir J;* 52(6). pii:1801278.

Bonella F, et al. *2016.* "European IPF Patient Charter: unmet needs and a call to action for healthcare policymakers." *Eur Respir J; 47(2):597-606.*

Burdon JG, et al. 1983. "Pattern of breathing during exercise in patients with interstitial lung disease." *Thorax*; 38(10):778-84.

Carvajalino S, et al. 2018. Symptom prevalence of patients with fibrotic interstitial lung disease: a systematic literature review. *BMC Pulm Med;* 18(1):78.

Corte TJ, et al. 2012. Elevated nocturnal desaturation index predicts mortality in interstitial lung disease. *Sarcoidosis Vasc Diffuse Lung Dis;* 29(1):41-50.

da Fontoura FF, et al. 2018. "Pulmonary Rehabilitation in Patients With Advanced Idiopathic Pulmonary Fibrosis Referred for Lung Transplantation." *Journal of Cardiopulmonary Rehabilitation and Prevention;* 38(2):131–134.

Dowman L, et al. 2014. "Pulmonary rehabilitation for interstitial lung disease." *Cochrane Database Syst Rev*; 10:CD006322.

Dowman L, et al. 2017 "Greater endurance capacity and improved dyspnoea with acute oxygen supplementation in idiopathic pulmonary fibrosis patients without resting hypoxaemia." *Respirology;* 22:957–964.

Dowman L, et al. 2017. "The evidence of benefits of exercise training in interstitial lung disease: a randomised controlled trial." *Thorax;* 72(7):610-9.

Fell CD, et al. 2009. "The prognostic value of cardiopulmonary exercise testing in idiopathic pulmonary fibrosis." *Am J Respir Crit Care Med*; 179:402-407.

Garber CE, et al. 2011. American College of Sports Medicine position stand. Quantity and quality of exercise for developing and maintaining cardiorespiratory, musculoskeletal, and neuromotor fitness in apparently healthy adults: guidance for prescribing exercise. *Med Sci Sports Exerc;* 43:1334–59.

Gläser S, et al. 2009. "Impact of pulmonary hypertension on gas exchange and exercise capacity in patients with pulmonary fibrosis. *Respir Med*; 103(2):317-24.

Greening N, et al. (2014) An early rehabilitation intervention to enhance recovery during hospital admission for an exacerbation of chronic respiratory disease: randomised controlled trial. *Brit Med J* 349: g4315.

Hansen JE, and Wasserman K. 1996. "Pathophysiology of activity limitation in patients with interstitial lung disease." *Chest*; 109(6):1566-76.

Heslop-Marshall K, et al. 2018. "Randomised controlled trial of cognitive behavioural therapy in COPD." *ERJ Open Res;* 4(4). pii: 00094-2018.

Higginson IJ, et al. 2014. "An integrated palliative and respiratory care service for patients with advanced disease and refractory breathlessness: a randomised controlled trial." *Lancet Respir Med;* 2(12):979-87.

Holland AE, et al. 2014. "Dyspnoea and comorbidity contribute to anxiety and depression in interstitial lung disease." *Respirology;* 19(8):1215-21.

Holland, AE, et al. 2012. "Predictors of benefit following pulmonary rehabilitation for interstitial lung disease." *Respir Med;* 106:429–435.

Holland, AE, et al. 2015. "Principles of rehabilitation and reactivation: interstitial lung disease, sarcoidosis and rheumatoid disease with respiratory involvement." *Respiration*; 89:89–99.

Holland, AE. 2010. "Exercise limitation in interstitial lung disease - mechanisms, significance and therapeutic options." *Chron Respir Dis*; 7(2):101-11

Horton MR, et al. 2012. "Thalidomide for the treatment of cough in idiopathic pulmonary fibrosis: a randomized trial." *Ann Intern Med;* 157(6):398-406.

Jo HE, et al. 2017. "Treatment of idiopathic pulmonary fibrosis in Australia and New Zealand: A position statement from the Thoracic Society of Australia and New Zealand and the Lung Foundation Australia." *Respirology;* 22(7):1436-58.

Kabitz HJ, et al. 2006. "Impact of impaired inspiratory muscle strength on dyspnea and walking capacity in sarcoidosis." *Chest*; 130:1496-1502.

Kenn K, et al. 2013. "Pulmonary rehabilitation in patients with idiopathic pulmonary fibrosis--a review." *Respiration*; 86(2):89-99.

Kenn, K, et al. 2015. "Predictors of success for pulmonary rehabilitation in patients awaiting lung transplantation." *Transplantation; 99(5):1072-7.*

Kozu, R, et al. 2011. "Differences in response to pulmonary rehabilitation in idiopathic pulmonary fibrosis and chronic obstructive pulmonary disease." *Respiration;* 81:196–205.

Lama VN, et al. 2003. "Prognostic value of desaturation during a 6-minute walk test in idiopathic interstitial pneumonia." *Am J Respir Crit Care Med*; 168:1084-1090.

Lederer DJ, et al. 2006. "Six-minute-walk distance predicts waiting list survival in idiopathic pulmonary fibrosis." *Am J Respir Crit Care Med*; 174:659-664.

Lindell KO, et al. 2018. "Randomised clinical trial of an early palliative care intervention (SUPPORT) for patients with idiopathic pulmonary fibrosis (IPF) and their caregivers: protocol and key design considerations." *BMJ Open Respir Res;* 5(1):e000272.

Marciniuk DD, et al. 1994. "Lung volumes and expiratory flow limitation during exercise in interstitial lung disease." *J Appl Physiol*; 77(2):963-973.

McDonald CF. 2018. "Exercise desaturation and oxygen therapy in ILD and COPD: Similarities, differences and therapeutic relevance." *Respirology*; 23(4):350-351.

Medical Research Council Working Party. 1981. "Long term domiciliary oxygen therapy in chronic hypoxic cor pulmonale complicating chronic bronchitis and emphysema." *Lancet;* 317(8222):681–686.

Nakazawa, A, et al. 2017. "Current best practice in rehabilitation in interstitial lung disease." *Ther Adv Respir Dis;* 11(2):115-128.

Nocturnal Oxygen Therapy Trial Group. 1981. "Continuous or Nocturnal Oxygen Therapy in Hypoxemic Chronic Obstructive Lung Disease: A Clinical Trial." *Ann Intern Med;* 93:391–398.

O'Donnell D, et al. 1988. "External mechanical loading in conscious humans: role of upper airway mechanoreceptors." *J Appl Physiol;65(2):541-8.*

Parshall MB, et al. 2012. "An official American Thoracic Society statement: update on the mechanisms, assessment, and management of dyspnea." *Am J Respir Crit Care Med;* 185(4):435-52.

Raghu G, et al. 2011. ATS/ERS/JRS/ALAT Committee on Idiopathic Pulmonary Fibrosis. An official ATS/ERS/JRS/ALAT statement: idiopathic pulmonary fibrosis: evidence-based guidelines for diagnosis and management. *Am J Respir Crit Care Med;* 183(6):788-824.

Risk C, et al. 1984."Exercise alveolararterial oxygen pressure difference in interstitial lung disease." *Chest*; 85:69-74.

Ryerson, C, et al. 2014 "Pulmonary rehabilitation improves long-term outcomes in interstitial lung disease: a prospective cohort study." *Respir Med;* 108:203–210.

Schaeffer MR, et al. 2017. "Effects of hyperoxia on dyspnoea and exercise endurance in fibrotic interstitial lung disease." *Eur Respir J.* 2017;49(5) pii:1602494.

Schiza S, et al. 2015. "Idiopathic pulmonary fibrosis and sleep disorders: no longer strangers in the night." *Eur Respir Re;* 24(136):327-39.

Schneeberger T, et al. 2017. "Pulmonary Rehabilitation Outcomes after Single or Double Lung Transplantation in Patients with Chronic Obstructive Pulmonary Disease or Interstitial Lung Disease." *Respiration;* 94(2):178-185.

Spagnolo P, et al. 2015. "Idiopathic pulmonary fibrosis: Recent advances on pharmacological therapy." *Pharmacol Ther*; 152:18-27.

Spruit MA, et al. 2005. "Skeletal muscle weakness in patients with sarcoidosis and its relationship with exercise intolerance and reduced health status." *Thorax*; 60:32-38.

Spruit MA, et al. 2013. ATS/ERS Task Force on Pulmonary Rehabilitation. An official American Thoracic Society/European Respiratory Society statement: key concepts and advances in pulmonary rehabilitation. *Am J Respir Crit Care Med*; 88(8):e13-64.

Sudduth CD, et al. 1993. "Failure of the circulatory system limits exercise performance in patients with systemic sclerosis." *Am J Med*; 95:413-418.

Swigris JJ, et al. 2011. "Benefits of pulmonary rehabilitation in idiopathic pulmonary fibrosis." *Respir Care*; 56(6):783-9.

Tashkin DP, et al. 2017. "Improved Cough and Cough-Specific Quality of Life in Patients Treated for Scleroderma-Related Interstitial Lung Disease: Results of Scleroderma Lung Study II." *Chest;* 151(4):813-20.

Troy LK, et al. 2016. "Exercise pathophysiology and the role of oxygen therapy in idiopathic interstitial pneumonia." *Respirology*; 21:1005–14.

Vainshelboim B, et al. 2017. "Supervised exercise training improves exercise cardiovascular function in idiopathic pulmonary fibrosis." *Eur J Phys Rehabil Med;* 53(2):209-218.

Vainshelboim B. 2016. "Exercise training in idiopathic pulmonary fibrosis: is it of benefit?" *Breathe (Sheff)*; 12(2):130-8.

Valapour M, et al. 2015. "OPTN/SRTR 2013 Annual Data Report: lung." *Am J Transplant. 2015 Jan; 15 Suppl 2():1-28.*

van Manen MJ, et al. 2016. "Cough in idiopathic pulmonary fibrosis." *Eur Respir Rev*; 25(141):278-86.

van Manen MJ, et al. 2017a. "Effect of pirfenidone on cough in patients with idiopathic pulmonary fibrosis." *Eur Respir J;* 50(4). pii: 1701157.

van Manen MJ, et al. 2017b. "What patients with pulmonary fibrosis and their partners think: a live, educative survey in the Netherlands and Germany." *ERJ Open Res;* 3(1). pii: 00065-2016.

Visca D, et al. 2018. "Effect of ambulatory oxygen on quality of life for patients with fibrotic lung disease (AmbOx): a prospective, open-label, mixed-method, crossover randomised controlled trial." *Lancet Respir Med;* 6(10):759-770.

Wijsenbeek M, et al. 2019. "Comprehensive supportive care for patients with fibrosing interstitial lung disease." *Am J Respir Crit Care Med;* 200(2):152-159.

Yusen RD, et al. *2014.* "The registry of the International Society for Heart and Lung Transplantation: thirty-first adult lung and heart-lung transplant report—2014." *J Heart Lung Transplant; 33(10):1009-24.*

In: Respiratory Ventilatory Strategies …
Editor: Antonio M. Esquinas
ISBN: 978-1-53617-847-0
© 2020 Nova Science Publishers, Inc.

Chapter 38

PULMONARY REHABILITATION IN IDIOPATHIC PULMONARY FIBROSIS. EVIDENCE-BASED GUIDELINES

Vânia Caldeira, MD
Pneumology Department, Hospital Santa Marta (CHLC),
Lisboa, Portugal

ABSTRACT

Pulmonary rehabilitation (PR) is a common practice in many respiratory diseases but most of the available evidence is limited to studies in Chronic Obstructive Pulmonary Disease (COPD) patients.

Thus, most centers have applied COPD programs to other respiratory diseases. Due to its different pathophysiology, as well as its rapid progression and poor prognosis, idiopathic pulmonary fibrosis (IPF) has a different evolution of COPD and certainly has different needs to a design of a PR program. Thus, the aim of this review was to gather some of the available evidence on the role of PR in IPF, its particularities and the impact of these studies on available guidelines.

Keywords: Pulmonary rehabilitation, IPF, guidelines, lung transplantation

MAIN TEXT

Pulmonary rehabilitation is widely recommended for patients with chronic lung diseases [1]. PR programs are a broad patient approach, which include aerobic conditioning, strength and flexibility training, educational lectures, nutritional interventions and psychological and social support. These interventions proved to be effective in reducing respiratory and non-respiratory symptoms (peripheral muscle fatigue), improving functional status and quality of life [2]. Besides optimizing functional capacity, PR also improves self-management of the disease [3].

Although the majority of evidence for PR comes from studies in COPD patients for whom PR have been widely assessed and validated [4], it could be expected that other patients diagnosed with respiratory disease with the same symptoms and functional limitations benefit from PR. Indeed, some of the mechanisms that cause the nuclear symptom of dyspnoea are common to IPF [5]. Both types of diseases share common clinical features, other than dyspnoea, like exercise intolerance, fatigue, persistent cough, low quality of life, anxiety and depression [3, 4].

However, while COPD patients are especially limited by impaired respiratory mechanics, hyperinflation and musculoskeletal dysfunction, in IPF patients, the impaired gas exchange is the major cause of exercise intolerance [1, 3]. Also, pulmonary hypertension is more commonly seen in IPF than in COPD and further impact on exercise tolerance [6]. Besides, the respiratory pathophysiology in IPF requires an increased breathing frequency, especially during physical activity, which leads to an unnecessary degree of hyperventilation in some patients, making strategies of breathing retraining central for them. Given the restrictive pattern of ventilation in this disease thoracic expansion exercises and stretching of the thoracic muscles may be also beneficial [3]. Finally, proper education about the disease, self-management plans, coping skills, strategies to control anxiety and end-of-life communication should be included in specific PR programs for IPF patients [3, 6].

In the natural evolution of interstitial lung diseases (ILDs), the patient's daily activities decline early following symptoms (shortness of breath, tiredness, muscle fatigue). With the progression of the disease and the escalation of respiratory functional restriction, there are additional physical and social limitations, which in turn have impact on quality of life [4]. The progressive course of disease also leads to premature disability and death, [3] being the optimal management of dyspnoea a central question in this group of patients [4].

In comparison with COPD, some studies showed that IPF patients had lower improvements in all outcome parameters [7]. However, this probably is the result of the absence of a specific program adapted for IPF characteristics. Further studies are needed to address which aims should be reached and which components should be included in an IPF-specific PR program [3, 6].

As a matter of fact, few trials have considered the real effect of PR in patients other than COPD. ILDs are a large group of restrictive diseases with different presentation and prognosis. Particularly, IPF is usually associated with progressive clinical and physiological deterioration over 6 - 12 months causing important desaturation on exercise [5].

Among the difficulties of implementing a PR program for IPF there are the lack of evidence for diseases other than COPD, the wide individual variation and the rapid progression of the disease with clinical deterioration, which makes it redundant in some patients (over the best supportive therapy and palliative care) [5]. Besides, the heterogeneous course of the disease in respect to progression, response to therapy and prognosis, also makes it difficult to decide the optimal timing for PR [3].

In the last years some trials had focused on the effect of PR in ILDs (and particularly IPF), the majority of them, uncontrolled studies and a pair of controlled trials [2, 6]. Most of the works published have small sample of patients, and there are large variations in scientific quality, local of PR (inpatient or outpatient), duration (6 - 12 weeks) and the training regimens [3].

The majority of studies showed improvements in walking distance on a 6-meter-walking test (6MWT) and in quality of life, but also demonstrate a loss of sustained benefit after 6 months [5], while in COPD the benefits can be maintained for up to 12 - 18 months [3]. In relation with this, the duration of PR programs seems to be a central question, and some authors propose to extend the PR program to 24 weeks [3].

Probably, the first and most important finding is that PR is safe and feasible in this group of patients, with no exercise-related adverse effects mentioned in any study [3, 5]. Tonelli and colleagues [4] concluded that patients with ILDs are likely to have benefit from PR in terms of exercise performance, symptoms and quality of life. ILD patients of different nature and severity could equally have gains with PR and the cause of fibrotic lung does not impact the positive effect of PR. On the contrary, in a systematic review, Holland et al. [8] showed that patients with IPF have lower improvement in functional capacity following PR in contrast with other forms of ILDs. On the other hand, Huppmann and colleagues [1] suggested that PR not only improve functional status and quality of life, but also improve lung function parameters.

In the majority of studies, benefits of PR seem to be greater in earlier stages of IPF with lower lung derangement, less desaturation and less severe pulmonary hypertension [4]. However, the studies of Ryerson [9], Tonelli [4] and Huppmann [1] suggested that patients with a lower baseline 6MWD and higher levels of dyspnoea could have larger improvement with PR.

Currently available pharmacological antifibrotic therapies (nintedanib,pirfenidone) are expected to slow disease progression and physical deterioration. In this sense, studies on the role of PR in patients under antifibrotic treatment are essential to give the best care possible for the patient in a progressive, severe and fatal disease [3].

Lung transplantation (LT) is also a viable treatment option in end-stage lung disease [3, 10]. As many patients with IPF are listing for LT, it is important to assure on-going support for exercise whilst on the waiting list [6]. Due to its rapid progressive nature and low survival, a transplant discussion with IPF patients is recommended from the moment that diagnosis be confirmed. PR programs play an essential role in LT candidates and recipients, improving physical function before surgery and facilitating post-LT recovery [11].

Usually, candidates for LT are markedly inactive in daily life in relation with peripheral muscle dysfunction and limitative symptoms like dyspnoea. Since impaired exercise capacity is a predictor of thoracic surgery outcome, PR prior to LT might maintain or optimize the functional status of patients before surgery, but also provide useful information about the upcoming surgery, potential complications and future management of care and medication [10]. In this period, patients could benefit from exercise training, aerobic, resistance and flexibility and oxygen supplementation should be considered [11]. Li and colleagues [12] showed a relation between an increase in 6MWD and a decrease in length of hospital stay. Florian and colleagues [13] found that a complete PR program pre-LT improved survival after unilateral LT in IPF patients, halving the risk of death after the surgery and reducing the time on invasive mechanical ventilation and the length of stay.

Despite near-normal lung function after surgery, many patients maintain exercise intolerance and decreasing quality of life in relation to limb muscle dysfunction, prolonged inactivity and nutritional depletion. To this problem, also contribute the extended hospital stay, immunosuppressive therapy and corticosteroids. To avoid these deleterious effects, PR seems essential. After LT, an early mobility is increasingly advised, even in the ICU, to prevent ICU-acquired weakness and its complications [10]. After ICU discharge, the aim is an increasing progression to independent function, with balance training, aerobic, resistance and flexibility exercises [11]. Increased activity after LT might improve exercise capacity and prevent frequent comorbidities after LT, such as osteoporosis, muscle dysfunction, metabolic and cardiovascular disorders [10].

As a result of the small available evidence, the guidelines are scarce in this matter. On the one hand, the ATS/ERS official statement on IPF [2] still provides a weak recommendation for PR. The expert panel advises that the majority of patients with IPF should be treated with PR, since it improves functional status and patient-centred outcome.

In the same document, it is highlighted that there is still uncertainty regarding duration of benefit and that a minority of patients will not benefit from this therapy and should instead have the best supportive care.

On the other hand, the BTS guideline about PR in adults [5] stated that patients with ILD benefit from PR and exercise training with improvements in capacity to exercise and quality of life, even though the gains are not sustainable over 6 months. This guideline also highlights the importance of exercising and maintaining an active life in disease management.

Although pre- and post-LT PR is a common practice in the majority of LT centers, there are currently no clinical practice guidelines with a tailored program for this special population [10, 11].

In conclusion, there is a growing body of evidence to support PR in patients with ILD, particularly in IPF. However, the results show positive short-term effects and most recent guidelines still provide a weak recommendation for PR in this group of patients. Besides, there is a lack of tailored PR programs for the specific needs of IPF patients, which could be the cause for the absence of benefit in some patients.

Further studies are needed, to address if there is a need for a standardized referentiation for PR programs, which is the optimal timing and duration of the program and what a specific IPF-PR program should be like.

Key Messages

- PR is a well-documented intervention in COPD, however, in IPF there are few studies of poor quality.
- Overall, most studies show that PR improves functional status and quality of life of IPF patients and increases survival after lung transplantation.
- The available guidelines attribute a weak recommendation to PR in IPF, but emphasizing that it may bring benefits to these patients.
- Further studies are needed to evaluate the role of PR in IPF and what a specific PR program should be for these specific patients.

References

[1] Huppmann, P. et al. 2013. "Effects of inpatient pulmonary rehabilitation in patients with interstitial lung disease". *Eur. Respir. J.,* 42:444 - 453.

[2] Raghu, G. et al. 2011. "An Official ATS/ERS/JRS/ALAT Statement: Idiopathic Pulmonary Fibrosis: Evidence-based Guidelines for Diagnosis and Management". *Am. J. Respir. Crit. Care Med.,* 183:788 - 824.

[3] Kenn, K. et al. 2013. "Pulmonary Rehabilitation in patients with Idiopathic Pulmonary Fibrosis – a review". *Respiration,* 86:89 - 99.

[4] Tonelli, R. et al. 2017. "Effectiveness of pulmonary rehabilitation in patients with interstitial lung disease of different etiology: a multicentre prospective study". *BMC Pulmonary Medicine,* 17:130.

[5] Bolton, C. et al. 2013. "British Thoracic Society guideline on pulmonary rehabilitation in adults". *Thorax,* 68:1 - 30.

[6] Holland, A. et al. 2013. "How to adapt the pulmonary rehabilitation programme to patients with chronic respiratory disease other than COPD". *Eur. Respir. Rev.,* 22:577 - 586.

[7] Kozu, R. et al. 2011. "Differences in response to pulmonary rehabilitation in idiopathic pulmonary fibrosis and chronic obstructive pulmonary disease". *Respiration,* 81:196 - 205.

[8] Holland, A. et al. 2008. "Physical training for interstitial lung disease". *Cochrane Database Syst. Rev.*, 4:CD006322.

[9] Ryerson, C. et al. 2014. "Pulmonary rehabilitation improves long-term outcomes in interstitial lung disease: a prospective cohort study". *Respir. Med.,* 108:203 - 210.

[10] Langer, D. 2015. "Rehabilitation in patients before and after lung transplantation". *Respiration,* 89:353 - 362.

[11] Wickerson, L. et al. 2016. "Physical rehabilitation for lung transplant candidates and recipients: an evidence-informed clinical approach". *World J. Transplant.,* 24:517 - 531.

[12] Li, M. et al. 2013. "Pulmonary rehabilitation in lung transplant candidates". *The Journal of Heart and Lung Transplantation,* 32:626 - 632.

[13] Florian, J. et al. 2019. "Pulmonary rehabilitation improves survival in patients with idiopathic pulmonary fibrosis undergoing lung transplantation". *Scientific Reports,* 9:9347. Accessed September 2019. doi: 10.1038/s41598-019-45828-2.

In: Respiratory Ventilatory Strategies …
Editor: Antonio M. Esquinas
ISBN: 978-1-53617-847-0
© 2020 Nova Science Publishers, Inc.

Chapter 39

PSYCHIATRIC AND PSYCHOLOGICAL DISORDERS IN IDIOPATHIC PULMONARY FIBROSIS

Rafael Soler**, MD
Department of Neurology, University Hospital, Melilla, Spain

ABSTRACT

Psychiatric and psychological disorders are very common in idiopathic pulmonary fibrosis. Although this topic is well-known among chronic lung diseases, specific reviews about patients suffering from idiopathic pulmonary fibrosis, are no very frequent.

The present analyses were performed to review the main diagnostic and therapeutic approaches in our patient population. Our final aim is to provide a better quality of life to our patients and it´s possible with current tools. However, further investigations are needed to in this area.

Keywords: idiopathic pulmonary fibrosis, anxiety, depression, psychological stress, psychiatric disorders

INTRODUCTION

Idiopathic pulmonary fibrosis (IPF) is a severe and chronic progressive lung disorder, of unknown cause, usually affecting adults, and limited to the lungs. It has been associated with a histopathologic and/or radiologic pattern of usual interstitial pneumonia [1].

* Corresponding Author's E-mail: rafael_soler_gonzalez@yahoo.es.

The prognosis is very poor, with a mean survival of about 2.5–5 years after definite diagnosis, but the median survival is under 3 years. Its prognosis can be worse than for many cancers, so it´s not accurate to refer to IPF as a benign disease [1].

The natural history is highly variable, so it´s not easy to predict the course of the disease for each individual patient. Sometimes patients progress slowly, sometimes experience a very quickly decline, while other patients suffer from acute deteriorations, that alternate with long periods of relative stability. However, it´s common to all type of patients, a serious fact: once an acute exacerbation occurs, recovery is extremely difficult.

The initial stages involve chronic inflammation; therefore, corticosteroids and other drugs that have anti-inflammatory and immunosuppressive actions were used. For a long time, it´s has been thought that this inflammation was the only cause of persistent fibrosis. However, the role of inflammation has been reviewed, paying special attention to the abnormal repair of alveolar epithelial injury, as the main reason for persistent fibrosis. This fact becomes the principal concern of disease management. So, pirfenidone, nintedanib and other antifibrotic agents have taken a very important role, and recently, we have observed how the use of agents targeting persistent fibrosis is increasing. Unfortunately, these drugs prevent deterioration but do not improve the disease, and other similar drugs were shown to be not efficacious [1].

Non-pharmacologic approaches are also very important: long-term oxygen therapy, pulmonary rehabilitation, and lung transplantation must be considered as additional treatment modalities, apart besides pharmacologic options.

Maybe, the final endpoint must be not only to reduce mortality. If we study how to keep and increase respiratory function and exercise tolerance, perhaps, in a second stage, we can improve mortality and final prognosis. In this way, forced vital capacity has often been used as the main end point in recent clinical studies.

Co-morbidities and multi-morbidity is very common in the older population, but not only [2].

We know very well some of these co-morbidities [2] such as: gastro-oesophageal reflux, pulmonary hypertension, chronic obstructive pulmonary disease, emphysema and obstructive sleep apnea, among others. Although treatment options in IPF are very limited, the study of co-morbidities and their treatments may improve the clinical disease course. Identification and treatment of co-morbidities is very important, in order to achieve quality of life in these patients. Eventually we can modify the outcome and the global survival, using a multimodal strategy. Actually, it is essential to understand not only the comorbidities, but also the specific approach in each individual case, paying special attention to the most prevalent conditions, but not underestimating the others.

Although comorbid conditions are well known in this population, electronic medical record data report lower prevalence when compared to prospective cohort studies. Among these conditions, psychological and psychiatric ones are specially underestimated.

Obviously, our final aim is to modify the clinical outcome in this patient population.

Depression is twice as likely, to develop in patients with chronic disease than in general population. Recent studies show an increasing incidence of depressive symptoms in patients with idiopathic pulmonary fibrosis, although we need more evidence.

We have studies about how psychological factors affect the health-related quality of life (HRQOL) or health status (HS) in chronic obstructive pulmonary disease patients, but this information is very limited for idiopathic pulmonary fibrosis patients. We need to use more psychological endpoints in research and clinical practice in this type of patients.

The health-related quality of life is one of the more important outcomes if we need to measure the effectiveness of therapeutic interventions in pulmonary disorders. However, whether or not psychological factors such as depression independently affect the HRQOL in patients with IPF remains unclear.

Recent studies have used the Japanese version of the Hospital and Anxiety Depression Scale, for psychological evaluation [3]. This test is reliable, valid, and useful as a screening tool for both anxiety and depression. This scale consists of 14 items, 7 of which comprise the anxiety subscale and another 7 of which comprise the depression subscale. These studies confirmed that the management of depression may improve the health-related quality of life in idiopathic pulmonary patients.

In order to diagnose psychiatric disorders, we need to perform structured interviews using the Diagnostic and Statistical Manual of Mental Disorder, 5th edition (DSM-V) criteria. The screening and management of depression should be considered clinically important in this population, even if their pulmonary function impairment is mild.

Even under conditions of mild-to-moderate pulmonary function impairment, anxiety and depressive symptoms were present in patients who were newly diagnosed.

Most of studies show that depression is very common in individuals.

Depression should be routinely screened in this type of patients. If we offer an appropriate supportive disease management, including antidepressants, psychological counseling, and pulmonary rehabilitation, the quality of life and the final outcome can improve.

Dyspnea is associated with depression in IPF subjects. Variables such as dyspnea, depression, and the health status are correlated with each other. So, we have an important problem to study the causality. We need to determine many confounding factors and it´s not simple. We can also assert that "depression symptoms" behave as an independent predictor for the health.

The etiology of the association between depression and idiopathic pulmonary fibrosis is not fully understood and it is not as obvious as we believe.

Physiological deregulation (activation of the sympathetic nervous system and hypothalamic-pituitary-adrenal axis) induced by chronic psychological stress may weaken the immune function and vulnerability to respiratory infection, in other pulmonary disorders. Biological changes induced by depression are speculated to be a potential pathway underlying the relationship between depression and respiratory exacerbations.

However, the exact mechanisms which relate idiopathic pulmonary fibrosis and the long-term impact of depression on this population have not been identified.

Not only depression and anxiety have been reported in these patients. Other psychiatric comorbidities affect this population, for example, bipolar affective disorders [4]. This is a very interesting association, because genetic factors are important both in bipolar patients and in pulmonary fibrosis.

However, as we have said previously, anxiety and depression are co-morbidities commonly find in patients with interstitial lung diseases including IPF [5]. Actually, both are the most frequent conditions among psychological disorders in IPF population. The prevalence of anxiety ranges from 30–50% while the prevalence of depression from 20–30. Obviously dyspnea and progression of the disease are aggravating factors. Also, it has a great impact on the quality of life of those patients [Figure 1].

Dyspnea is a major contributor for both anxiety and depression. There is still some doubt about the directionality of this relationship, between IPF and symptoms of anxiety and depression. However, it´s clear that the need for pharmacological or behavioral therapy must be detected early and assessed individually, in order to improve global management of patient's IPF and quality of life.

Depression is a well-known co-morbidity in these patients and carries enormous global morbidity and is about 2 times likelier to occur in individuals with chronic illness than in the general population. IPF has a severe impact on quality of life. The prevalence of depression in this group is therefore of paramount interest. A prospective study [6] was performed in Scotland, using the Wakefield Self-assessment of Depression Inventory (scores ≥15 denote a depressed state). Pulmonary function tests were measured to correlate disease severity with depression scores. More than fifty percent patients had significant depressive symptoms scoring ≥15; but only ten percent of them were taking antidepressant medication and receiving specific treatment. So, after IPF diagnosis, we must not only treat the lung disease but other comorbidities such depression should be actively screened in patients with IPF.

Also female patients were found to be more depressed than male patients, though this was not statistically significant [6], [Figure 2]. Statistically significant negative correlations were found between depression scores and gas transfer factor measurements, FEV1 and FVC. There was also no significant correlation between depression score and duration since diagnosis, age and number of co-morbidities.

Many studies show that Depression is under-recognized in the IPF patient population [7]. In some cohorts, depression prevalence was under 5%, but after exploring comorbidity by the mean of accurate tests, the prevalence range was between 25% and 50%. Unlike depression in general population, depression among IPF patients is equally common in women and men. Further, these symptoms appear to persist over time.

Independent predictors of depression included dyspnea, pain, sleep quality and decreased FVC. There are no IPF-specific screening tools for depression, but in general, the threshold to screen patients for depression should be low. Increased attention to screen for the presence of depression in this patient population is needed, given its impact on QOL for the patient. Treatment includes pharmacotherapy with anti-depressants, cognitive behavioral therapy and other adjunctive treatments. Moreover, as the relationship between degree of dyspnea and depression severity is fully accepted, the specific management of dyspnea may improve depression in these patients. Also pulmonary rehabilitation is very useful and has influence in depressive symptoms.

The effective management of depression may improve the HRQOL in IPF patients [8]. Depression symptoms act as an independent predictor for the health status, in addition to dyspnea and exercise impairment. The etiology of the association between depression and IPF is still not fully understood. Physiological deregulation induced by chronic psychological stress may weaken the immune function and vulnerability to respiratory infection, as we commented previously. In COPD patients, the potential pathway is not the same. However, the exact mechanisms linking IPF with depression and the long-term impact of depression on IPF have not been identified.

Although relationship between chronic lung diseases and psychiatric disorders are widely studied, the complex interplay between psychiatric issues and pulmonary diseases, usually are not well defined, including for all the chronic diseases, but few specific studies about IPF have been performed so far [9]. Usually, the studies involve all the pulmonary spectrum diseases, including chronic obstructive pulmonary disease, asthma, restrictive lung disease, and cystic fibrosis.

Cognitive impairment probably is underestimated [10] and it´s due to many reasons specially not being the usual main endpoint. Results from a recent study show that neuropsychological problems are linked to IPF, proportional to severity scale [10]. In this study, participants completed five neuropsychological tests: Trail Making Test (TMT) A and B, Stroop Color Word (1, 2, 3), Hopkins Verbal Learning, Boston Naming and Grooved Pegboard tests, additionally, the short form-36 and Beck Depression Index. Controlling for gender and age, the severe group had a significantly longer mean TMT B time (69.4, 135.9 seconds) than the mild group and the control group, suggesting inferior performance on tasks requiring speed divided attention. In addition, the severe group had a significantly lower number of correctly identified colors in the Stroop 3 test, suggesting slower processing speeds when requiring suppression of a familiar response. Patient subgroup with severe IPF had worse cognitive function than mild IPF or control subjects. Although further research is needed to explain these findings, it seems there is a linear correlation between IPF severity and cognitive decline.

Sleep quality and associate daytime consequences need to be described in idiopathic pulmonary fibrosis, although sleep disorders are usually related to neurologic diseases (we recommend you to review the specific chapter in this book), we see in clinical practice that are more frequently associated with psychiatric items than neurological ones. In an interesting study, patients suffering from IPF were examined [11]. Sleep quality and its daytime consequences were assessed by clinical interview, the Pittsburgh Sleep Quality Index (PSQI), the Functional Outcomes in Sleep Questionnaire (FOSQ), the Fatigue Severity Scale (FSS), the Epworth Sleepiness Scale and attended all-night polysomnography (PSG). PSG revealed a decrease in sleep efficiency and slow wave sleep, and an increase in stage 1 sleep and arousal index in IPF patients compared to controls. Daytime tachypnea persisted during sleep. Quality of sleep and daytime function were moderately to significantly deteriorated, based on the PSQI and FOSQ. These data suggest significant sleep disruption and impairment of physical and social functioning in these patients. Decrease in REM sleep, marked sleep fragmentation and nocturnal hypoxemia are common in IPF. Nocturnal hypoxemia and its negative impact on health-related quality also contribute to psychological status. This study [11] confirms that sleep disturbances in IPF are different, compared to other interstitial lung diseases. For example, significant sleep disruption was observed in IPF patients, with alterations in sleep macro-architecture (decrease in stage 1 and slow wave sleep) and micro-architecture (sleep fragmentation due to an increased arousal index). An interesting feature was the sleep breathing pattern of these patients, namely the maintenance of daytime tachypnea during sleep. This finding was observed in all patients, independently of disease severity. Normal sleep is associated with a reduction in minute ventilation due to a decrease in the tidal volume and respiratory frequency. The maintenance of increased respiratory rate during sleep in IPF patients suggested that reflexes causing the rapid shallow breathing during wakefulness are active during the sleep phase as well.

Nocturnal hypoxemia parameters (mean oxygen saturation and TST % with oxygen saturation below 90%) showed a significant correlation with FSS scores. Daytime fatigue was the most common and probably the most disabling clinical symptom in our patients. Nocturnal hypoxemia and alterations in sleep macro- and micro-architecture might represent two crucial etiologic factors for daytime fatigue.

Based on these features, nocturnal hypoxemia appears to be associated with a reduction in energy levels and impairment of social and physical functioning. A 'poor' sleep quality and its consequences in daytime function and overall quality of life may be markedly under-diagnosed in IPF patients. The early recognition and treatment of sleep disturbances in these patients might be a primary goal since there is no effective treatment for IPF so far. This objective contributes to improve the final psychological status in our IPF patients, are necessary both pharmacologic and behavioral treatment. In addition the observed association between nocturnal oxygen de-saturation parameters and daytime functional and social factors may support the recommendation of supplemental oxygen during sleep in IPF patients.

In fact, sleep is reported to be markedly disturbed in patients with IPF [12]. The possible lack of body and brain recovery during sleep in patients with IPF might be related to the negative consequences of the disease that take place both during wakefulness and during sleep time. Moderate-to-severe obstructive sleep apnea (OSA) syndrome, defined by an apnea–hypopnea index (AHI) > 15 events per hour, is frequent in patients with IPF. Moreover, although the increase of central respiratory drive in IPF is thought to be a protective factor for the development of sleep disorders, OSA has been recognized as an important, high-prevalence co-morbidity in the latest official guidelines for the diagnosis and management of IPF. There is a positive correlation between the AHI and body mass index values. REM AHI and total AHI were negatively correlated with FEV1 and FVC percentages. Most studies agreed on the finding of disturbance of sleep architecture. The abnormal sleep macro-architecture in patients with IPF is characterized by abnormal sleep stage distribution with reduced slow-wave and REM sleep, increased stage 1 sleep, multiple awakenings, decreased percentage of total sleep time, low sleep efficiency, and increased wake time after sleep onset. These patients also have an altered micro-architecture, as they present with an increased number of sleep micro-arousals resulting in sleep fragmentation. Therefore, these disorders in sleep architecture and the resulting poor quality of sleep impair the quality of life in patients. Another issue to take into account is that IPF patients present an altered sleep breathing pattern. IPF patients exhibit an increased respiratory frequency during wakefulness that persists during sleep. In conclusion, alterations in sleep architecture, breathing pattern, and de-saturations in IPF patients, especially during REM sleep, as well as coexisting OSA, might have a significant negative impact on the sleep quality of these patients. Physicians should ask the patient for symptoms during the night and should maintain a high degree of clinical suspicion for the presence of possible comorbid sleep disorders. As IPF is a progressive and life-threatening disease, the role of the poor quality of sleep as a significant comorbidity must be reconsidered. The effective treatment of co-morbidities in IPF patients, such as sleep disorders, should be a field of future research. All these sleep disturbances have a great impact on individual´s psychological status and can cause anxiety and mood disorders. In the other hand, anxiety and depression impair affect in sleep quality. So, both factors are intimately related. In this way, it´s worth checking sleep status in these patients, and, on the other way, testing psychological situation.

Apart from pharmacological approaches, obviously, educational and psychotherapeutic protocols seem to be useful in this special population. To empower psychological status in these patients is very important, as we fight against a quickly progressive, deadly disease with a devastating impact on patients and their partners' quality of life (QoL). Although we know, through many studies, the need for support groups, better information resources and disease education in IPF, few studies currently exist concerning interventions that can fulfill them and possibly improve QoL for patients and their partners. In a Dutch study [12], a short multidisciplinary empowerment program on the QoL for patients with IPF and their partners, was evaluated. A multidisciplinary team, led by an expertise psychologist and composed by a pneumologist, a specialised interstitial lung disease nurse, an oxygen supplier, a social worker and physiotherapists, had the responsibility for this aim. Patients were divided in groups, depending on severity. The study had three arms (two groups according the severity, and one placebo group). Previously, patients were asked to fill in some questionnaires at baseline, after 3 weeks and after 3 months. All participants filled in the Hospital Anxiety and Depression Scale (HADS), Perceived Stress Scale (PSS) and a knowledge quiz about IPF. Furthermore, patients completed the King's Brief Interstitial Lung Disease health status questionnaire (K-BILD), the Euroqol5D5L (EQ5D5L) and the Medical Research Council (MRC) dyspnea scale, while their partners completed the Carer Quality of Life instrument (CarerQoL). We also asked participants to complete an evaluation form after PPEPP. Questionnaire scores significantly improved after 3 weeks of PPEPP in the intervention group only. After a 3-month follow-up, no significant changes in questionnaire scores compared. This study showed that a short multidisciplinary empowerment program improved QoL for patients with IPF and their partners and demonstrated a positive effect on the wellbeing of patients and their partners.

Following the World Health Organization rules, control of psychiatric symptoms and psychological care is very important in any disorder, but specially in progressive and life threatening diseases, through the prevention and alleviation of suffering through the early identification and impeccable evaluation and treatment of pain and other physical, psychological and spiritual problem" [5]. It is evident that this is the situation of many patients affected by IPF, given the evolution and progression of this disease.

Depression and anxiety, related to the diagnosis and prognosis, is prevalent in patients with IPF. It has a significant impact on QOL. So, it is important to perform a psychological assessment regularly in these patients. Short-comings in the control of symptoms, psychological care and the planning of last wills are special items in this population. Effective communication is also crucial to assess and readjust patient's therapies throughout the whole process. All these actions must be integrated in a multidisciplinary care model. Its implementation empowers the patients not only to bear the disease, but to improve their quality of life. Although it´s not the main aim, this integral care model, in IPF patients, is associated with a decrease in the number of admissions, as well as in the consumption of health care resources. Patients are encouraged to deal with some difficult situations as: use of life-supporting interventions, the place to die. In conclusion, the early inclusion of patients with IPF in an advanced phase in a multidisciplinary care program helps to adequately control symptoms, psychological support and makes decisions regarding the end of life, with the aim of maintaining the quality of life during the whole process of the disease.

In a recent work [13], we can observe that anxiety and depression were not related to physiological parameters; however, dyspnea and a number of co-morbidities were important contributors. 21% of the patients had prolonged anxiety, of which 75% were not taking an anxiolytic medicine. There was no association between prolonged anxiety and mortality. However, prolonged anxiety was associated with more severe baseline dyspnea, supplemental oxygen use at baseline, suffering more co-morbidities and more severe baseline cough. There was no relationship with forced vital capacity (FVC) decline. Pharmacologic therapy for anxiety and depression was being received in only approximately a quarter of cases, suggesting a large proportion of them remain untreated. The strong relation seen between IPF symptoms and anxiety and depression, raises the question of the direction of that relationship. Whether the treatment of anxiety and depression might provide a route to the palliation of cough or dyspnea remains an important question to explore. Further research should examine the basis to prolonged anxiety and depression among sufferers of IPF. Any under recognition of anxiety and depression, or nihilism about their therapy should be addressed, given its strong linkage with IPF symptoms and health-related quality of life. Given the incomplete response of dyspnea and cough to current palliative approaches, these study´s findings suggest a further avenue for symptom control research via the treatment of anxiety and depression.

Therefore, management of depression may be critical in improving QOL in patients with IPF [3]. Some authors have suggested that treatment of depression in patients with ILD may improve not only mood, but also dyspnea. However, there is a poor compliance with prescribed medical treatments. Although neither depression nor anxiety exerted a significant influence on mortality or hospital admission rates, both depression and anxiety significantly influenced patient QOL.

In conclusion, psychiatric and psychological disorders are very common in idiopathic pulmonary fibrosis. Unfortunately, most of studies about psychiatric disorders in this type of patients are not focused in idiopathic pulmonary fibrosis, as they are referred to the pulmonary diseases as a global target.

What we now about IPF and psychiatric disorders is limited to a small number of well-designed studies. Although we have specific works about IPF and bipolar disorders, or cognitive impairment, or sleep disorders (related to psychiatric problems, as a causal relation), and others, most of studies are focused on depression and/or anxiety.

Unfortunately, although co-morbidities are well known in IPF [14], our knowledge about this spectrum of items is very limited. We know both anxiety and depression are prevalent and have an enormous impact on quality of life in this population, but further studies are required to determine whether psychological and pharmacological treatment for depression and/or anxiety can improve health outcomes such as QOL, mortality, hospitalization, and exacerbation of symptoms in patients with IPF.

It´s true that cognitive behavioral therapy and counseling by qualified healthcare professionals, and multidisciplinary teams, can modify some psychological aspects in these patients. It´s true that pharmacologic therapy can help to improve some psychological items, but we need further studies to investigate the effect of antidepressants and anxiolytic treatments on QOL and determine the prognostic significance of depression and anxiety in patients with IPF.

Finally, in spite of accumulated knowledge about this topic, we need specific tools for IPF patients, not only diagnostic, but therapeutic. We need to understand better the mechanisms of psychological disorders in these patients, and we need new approaches to these topics, not only to improve quality of life, but to improve prognosis.

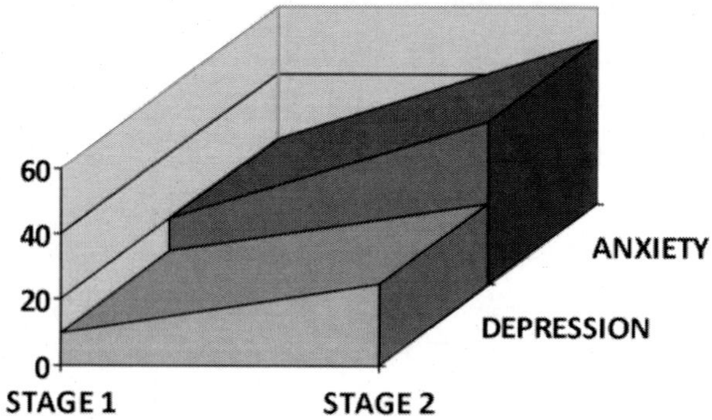

Own elaboration.

Figure 1. Prevalence of Anxiety and Depression in IPF: Increasing along the Natural Evolution.

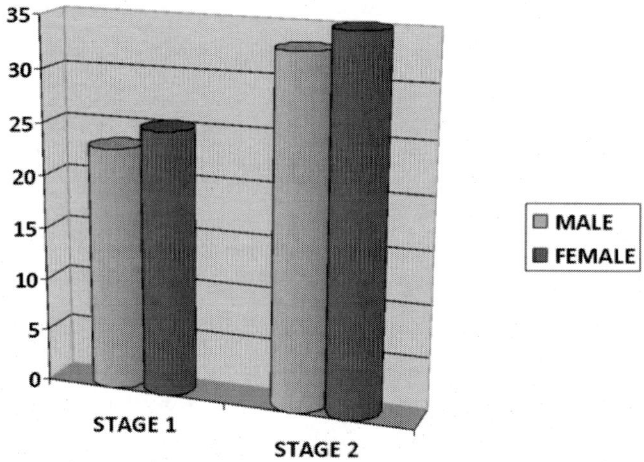

Own elaboration.

Figure 2. Prevalence of Psychiatric Disorders in IPF, Depending on Gender.

References

[1] Fujimoto et al. Idiopathic Pulmonary Fibrosis: Treatment and Prognosis. *Clinical Medicine Insights: Circulatory, Respiratory and Pulmonary Medicine* 2015:9(S1) 179-185 doi: 10.4137/CCRPM.S23321.

[2] Raghu G, Amatto V, Behr J, Stowasser S. Comorbidities in idiopathic pulmonary fibrosis patients: a systematic literature review. *Eur. Respir. J.* 2015; 46: 1113-1130 | doi: 10.1183/13993003.02316-2014.

[3] Matsuda T, Taniguchi H, Ando M, Kondoh Y, Kimura T, Kataoka K, Nishimura K, et al. Depression Is Significantly Associated with the Health Status in Patients with Idiopathic Pulmonary Fibrosis. *Intern. Med.* 56: 1637-1644, 2017.

[4] Bhandari S, Samellas D. Bipolar affective disorders and Idiopathic pulmonary fibrosis. *J. Clin. Psychiatry* 2001; 62 (7): 574-5.

[5] Millan-Billi P, Serra C, Alonso-León A, Castillo D. Comorbidities, Complications and Non-Pharmacologic Treatment in Idiopathic Pulmonary Fibrosis. *Med. Sci.* 2018, 6, 59.

[6] Akhtar AA, Ali MA, Smith RP. Depression in patients with idiopathic pulmonary fibrosis. *Chron. Respir. Dis.* 2013 Aug; 10(3):127-33.

[7] De Boer, K, Lee JS. Under-recognised co-morbidities in idiopathic pulmonary fibrosis: A review. *Respirology* (2016) 21, 995-1004.

[8] Glaspole IN, Watson AL, Allan H, et al. Determinants and outcomes of prolonged anxiety and depression in idiopathic pulmonary fibrosis. *Eur. Respir. J.* 2017; 50: 1700168.

[9] Jain A, Lolak S. Psychiatric aspects of chronic lung disease. *Curr. Psychiatry Rep. 2009* Jun; 11(3):219-25.

[10] Bors M, Tomic R, Perlman DM, Kim HJ, Whelan TP. Cognitive function in idiopathic pulmonary fibrosis. *Chron. Respir. Dis.* 2015; Nov; 12(4): 365-72.

[11] Mermigkis E, Stagaki A, Amfilochiou V, Polychronopoulos P, Korkonikitas D, Mermigkis M, et al. Sleep Quality and Associated Daytime Consequences in Patients with Idiopathic Pulmonary Fibrosis. *Med. Princ. Pract.* 2009; 18:10-15.

[12] Van Manen MJG, Van't Spijker A, Tak NC, et al. Patient and partner empowerment programme for idiopathic pulmonary fibrosis. *Eur. Respir. J.* 2017; 49: 1601596.

[13] Lee YJ, Choi SM, Lee YJ, Cho YJ, Yoon HI, Lee JH, et al. Clinical impact of depression and anxiety in patients with idiopathic pulmonary fibrosis. *PLoS ONE* (2017); 12(9): e0184300.

[14] Cano-Jiménez E, Hernández-González F, Bermudo-Peloche, G. Comorbidities and Complications in Idiopathic Pulmonary Fibrosis. *Med. Sci.* 2018, 6, 71.

In: Respiratory Ventilatory Strategies …
Editor: Antonio M. Esquinas
ISBN: 978-1-53617-847-0
© 2020 Nova Science Publishers, Inc.

Chapter 40

IDIOPATHIC PULMONARY FIBROSIS (IPF) AND EVIDENCE-BASED GUIDELINES

Mehmet Selim Comez*
MD, Anesthesiology and Reanimation Department,
Tayfur Ata Sökmen Faculty of Medicine,
Hatay Mustafa Kemal University,
Hatay, Turkey

ABSTRACT

Idiopathic pulmonary fibrosis (IPF) is defined as a specific form of chronic, progressive fibrosing interstitial pneumonia of unknown cause. The first guideline on IPF management, published in 2000, is based on the consensus of an international group of experts in the field. The guideline, created by hard work by the American Thoracic Society (ATS), European Respiratory Society (ERS), Japanese Respiratory Society (JRS), and Latin American Thoracic Society (ALAT) in 2011, reviewed all available evidence, clarified the definition of IPF, provided precise diagnostic criteria, described the natural course of the disease, and provided evidence-based recommendations for treatment.

In 2015, recommendations for the treatment of IPF were updated on the basis of new scientific evidence.

No pharmacological intervention has received strong recommendations for treatment. Clinicians should make individualized decisions based on conditional recommendations in the treatment of patients with IPF.

* Corresponding Author's E-mail: drmcomez313@gmail.com, phone: +090 506 509 09 53.

PURPOSE OF REVIEW

Idiopathic pulmonary fibrosis (IPF) is defined as a specific form of chronic, progressive fibrosing interstitial pneumonia of unknown cause, occurring primarily in older adults, and limited to the lungs. It is characterized by progressive worsening of dyspnea and lung function and is associated with a poor prognosis. Radiologic and/or histopathologic patterns are consistent with usual interstitial pneumonia (UIP) [1].Although the first guideline on management of IPF, published in 2000, was based on the consensus of a group of international experts in the field [2], the 2011 guideline represented a rigorous joint effort by the American Thoracic Society (ATS), European Respiratory Society (ERS), Japanese Respiratory Society (JRS), and Latin American Thoracic Society (ALAT).It reviewed all available evidence, clarified the definition of IPF, provided precise diagnostic criteria, described the natural course of the disease, and provided evidence-based recommendations for treatment [3]. The 2011 guideline also stated that updates would be provided based on pertinent new evidence [4]. Finally, in 2015, recommendations for the treatment of IPF were updated on the basis of new scientific evidence.The purpose of this chapter is to review the 2015 update of the guideline that allows for the inclusion of new evidence as possible, with periodic updates to guide clinical management based on the best available evidence.

RECENT FINDINGS

For the diagnosis and treatment sections in the guidelines, pragmatic GRADE evidence-based methodology was applied in a question-based format. For each diagnosis and treatment question, the committee graded the quality of the evidence available (high, moderate, low, or very low), and made a recommendation (yes or no, strong or weak) [3].

Diagnostic Criteria with 2015 Update

The diagnosis of IPF requires the following:

1. Exclusion of other known causes of interstitial lung disease (ILD) (e.g., domestic and occupational environmental exposures, connective tissue disease, and drug toxicity).
    - Question 1: Should BAL cellular analysis be performed in the diagnostic evaluation of suspected IPF?

Recommendation: BAL cellular analysis should not be performed in the diagnostic evaluation of IPF in the majority of patients, but may be appropriate in a minority (weak recommendation, low-quality evidence).

- Question 2: Should transbronchial lung biopsy be used in the evaluation of suspected IPF?
  Recommendation: Transbronchial biopsy should not be used in the evaluation of IPF in the majority of patients, but may be appropriate in a minority (weak recommendation, low-quality evidence).
- Question 3: Should serologic testing for connective tissues disease be used in the evaluation of suspected IPF?
  Recommendation: Serologic testing for connective tissue disease should be performed in the evaluation of IPF in the majority of patients, but may not be appropriate in a minority (weak recommendation, very low-quality evidence).
  Note: This recommendation places a high value on distinguishing connective tissue disease from IPF and low value on cost.
- Question 4: Should a multi-disciplinary discussion (MDD) be used in the evaluation of suspected IPF?
  Recommendation: The committee recommend that a multi-disciplinary discussion should be used in the evaluation of IPF (strong recommendation, low-quality evidence).

2. The presence of a UIP pattern on High- Resolution Computed Tomography (HRCT) in patients not subjected to surgical lung biopsy.
3. Specific combinations of HRCT and surgical lung biopsy pattern in patients subjected to surgical lung biopsy [4].

Thus, the accuracy of diagnosis of IPF increases with clinical, radiologic, and histopathologic correlation and can be accomplished with a multidisciplinary discussion among experienced clinical experts in the field of interstitial lung diseases (ILD) (Figure 1) [5].

TREATMENT

Pharmacological Therapies

- Question 1: Should patients with IPF be treated with corticosteroid monotherapy?Recommendation: The committee recommend that patients with

IPF should not be treated with corticosteroid monotherapy (strong recommendation, very low-quality evidence).
Note: The 2011 guideline

- Question 2: Should patients with IPF be treated with colchicine?
Recommendation: The committee recommend that patients with IPF should not be treated with colchicine (strong recommendation, very low-quality evidence).
Note: The 2011 guideline
- Question 3: Should patients with IPF be treated with cyclosporin A?

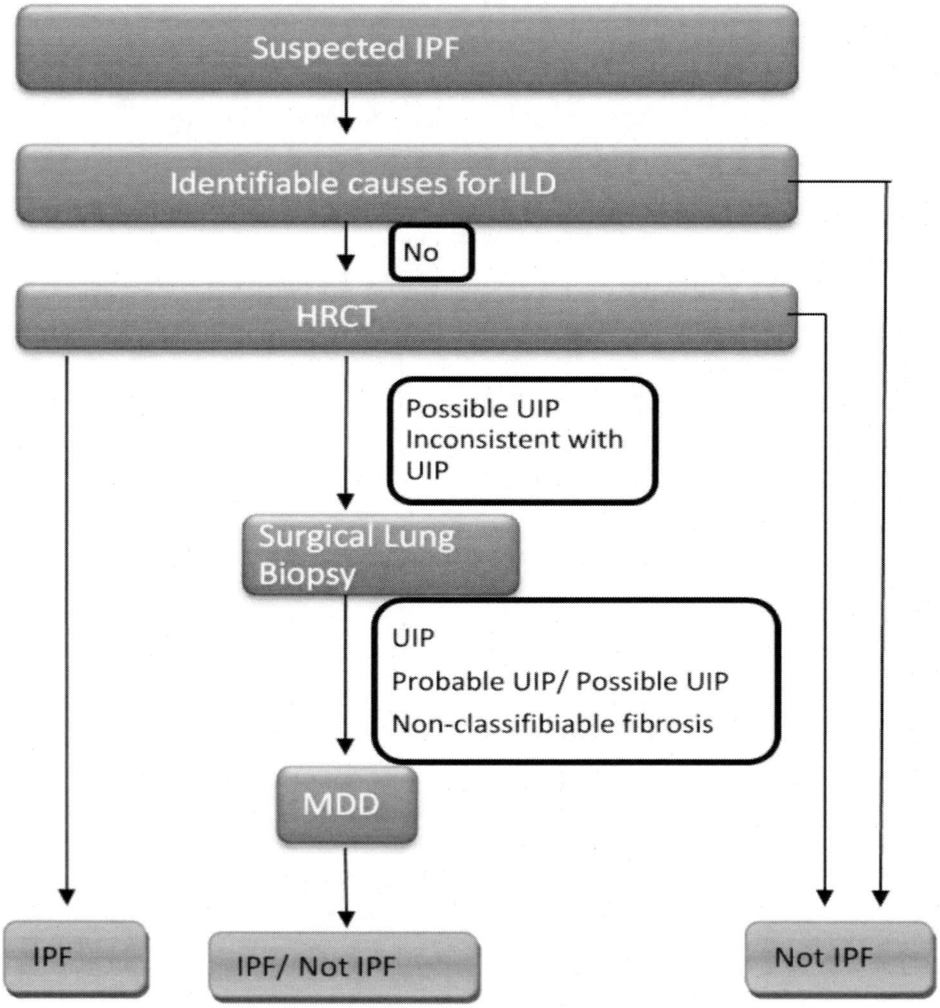

IPF: Idiopathic Pulmonary Fibrosis, ILD: Interstitial Lung Disease, HRCT: High-Resolution Computed Tomography, UIP: Usual Interstitial Pneumonia, MDD: Multidisciplinary Discussion.

Figure 1. Diagnostic algorithm for IPF.

Recommendation: The committee recommend that patients with IPF should not be treated with cyclosporine A (strong recommendation, very low quality evidence).
Note: The 2011 guideline

- Question 4: Should patients with IPF be treated with combination corticosteroid and immunomodulator therapy (e.g., azathioprine or cyclophosphamide)?
  Recommendation: The committee recommend that patients with IPF should not be treated with combination corticosteroid and immunomodulator therapy (strong recommendation, low-quality evidence).
  Note: The 2011 guideline
- Question 5: Should patiets with IPF be treated with combination corticosteroid, azathioprine, and acetylcysteine therapy?
  Recommendation: The committee recommend that clinicians not use the combination therapy of N-acetylcysteine, azathioprine, and prednisone in patients with IPF (strong recommendation, low confidence in estimates of effect).
  Note: The2015 guideline (Recommendation of the 2011 guideline was weak recommendation, low quality evidence).
- Question 6: Should patients with IPF be treated with acetylcysteine monotherapy?
  Recommendation: The majority of patients with IPF should not be treated with acetylcysteine monotherapy, but this therapy may be a reasonable choice in a minority (weak recommendation, low-quality evidence).
  Note: The 2015 guideline (unchanged recommendation)
- Question 7: Should patients with IPF be treated with interferon-g 1b?
  Recommendation: The committee recommend that patients with IPF should not be treated with IFN-g (strong recommendation, high-quality evidence).
  Note: The 2011 guideline
- Question 8: Should Patients with IPF Be Treated with Bosentan or Macitentan, Dual Endothelin Receptor Antagonists (ER-A and ER-B)?
  Recommendation: The committee suggest that clinicians not use bosentan or macitentan, both dual ER-A and ER-B endothelin receptor antagonists, for the treatment of IPF (conditional recommendation against, low confidence in estimates of effect).
  Note: The 2015 guideline (Recommendation of the 2011 guideline was strong recommendation against bosentan use).
- Question 9: Should patients with IPF be treated with etanercept?
  Recommendation: The committee recommend that patients with IPF should not be treated with etanercept (strong recommendation, moderate-quality evidence).
  Note: The 2011 guideline
- Question 10: Should patients with IPF be treated with anticoagulants?

Recommendation: The committee recommend that clinicians not use warfarin anticoagulation in patients with IPF who do not have a known alternative indication for its use (strong recommendation against, low confidence in estimates of effect).Note: The 2015 guideline (Recommendation of the 2011 guideline was weak recommendation, very low-quality evidence)

- Question 11: Should patients with IPF be treated with pirfenidone?
  Recommendation: The committee suggest that clinicians use pirfenidone in patients with IPF (conditional recommendation, moderate confidence in estimates of effect).
  Note: The 2015 guideline (Recommendation of the 2011 guideline was weak recommendation, low- to moderate-quality evidence against use).
- Question 12: Should Patients with IPF Be Treated with Ambrisentan, a Selective ER-A Endothelin Receptor Antagonist?
  Recommendation: The committee recommend that clinicians not use ambrisentan, a selective ER-A endothelin receptor antagonist, in patients with IPF, regardless of the presence or absence of PH (strong recommendation against, low confidence in estimates of effect).
  Note: The 2015 guideline (No recommendation was offered in the 2011 guideline)
- Question 13: Should Patients with IPF Be Treated with Nintedanib, a Tyrosine Kinase Inhibitor?
  Recommendation: The committee suggest that clinicians use nintedanib in patients with IPF (conditional recommendation, moderate confidence in estimates of effect).
  Note: The 2015 guideline (No recommendation was offered in the 2011 guideline)
- Question 14: Should Patients with IPF Be Treated with Sildenafil, a Phosphodiesterase-5 Inhibitor?
  Recommendation: The committee suggest that clinicians not use sildenafil, a phosphodiesterase-5 inhibitor, for treatment of IPF (conditional recommendation against, moderate confidence in estimates of effect).
  Note: The 2015 guideline (No recommendation was offered in the 2011 guideline)
- Question 15: Should Patients with IPF Be Treated with Imatinib, a Tyrosine Kinase Inhibitor?
  Recommendation: The committee recommend that clinicians not use imatinib in patients with IPF (strong recommendation, moderate confidence in estimates of effect).
  Note: The 2015 guideline (No recommendation was offered in the 2011 guideline)

Nonpharmacologic Therapies

- Question 1: Should patients with IPF and resting hypoxemia receive long-term oxygen therapy?
  Recommendation: The committee recommend that patients with IPF and clinically significant resting hypoxemia should be treated with long-term oxygen therapy (strong recommendation, very low-quality evidence).
  Note: The 2011 guideline (Recommendation was not prioritized for an update in the 2015 guideline).
- Question 2: Should appropriate patients with IPF undergo lung transplantation?
  Recommendation: The committee recommend that appropriate patients with IPF should undergo lung transplantation (strong recommendation, low-quality evidence).
  Note: The 2011 guideline (Recommendation was not prioritized for an update in the 2015 guideline).
- Question 3: Should patients with respiratory failure due to IPF receive mechanical ventilation?
  Recommendation: The majority of patients with respiratory failure due to IPF should not receive mechanical ventilation, but mechanical ventilation may be a reasonable intervention in a minority (weak recommendation, lowquality evidence). Note: The 2011guideline(Recommendation was not prioritized for an update in the 2015 guideline).
- Question 4: Should patients with IPF receive pulmonary rehabilitation?
  Recommendation: The majority of patients with IPF should be treated with pulmonary rehabilitation, but pulmonary rehabilitation may not be reasonable in a minority (weak recommendation, low-quality evidence).
  Note: The2011 guideline (Recommendation was not prioritized for an update in the 2015 guideline).
- Question 5: Should Patients with IPF Be Treated with Bilateral Lung Transplantation versus Single-Lung Transplantation?
  Recommendation: The committee did not make a recommendation regarding single versus bilateral lung transplantation in patients with IPF.Note: The 2015 guideline (No recommendation was offered in the 2011 guideline)

Treatment of Comorbidities

- Question 1: Should patients with acute exacerbation of IPF be treated with corticosteroids?

Recommendation: The majority of patients with acute exacerbation of IPF should be treated with corticosteroids, but corticosteroids may not be reasonable in a minority (weak recommendation, very low-quality evidence).
Note: The 2011 guideline (Recommendation was not prioritized for an update in the 2015 guideline).

- Question 2: Should pulmonary hypertension (PH) be treated in patients with IPF?
  Recommendation: Pulmonary hypertension should not be treated in the majority of patients with IPF, but treatment may be a reasonable choice in a minority (weak recommendation, very low-quality evidence).
  Note: The 2011 guideline (The committee did not make a recommendation regarding treatment of PH in patients with IPF).
- Question 3: Should asymptomatic gastroesophageal reflux disease be medically treated in patients with IPF?
  Recommendation: The committee suggest that clinicians use regular antiacid treatment for patients with IPF (conditional recommendation, very low confidence in estimates of effect).
  Note: The 2015 guideline (unchanged recommendation) [4].

Table 1. IPF Guidelines

Pharmacological Therapies	**2011**	**2015**
Q1: Corticosteroid (CS) monotherapy	Strong recommendation against use	-
Q2: Colchicine	Strong recommendation against use	-
Q3: Cyclosporin A	Strong recommendation against use	-
Q4: Combination corticosteroid and immunomodulator therapy	Strong recommendation against use	-
Q5: Combination CS, Azothioprine, and NAC therapy	Conditional recommendation against use	Strong recommendation against use
Q6: NAC monotherapy	Conditional recommendation against use	Unchanged recommendation
Q7: INF-g 1b	Strong recommendation against use	-
Pharmacological Therapies	2011	2015
Q8: Bosentan	Strong recommendation against use	Conditional recommendation against use
Q9: Etanercept	Strong recommendation against use	-
Q10: Anticoagulants	Conditional recommendation against use	Strong recommendation against use

Pharmacological Therapies	**2011**	**2015**
Q11: Pirfenidone	Conditional recommendation against use	Conditional recommendation foruse
Q12: Ambisertan	Not adressed	Strong recommendation against use
Q13: Nintedanib	Not adressed	Conditional recommendation foruse
Q14: Lung transplantation: single vs. bilateral	Not adressed	Deferred
Q15: Sildenafil	Not adressed	Conditional recommendation against use
Q16: İmatinib	Not adressed	Strong recommendation against use
Nonpharmacologic Therapies	2011	2015
Q1: Oxygen supplementation	Strong recommendation for use	Not prioritized
Q2:Lung transplantation	Strong recommendation for use	Not prioritized
Q3:Mechanical ventilation	Conditional recommendation against use	Not prioritized
Q4:Pulmonary rehabilitation	Conditional recommendation foruse	Not prioritized
Treatment of comorbities	2011	2015
Q1: Treatment of acute exacerbation of IPF with CS	Conditional recommendation foruse	Not prioritized
Q2: Treatment of pulmonary hypertension	Conditional recommendation against use	Deferred
Q3: Antiacid treatment	Conditional recommendation foruse	Unchanged

SUMMARY

IPF is idiopathic, chronic, progressive fibrosing interstitial pneumonia, occuring primarily in older adults. Because diagnosis of IPF requires a high level of clinical suspicion and consideration of other possible causes, thorough history, physical examination and serological studies must be obtained.

The diagnosis of IPF requires [3]:

a. Exclusion of other known causes of interstitial lung disease (ILD) (e.g., domestic and occupational environmental exposures, connective tissue disease, and drug toxicity).
b. The presence of a UIP pattern on high-resolution computed tomography (HRCT) in patients not subjected to surgical lung biopsy.

c. Specific combinations of HRCT and surgical lung biopsy pattern in patients subjected to surgical lung biopsy.

The accuracy of the diagnosis of IPF increases with multidisciplinary discussion between pulmonologists, radiologists, and pathologists experienced in the diagnosis of ILD.

In 2015, recommendations for the treatment of IPF were updated on the basis of new scientific evidence that emerged after the first diagnostic-therapeutic guidelines were published in 2011[3,4].

Treatment Recommendations (2011-2015 Guidelines):

The following recommendations are new or revised from the 2011 guideline

1. Agents with strong recommendation against use: Anticoagulation (warfarin), imatinib, ambrisentan and combination prednisone, azathioprine, and N-acetylcysteine.
2. Agents with conditional recommendation for use: Nintedanib and pirfenidone.
3. Agents with conditional recommendation against use: Sildenafil, macitentan, bosentan.

The following recommendations are unchanged from the 2011 guideline

1. A conditional recommendation against N-acetylcysteine monotherapy and a conditional recommendation for antiacid therapy.
2. A conditional recommendation against the treatment of pulmonary hypertension use.
3. A strong recommendation for the use ofoxygen supplementation and lung transplantation.
4. A conditional recommendationagainstthe use of mechanical ventilation.
5. A conditional recommendationforthe use of pulmonary rehabilitation and treatment of acute exacerbation of IPF with corticosteroids.

An evidence synthesis was also performed for a new question about single versus bilateral lung transplantation, but decisions regarding a recommendation were deferred until the next version of the guideline to gather additional information that was felt necessary before formulating a recommendation. Questions regarding newer treatments (e.g., antibiotics) were not addressed and were deferred until the next version of the guideline because of resource constraints [4].

No pharmacologic interventions have received strong recommendations for treatment, but conditional recommendations have been made for treatment with pirfenidone,nintedanib and antiacid treatment. Clinicians confronted with treating patients with IPF should individualize decisions with their patients, as suggested by the conditional recommendations, and they should be cautious in comparing the relative net benefit of one intervention with another [4].

REFERENCES

[1] Luppi, F., Spagnolo, P., Cerri, S., Richeldi, L. The big clinical trials in idiopathic pulmonary fibrosis. *Curr. Opin. Pulm. Med.,* 2012;18: 428 - 432.

[2] American Thoracic Society; European Respiratory Society. American Thoracic Society: idiopathic pulmonary fibrosis: diagnosis and treatment: international consensus statement. *Am. J. Respir. Crit. Care Med.,* 2000;161:646 - 664.

[3] Raghu, G., Collard, H. R., Egan, J. J., Martinez, F. J., Behr, J., Brown, K. K., Colby, T. V., Cordier, J. F., Flaherty, K. R., Lasky, J. A. et al.; ATS/ERS/JRS/ALAT Committee on Idiopathic Pulmonary Fibrosis. An official ATS/ERS/JRS/ALAT statement: idiopathic pulmonary fibrosis: evidence-based guidelines for diagnosis and management. *Am. J. Respir. Crit. Care Med.,* 2011; 183:788 - 824.

[4] Raghu, G., Rochwerg, B., Zhang, Y., Garcia, C. A., Azuma, A., Behr, J. et al. An official ATS/ERS/JRS/ALAT clinical practice guideline: treatment of idiopathic pulmonary fibrosis. An update of the 2011 clinical practice guideline. *Am. J. Respir. Crit. Care Med.,* 2015;192:e3 - 19.

[5] Flaherty, K. R., King, T. E. Jr., Raghu, G., Lynch, J. P. III, Colby, T. V., Travis, W. D., Gross, B. H., Kazerooni, E. A., Toews, G. B., Long, Q. et al. Idiopathic interstitial pneumonia: what is the effect of a multidisciplinary approach to diagnosis? *Am. J. Respir. Crit. Care Med.,* 2004;170:904 - 910.

ABOUT THE EDITOR

Antonio M. Esquinas is a 54 year old critical care MD in Intensive Unit at Hospital Morales Meseguer, Murcia (Spain). He holds a PhD in Medicine (University of Murcia) and BA in Pulmonary and Critical Care Medicine (University of Granada). He has taken part in many academic and research activities in the field of mechanical ventilation, with special focus on Noninvasive Mechanical Ventilation and weaning from mechanical ventilation, COPD exacerbation and acute hypoxemic respiratory failure.

Furthermore, Antonio M. Esquinas MD, PhD has contributed to research as author of 648 articles indexed, 550 chapters and as editor in chief of 55 books edited in the field of related mechanical ventilation, invasive (weaning mechanical ventilation) and noninvasive ventilation approach in acute hypoxemic and chronic respiratory failure (COPD, idiopathic pulmonary fibrosis, sleep breathing disorders) in pulmonary, critical care and sleep medicine.

He is recognized as International Fellow from the American College Chest Physicians (FCCP), International Fellow American Association Respiratory Care (AARC) and Fellow Noninvasive Ventilation by International Association of Noninvasive Ventilation. Besides, Antonio M. is an active member in many educational postgraduate programs in pulmonary and critical care as he is the Director of International School of Noninvasive Ventilation and of the program of Fellowship Noninvasive Ventilation, as well as President of the International Association of Noninvasive Ventilation.

INDEX

A

D

E

F

G

H

N

O

P

Q

R

S

T

U

V

W

X